ABDOMINAL
EMERGENCIES

ABDOMINAL EMERGENCIES

Edited by

David M. Cline, MD
Associate Professor of Emergency Medicine
Director of Research
Department of Emergency Medicine
Wake Forest University Health Sciences
Medical Center Boulevard
Winston-Salem, North Carolina

Latha G. Stead, MD, FACEP
Chair, Division of Emergency Medicine Research
Associate Professor
Mayo Clinic College of Medicine
Rochester, Minnesota

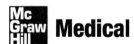

New York   Chicago   San Francisco   Lisbon   London   Madrid   Mexico City   Milan
New Delhi   San Juan   Seoul   Singapore   Sydney   Toronto

Abdominal Emergencies

1 2 3 4 5 6 7 8 9 0   FG/FG   0 9 8 7

ISBN 978-0-07-146861-9
MHID 0-07-146861-7

This book was set in Times by International Typesetting and Composition.
The editor was Anne Sydor.
The production supervisor was Thomas Kowalczyk.
The cover designer was Mary Mckeon.
The indexer was Robert Swanson.
Quebecor World/Fairfield Graphics was printer and binder.

This book is printed on acid-free paper.

Cataloging-in-Publication Data for this title is on file with Library of Congress.

I would like to dedicate this work to my family who support me in all that I do: Joseph, Paul, Olivia, Jill, and Lisa.

David M. Cline

I would like to dedicate this work to Dr. Wyatt Decker for making the job a true pleasure every day and to my family—Mom, Dad, Matt, Thor, Tej, Trilok, and Karthik—for making the household so much fun.

Latha G. Stead

CONTENTS

CONTRIBUTORS

Roy L. Alson, MD, PhD [13]
Associate Professor
Wake Forest University Health Sciences
Department of Emergency Medicine
Winston-Salem, North Carolina

Kim Askew, MD [37]
Fellow Pediactric Emergency Medicine
Inova Fairfax Hospital for Children
Falls Church, Virginia

David M. Barrett, MD [11]
Assistant Professor
Department of Emergency Medicine
Baystate Medical Center
Tufts University School of Medicine
Springfield, Massachusetts

M. Fernanda Bellolio, MD [40, 43]
Instructor of Emergency Medicine
Mayo Clinic College of Medicine
Rochester, Minnesota

Anjali Bhagra, MBBS [27]
Research Fellow
Department of Emergency Medicine
Mayo Clinic College of Mediicne
Rochester, Minnesota

Joshua Broder, MD [15]
Assistant Professor
Division of Emergency Medicine
Department of Surgery
Duke University
Durham, North Carolina

Thomas A. Brunell, MD [19]
Director of Emergency Medicine Education
St. Francis Hospital and Medical Center
Department of Emergency Medicine
Hartford, Connecticut

Esther H. Chen, MD [20]
Assistant Professor
University of Pennsylvania
Emergency Medicine Department
Philadelphia, Pennsylvania

Phillip A. Clement, MD [7]
Clinical Assistant Professor
Department of Emergency Medicine
East Carolina University
The Brody School of Medicine
Greenville, North Carolina

David M. Cline, MD [1, 2, 3, 6, 8, 13, 23]
Associate Professor of Emergency Medicine
Director of Research
Department of Emergency Medicine
Wake Forest University Health Sciences
Medical Center Boulevard
Winston-Salem, North Carolina

Kevin J. Corcoran, DO [7]
Clinical Associate Professor
Department of Emergency Medicine
East Carolina University
The Brody School of Medicine
Greenville, North Carolina

Melissa W. Costello, MD [34]
Assistant Professor of Emergency Medicine
Clinical Instructor of Pediatric Emergency Medicine
University of South Alabama
Mobile, Alabama

Heather L. Farley, MD [33]
Department of Emergency Medicine
Christiana Care Health System
Newark, Delaware

Michael T. Fitch, MD [4]
Assistant Professor
Wake Forest University Health Sciences
Department of Emergency Medicine
Winston-Salem, North Carolina

J. Christian Fox, MD [22]
Associate Clinical Professor
Department of Emergency Medicine
University of California, Irvine
Orange, California

Christopher J. Fullagar, MD [24]
Assistant Professor
Department of Emergency Medicine
SUNY Upstate Medical University at Syracuse
Syracuse, New York

Rachel M. Gilmore, MB, MRCPI [16]
Research Fellow
Department of Emergency Medicine
Mayo Clinic College of Medicine
Rochester, Minnesota

Alan Heins, MD [26, 39]
Clinical Assistant Professor of Emergency Medicine
University of South Alabama
Mobile, Alabama

Douglas K. Holtzman, MD [36]
Assistant Professor
Department of Emergency Medicine
Wake Forest University Health Sciences
Winston-Salem, North Carolina

Randall W. King, MD [10]
Residency Director
Division of Emergency Medicine
Department of Surgery
Medical College of Ohio
Toledo, Ohio

Christopher C. Kwon, MD, MPH [45]
Department of Emergency Medicine
Mayo Clinic College of Medicine
Rochester, Minnesota

Bruce Y. Lee, MD [20]
Assistant Professor
Section of Decision Sciences and Clinical Systems
  Modeling
Department of Medicine
University of Pittsburgh
Pittsburgh, Pennsylvania

Lawrence M. Lewis, MD [5]
Professor of Emergency Medicine
Department of Emergency Medicine
Washington University School of Medicine
St. Louis, Missouri

Charles L. Maddow, MD, FACEP [47]
Assistant Professor
Department of Emergency Medicine
University of Rochester School of Medicine & Dentistry
Rochester, New York

David Magilner, MD [35, 38]
Assistant Professor
Wake Forest University Health Sciences
Department of Emergency Medicine
Winston-Salem, North Carolina

Simon A. Mahler, MD [18, 29]
Clinical Instructor of Emergency Medicine
Department of Emergency Medicine
Louisiana State University Health Science Center
  Shreveport
Shreveport, Louisiana

David E. Manthey, MD [25]
Associate Professor
Wake Forest University Health Sciences
Department of Emergency Medicine
Medical Center Boulevard
Winston-Salem, North Carolina

Catherine A. Marco, MD [10]
Clinical Professor
Division of Emergency Medicine
Department of Surgery
Medical College of Ohio
Toledo, Ohio

Henderson D. McGinnis, MD [3]
Clinical Instructor
Wake Forest University Health Sciences
Department of Emergency Medicine
Winston-Salem, North Carolina

Howard K. Mell, MD, MPH, EMT-P(IL) [30, 41]
Assistant Professor of Emergency Medicine
Ohio State University
Columbus, Ohio

Angela M. Mills, MD [12]
Assistant Professor
University of Pennsylvania
Emergency Medicine Department
Philadelphia, Pennsylvania

Milan D. Nadkarni, MD [37]
Assistant Professor
Wake Forest University Health Sciences
Department of Emergency Medicine
Medical Center Boulevard
Winston-Salem, North Carolina

W. Scott McNair, MD [34]
Assistant Professor of Emergency Medicine
Assistant Professor of Pediatrics
University of South Alabama
Mobile, Alabama

Bret A. Nicks, MD [17, 25]
Assistant Professor
Wake Forest University Health Sciences
Department of Emergency Medicine
Winston-Salem, North Carolina

Mary C. O'Brien, MD [2]
Associate Professor
Wake Forest University Health Sciences
Department of Emergency Medicine
Medical Center Boulevard
Winston-Salem, North Carolina

Michael C. Plewa, MD [16]
Clinical Assistant Professor
Division of Emergency Medicine
Department of Surgery
Medical College of Ohio
Toledo, Ohio

Christopher Reynolds, MD [15]
Attending Physician
Mid-Atlantic Emergency Physicians
Charlotte, North Carolina

Joseph C Schmidt, MD [14]
Assistant Professor
Department of Emergency Medicine
Baystate Medical Center
Tufts University School of Medicine
Springfield, Massachusetts

William P. Scruggs, MD [22]
Clinical Instructor
Department of Emergency Medicine
University of California, Irvine
Orange, California

Kim Ryan Schutterle, MS, MD [42]
Department of Emergency Medicine
Mayo Clinic College of Medicine
Rochester, Minnesota

Manish N. Shah, MD, FACEP [47]
Assistant Professor
Departments of Emergency Medicine & Community
    and Preventive Medicine
University of Rochester School of Medicine & Dentistry
Rochester, New York

Sara R. Shimmin, MD [44]
Instructor, Department of Emergency Medicine
Mayo Clinic Arizona
Scottsdale, Arizona

Scott M. Silvers, MD [31]
Assistant Professor of Medicine (Emergency Medicine)
Associate Chair of Education
Division of Emergency Medicine
Mayo Clinic-Jacksonville
Jacksonville, Florida

Mitchell C. Sokolosky, MD [9]
Associate Professor
Department of Emergency Medicine
Wake Forest University Health Sciences
Winston-Salem, North Carolina

Latha G. Stead, MD, FACEP [27, 40, 43, 46]
Chair, Division of Emergency Medicine Research
Associate Professor
Mayo Clinic College of Medicine
Rochester, Minnesota

Kristine Thompson, MD [28]
Instructor of Medicine (Emergency Medicine)
Division of Emergency Medicine
Mayo Clinic-Jacksonville
Jacksonville, Florida

Susan P. Torrey, MD [21]
Assistant Professor
Department of Emergency Medicine
Tufts University School of Medicine
Baystate Medical Center
Springfield, Massachusetts

Lekshmi Vaidyanathan, MBBS [29, 46]
Instructor of Emergency Medicine
Mayo Clinic College of Medicine
Rochester, Minnesota

Larry F. Vukov, MD [42]
Associate Professor of Emergency Medicine
Mayo Clinic College of Medicine
Rochester, Minnesota

Johnny J. Vazquez, MD [45]
Instructor of Emergency Medicine
Mayo Clinic College of Medicine
Rochester, Minnesota

Stacy Zelman, MD [32]
Assistant Professor
Department of Emergency Medicine
Wake Forest University Health Sciences
Medical Center Boulevard
Winston-Salem, North Carolina

Advances in the Care of Patients with Abdominal Pain–From Babe Ruth, to the Beatles, and Beyond.

During spring training in 1925, at the age of 30 years the famous ball player, George "Babe" Ruth began having stomach cramps and fever. On April 7, 1925, following an exhibition game in Asheville North Carolina, Ruth suffered a syncopal episode while in the bathroom of a hotel. The collapse prompted one London paper to falsely report Ruth had died. Paul Krichell, a scout for the Yankees, was given the responsibility of taking Ruth back to New York for diagnosis and treatment. By the time the train reached New York, Ruth was unconscious and was observed to shake uncontrollably, flailing his arms and legs; he required physical restraint. He was taken to St. Vincent's hospital where he sustained several more "convulsive attacks." Ruth's personal physician, Dr. Edward Kinder, examined him and made the diagnosis of "a touch of flu" and "an intestinal attack." Dr. Kinder at the time stated that part of the problem was Babe's diet, which included frequent binging, and his weight had increased to 256 pounds. W.O. McGeehan created the popular story stating the problem was caused by too many hot dogs and bottles of soda pop. McGeehan coined the phrase—a bellyache heard "round the world"—to describe the incident.

After a brief initial hospital stay, Babe Ruth was back on the ball field, but a week later he once again had fever and recurrent abdominal pain. Dr. Kinder reexamined Ruth and diagnosed him with "an intestinal abscess." On April 17, 1925, Ruth underwent surgery, which reportedly only lasted 20 minutes. "Intestinal abscess" was the postoperative diagnosis released to the press. These official reports were clouded by rumors that the real problem was gonorrhea, an assertion never confirmed by his physician or Ruth or any other reliable report. Although Ruth was reported to have recovered completely, 1925 was the worst year he had in the major leagues, especially compared to the superlative years he enjoyed immediately prior.

In 1925, the diagnosis of abdominal pain was almost entirely clinical. Although plain film X-rays were available to physicians, there is no report that X-rays were used to diagnose Babe Ruth's condition. It wouldn't be until four years later that Victor Schilling published his book, *The Blood Picture and its Clinical Significance*, which popularized the use of differential white blood counts to help diagnose many medical conditions, including, eventually the acute abdomen. It is no wonder that Ruth's condition was incompletely diagnosed on first assessment, and he developed an abscess from some unknown primary condition at the age of 30 years. As the twentieth century continued, more and more tests became available to clinicians to evaluate patients with abdominal pain, including urinalysis, amylase, liver function tests, lipase, renal function tests, pregnancy tests, and other blood tests, all increasing the importance of using the laboratories of hospitals and emergency departments to facilitate a diagnosis in patients with acute abdominal pain.

Ultrasound techniques were described in the 1940s, but would not impact decision making in the evaluation of abdominal pain until decades later. The first application of ultrasound in clinical evaluations of patients with abdominal pain was for pregnant females in the 1960s and 1970s, but usually this was not used on an emergency basis. Bedside emergency applications would not begin until two decades later. Barium was discovered as a potential contrast material to diagnose hollow viscus diseases, and was reported to be helpful in the diagnosis of appendicitis in 1968. Typically, these tests were ordered by the surgeon and done after admission to the hospital.

In the late 1960s and early 1970s, research laid the foundation for one of the biggest innovations in the diagnosis of abdominal pain: computed tomography (CT). EMI corporation (Electric and Musical Industries Ltd.) published the Beatles' recordings and profited by approximately $200 million. According to Sir Godfrey Hounsfield, the profit from the Beatles' recordings allowed EMI to fund his research in the late 1960s that led to the development of the CT scanner, which was made available in a commercial form in the mid- to late-1970s. Initially, it was designed for head examinations only, but in time, was used for chest and abdomen evaluations.

However, the frequent use of CT in the diagnosis of abdominal emergencies occurred in the 1990s with the advent of spiral CT. This modality has revolutionized the emergency practitioner's approach to abdominal pain. At the same time the use of ultrasound to diagnose emergency abdominal conditions has become more refined, if somewhat specialized to individual expertise at each institution. The reliability of imaging to rule out and rule in surgical conditions has changed the nonsurgeon's approach to the evaluation of abdominal pain. Which patients require surgical consultation may not be an issue that has been resolved, but certainly this question has different answers than a few decades ago. Another development that has changed the clinician's approach to abdominal pain is "evidence-based medicine" and the application of meta-analysis to determine the reliability of diagnostic techniques. Clinicians are faced with an ever increasing number of articles in the literature that challenge or better define the validity of previously recommended diagnostic algorithms as new information is elucidated.

All these changes have contributed to the need for this book on the evaluation and management of patients with abdominal pain. Latha Stead and I have attempted to bring together new information on diagnostic techniques, and the reliability of those techniques. We have asked our individual chapter authors to compile diagnostic images that characterize the clinical conditions being discussed in each section, including CT images, as well as plain film and ultrasound images as appropriate to each chapter. We have included in the book greater detail on conditions that yield abdominal pain, and which should be considered in the differential diagnosis, but rarely get the thorough discussion as included in this book, for example, metabolic causes of abdominal pain. It is our sincere hope that this book provides insight to the clinician responsible for the initial evaluation and management of patients presenting with abdominal pain.

We thank Dr M. Fernanda Bellio, Dr Rahul Kashyap and Ms Cameron Rowe for the cover pictures.

David M. Cline, MD

Latha G. Stead, MD, FACEP

1

Mechanisms of Abdominal Pain

David M. Cline

HIGH YIELD FACTS

- Understanding the mechanisms by which abdominal pain is perceived by the patient helps the clinician to understand the course of the disease process.
- There are anatomic and pathophysiologic concepts that explain some of the atypical presentations of known diseases, such as sterile pyuria associated with appendicitis.

INTRODUCTION

The mechanisms by which the patient perceives abdominal pain helps the clinician understand the course of the disease process. However, the course of many patients is atypical and confusing to clinicians. Many atypical presentations can also be explained by anatomical and pathophysiologic concepts described in this chapter.

Pathophysiology and Anatomy

Visceral Pain Fibers

Abdominal visceral pain fibers originate in the organs of the abdomen and enter the spinal cord at more than one vertebral level.[1] Pain can be produced by inflammation or ischemia, but more commonly it occurs when hollow organs are distended, as in small bowel obstruction or when the capsules of solid organs are stretched, as in the distension of the spleen with contusion or fracture. In contrast to the nerve fibers that transmit somatic pain, these fibers are unmyelinated and bilateral. These facts help to explain why pain originating from organ involvement early in the course of many abdominal diseases begins as poorly localized pain. Patients may describe this pain with vague terms or as crampy pain. The pain may range in severity from mild to excruciating. If the affected organ is hollow, continued peristalsis frequently affects the pain, making it intermittent and colicky in nature.

Correlating to their embryonic origins, pain from these grouped abdominal organs manifests in similar locations. The stomach, duodenum, liver, gallbladder, and pancreas are foregut structures. Pain originating from these structures typically is perceived as emanating from the epigastrium. The small bowel, the cecum and proximal portion of the large bowel, and the appendix are midgut structures. Pain originating from these structures produces periumbilical pain. The distal large bowel and the genitourinary systems are hindgut structures. Pain originating from these structures is perceived in the lower abdomen. These concepts provide a guideline; individual patient variation exists.

Somatic Pain Fibers

Somatic or parietal pain arises from noxious stimulation of the parietal peritoneum.[1] Parietal pain is transmitted by myelinated fibers to specific dorsal root ganglia on the ipsilateral side of the spinal cord along known dermatomes yielding a better localized perception of pain from the source of the stimuli. The perception of pain can be initiated by a variety of stimuli including stretching, ischemia, or inflammation. Patients typically describe the pain from a somatic source as being sharp, like a knife. Movement commonly aggravates this pain. Rebound tenderness and involuntary guarding are phenomena associated with somatic pain as the parietal peritoneum becomes increasingly affected during intra-abdominal diseases, typically secondary to an inflammatory process.

Clinical Applications

Referred Pain

Referred pain is defined as pain that is perceived at a distance from the diseased organ. This phenomenon occurs due to shared pain pathways for afferent neurons from different sources beginning in distinct locations. There are multiple examples. The T9 dermatome carries afferent pain fibers from both the lung and the abdomen. Patients may complain of abdominal pain when they have pain associated with lower lobe pneumonia. The pain of inferior wall myocardial infarction may be perceived as originating from the stomach. Shoulder pain may be perceived when irritation of the diaphragm results from an intraperitoneal bleed; for example a patient with traumatic splenic bleeding may complain of left-shoulder pain. Other examples include testicular pain associated with ureteral obstruction, and infrascapular pain associated with biliary colic.

Appendicitis Course and Signs

The classic course of appendicitis illustrates the pathophysiology of visceral, somatic, and referred pain. Initially the pain of appendicitis, a midgut structure, is perceived in the periumbilical region and is typically a vague pain. As the disease progresses, the parietal peritoneum becomes affected by the inflammation, and the pain migrates to the right lower quadrant. The increasing inflammation results in rebound tenderness; when the examiner rapidly releases pressure on the abdomen, movement of the parietal peritoneum over the inflamed appendix results in pain. Rovsing sign is another application; pressure on the left lower quadrant moves the parietal peritoneum, including the right lower quadrant, over the inflamed appendix and results in pain there rather than the left lower quadrant where there is no primary source of inflammation. Eventually the inflammation stimulates the abdominal wall muscles to be held in sustained contraction (involuntary guarding) to reduce movement of the parietal peritoneum and reduce the severity of the pain perceived by the patient. The variability of patient presentation in large part reflects the fact that patients present at varying points on this continuum from early vague visceral pain to late pain with involuntary guarding. Furthermore, patients' individual reactions to these pathophysiologic processes are different and therefore may manifest different signs at different points in the process. This explains the occasional occurrence of a patient without rebound tenderness or involuntary guarding found to have a perforation at the time of surgery.

The appendix varies in length from several centimeters up to 30 cm. When an inflamed appendix rests over the ureter, it can produce pyuria (sterile), which may confuse the clinician. A retrocecal appendix may come to rest over the psoas muscle yielding a positive psoas sign or may yield tenderness on rectal exam. See Chapter 9 for further discussion of the clinical application of these pathophysiologic processes.

Extra-abdominal Sources of Pain

Pain originating from the abdomen may be perceived as being intra-abdominal by the patient. This is due to the fact that superficial skin innervation from the lower thoracic nerve roots enters the spinal cord via the same dorsal horn as the deeper visceral fibers. Careful examination of the abdominal wall will help differentiate these processes (see Chapter 40).

Infectious agents may cause crampy abdominal pain by their affects on the mucosa of the bowel wall. However, because simple infections are limited to the mucosa, the pain should not be severe, and no peritoneal signs should be present as mucosal disease does not irritate the parietal peritoneum. In contrast, infections that become invasive can lead to infarction or perforation and yield peritoneal signs. Therefore, abdominal pain of any significance should not be attributed to simple gastroenteritis.

Several toxic agents can cause significant abdominal pain. One example is a black widow spider bite, which causes significant muscle cramping and pain. Rarely is the abdominal wall the only muscle group involved. Metabolic acidosis (from whatever the underlying cause) may present with abdominal pain, as in diabetic ketoacidosis (DKA). The mechanism of these phenomena is not clear, although it has been blamed on gastric distention and paralytic ileus. These symptoms should improve with treatment of the underlying cause; in the example of DKA, fluids and insulin. However, the possibility that the episode of DKA was initiated by an acute intra-abdominal process should be kept in mind.

Emergency Department Care and Disposition

This book contains more than forty chapters that describe the management of patients presenting with abdominal pain.

PITFALLS

- Attempting to categorize a patient's presentation into a classic disease pattern that follows strict anatomical concepts and pathophysiologic processes may lead to misdiagnosis.

REFERENCE

1. Bockus HL. Mechanism of abdominal pain. *J Lancet* 1956:76:31.

2

Approach to Abdominal Pain

Mary Claire O' Brien
David M. Cline

"It is much more important to know what sort of patient has a disease than what sort of disease a patient has."   Sir William Osler

More patients visit emergency departments (EDs) annually in the United States for "stomach and abdominal pain, cramps or spasms" than for any other chief complaint. In 2003, 6.7% of ED visits—7.63 million patient encounters—were for abdominal pain.[1] Demographics (age, gender, ethnicity, family history, sexual orientation, cultural practices, geography) influence both the incidence and the clinical expression of abdominal disease. The patient's history, vital signs, and physical findings may not point to a specific diagnosis. Routine laboratory testing is often not helpful. In the era before computed tomography (CT), a study of 8500 patients found that 40% of patients seen in the emergency department with acute abdominal pain were discharged with a diagnosis of "undifferentiated" or "nonspecific" disease.[2] A recent small study found nonspecific abdominal pain to account for as little as 9% of patients presenting with abdominal pain, but the group of patients under study were deemed to be in need of a CT scan for management.[3] While we cannot always identify the exact cause of the patient's pain, we do seek to exclude life-threatening disease and to narrow the list of diagnostic possibilities for further workup. Notwithstanding our best efforts, missed diagnoses for acute abdominal pain are a continued source of malpractice litigation.[4–8] On the whole, clinical suspicion is paramount, in other words, knowing "what sort of patient has the disease."

There are diverse conceptual frameworks with which to approach a chief complaint of abdominal pain (Table 2-1). The goal of this chapter is to present a pragmatic scheme based on patient acuity and the presence or absence of modifying factors that identify special populations of patients with abdominal pain. We suggest that the clinical answers to the questions below be used to determine the urgency and method of the diagnostic approach.

1. Is this patient critically ill?
2. Does the patient have a constellation of symptoms that fit a known disease pattern?
3. Are there special conditions (risk factors) that would make it difficult to identify the critical illness or known disease process?

Patients with abdominal pain who present with critical illness require simultaneous resuscitation and rapid evaluation. Stable patients undergo standard assessments with the history and physical exam being used to guide their workup. If special modifying factors are noted during the assessment, such as an immunocompromised state, alternative testing or diagnostic evaluation may be needed.

IS THIS PATIENT CRITICALLY ILL?

Critically ill patients need stabilization before diagnosis. Red flags indicating that a patient is "sick" include extremes of age, severe pain of rapid onset, abnormal vital signs, dehydration, and evidence of visceral involvement (i.e., pallor, diaphoresis, and vomiting).[9–12] The general appearance of a patient is an important guide: critically ill patients are in distress. They are wide-eyed, anxious, agitated, or obtunded. They may be pale, flushed, or icteric. Their skin may be hot and dry or cold and clammy. To the experienced clinician, it is usually obvious that something is seriously wrong. Within moments, the patient's vital signs (temperature, pulse, blood pressure, respiratory rate, and pulse oximetry) must be assessed. While vital signs are frequently abnormal in critically ill patients,[13] normal vital signs do not preclude serious illness, particularly in high risk groups such as neonates, the elderly, and the immune suppressed.[14–18] Temperature is neither sensitive nor specific for disease process or patient condition, and the presence or absence of fever cannot be used to distinguish surgical from medical disease. Blood pressure and pulse suggest the severity of the underlying process and/or blood or fluid loss. Frank shock, which develops rapidly following the onset of acute abdominal pain, is usually the consequence of intraabdominal hemorrhage. Do not perform "orthostatics" in patients who are already hypotensive or tachycardic. Tachypnea may indicate a cardiopulmonary process, metabolic acidosis, anxiety, or pain.

Table 2-1. Traditional Approaches to Acute Abdominal Pain

Neuroanatomic:	Visceral, parietal, referred
Four quadrants:	RUQ, RLQ, LUQ, LLQ; diffuse
Temporal characteristics:	Sudden versus gradual, constant versus colicky
Threat to life:	Acute MI, perforated viscus, acute mesenteric ischemia, ruptured ectopic pregnancy, ruptured abdominal aortic aneurysm, intestinal obstruction, ruptured esophagus, hemorrhagic pancreatitis
Etiology:	Infectious, inflammatory, traumatic, obstructive, toxic
Body systems:	Gastrointestinal, hepatobiliary, urinary, uterine, vascular, genital, endocrine, hematologic
Pragmatic:	Critically ill? Known disease? Special risk?

Abbreviation: MI, myocardial infarction.

Simultaneous Resuscitation and Assessment of the Critically Ill Patient

Resuscitation of the critically ill patient with abdominal pain includes: a cardiac monitor, oxygen (2 to 4 L/min via nasal cannula or mask), large bore intravenous (IV) access, and an isotonic fluid bolus adjusted for age, weight, and cardiovascular status. A "rainbow" of blood samples should be drawn at the time of IV insertion including, at minimum: electrolytes, BUN and creatinine, complete blood count (CBC) with platelets, clotting studies, and a type and screen. Blood should be cross matched if the initial diagnostic impression suggests a hemorrhagic etiology or if it is believed that the patient will require urgent surgery. In addition to obtaining a clear description of the pain itself ("PPQRSTT:" provocative/palliative factors, quality, radiation, associated symptoms, timing, and what the patient has taken for the pain), the brief history must address pertinent past medical illness (diabetes, heart disease, hypertension, liver disease, renal disease, pregnancies, sexually transmitted diseases); previous abdominal surgeries; medications (steroids, immune suppressants, ASA/NSAIS, antibiotics, laxatives, narcotics, fertility agents, intrauterine devices, chemotherapeutic agents); allergies; and the last menstrual period. The patient

should also be asked about previous episodes of similar abdominal pain including any prior doctor or ED visits, diagnostics, and treatments. If available, previous test results and physician impressions should be sought, but should not delay resuscitation.

Observe the patient's general appearance, level of consciousness, and posture. Take a moment to gain the patient's trust before you begin a complete physical examination. Explain what you intend to do and expose only what you need to see, exposing then recovering the patient sequentially, assuring as much privacy as possible. Note the patient's skin (color, temperature, turgor, perfusion status) and include a brief heart and lung exam. Determine immediately whether the abdomen is "acute," as indicated by the presence of peritoneal findings: rebound tenderness, guarding, and rigidity. Rebound has been shown to have better interexaminer reliability than tenderness to palpation, distension, bowel sounds, and guarding in the evaluation of pediatric patients with acute abdomen pain.[19] However, a recent study of interrater variation of adult ED patients with acute abdominal pain found only moderate levels of agreement for the individual components of the physical examination, including the presence of a surgical abdomen.[20] No single physical finding accurately predicts the presence of appendicitis.[21] An acute abdomen warrants a more aggressive approach and urgent surgical consultation. Look at the abdomen for signs of distension (ascites, ileus, obstruction, volvulus), obvious masses (hernia, tumor, aneurysm), surgical scars (adhesions), ecchymoses (trauma, bleeding diathesis), and stigmata of liver disease (spider angiomata, caput medusa.) Next, listen. Absence of bowel sounds suggests peritonitis, ileus, mesenteric infarct, or narcotic use. Hyperperistalsis with a history of diarrhea suggests gastroenteritis. High-pitched bowel sounds suggest small bowel obstruction. Percuss the abdomen. Liver size can be estimated by the presence of dullness in the midclavicular line, except in cases of severe bowel distension. A fluid wave suggests ascites; tympany suggests dilated loops of bowel. Palpate the abdomen, saving the painful area for last. Check for hernias (inguinal, femoral, obturator, umbilical, ventral). Assess the femoral pulses. Evaluate the aorta. Palpation cannot reliably exclude abdominal aortic aneurysm (AAA),[22,23] but ultrasound of the aorta by emergency physicians can accurately identify the presence of AAA.[24–27] In the presence of circulatory collapse, patients with AAA require immediate surgical exploration. Characterize any guarding as "voluntary" or "involuntary." Note rebound tenderness, but remember that more than one-third of patients with surgically proven appendicitis do not have rebound tenderness.[28] Perform a thorough genito-urinary exam, including a pelvic exam for females and a testicular exam for males. While not specific, peritoneal signs, cervical motion tenderness, and unilateral or bilateral abdominal/pelvic tenderness increase the likelihood of ectopic gestation in pregnant patients with acute abdominal pain.[29] Except in rare circumstances, all patients require a rectal examination. Males may have lower abdominal pain with prostatitis, and patients of either gender with appendicitis may have tenderness on the lateral aspect of the rectum. If stool is present, it should be checked for occult blood. Failure to perform a rectal exam has been cited successfully in malpractice litigation for missed appendicitis.[7]

Following the initial stabilization, a more thorough history can be obtained, including a full review of symptoms, a social history, and a family history (kidney stones, gallbladder problems, AAA, inflammatory bowel disease). If possible, old records should be reviewed. The patient's family members may give a more accurate answer to questions regarding a patient's alcohol use. Additional information may be available from paramedics, family members or primary caregivers, and nursing home personnel. At this point in the diagnostic process, offer symptomatic relief. Judicious use of narcotic analgesia (such as small doses of IV morphine) relieves pain and will not obscure abdominal findings, delay diagnosis, or lead to increased morbidity/mortality.[30–33] Consider IV antiemetics. Nasogastric suction may relieve patients with intractable vomiting, suspected bowel obstruction, or severe pancreatitis. Nasogastric aspirate may confirm upper gastrointestinal (UGI) bleeding. A urinary catheter will relieve bladder obstruction; hourly urine output helps gauge renal perfusion.

DOES THE PATIENT HAVE A CONSTELLATION OF SYMPTOMS THAT FIT A KNOWN DISEASE PATTERN?

Abdominal crises present with one or more of the following: pain, vomiting, abdominal distension, muscular rigidity, and or shock. The grouping of these symptoms helps to differentiate among known diseases.[34] See Table 2-2 for more information. This table is a guideline and not intended to be a rule. Another commonly used approach is to use the location of pain (diffuse, left upper quadrant, right upper quadrant, left lower quadrant, right lower quadrant, see Table 2-3) to guide differential diagnosis generation. Both approaches should be used first to determine the likelihood of life-threatening illness, then to generate a differential diagnosis to guide the workup.

Laboratory Testing

Laboratory testing does not take the place of a conscientious history and physical examination. For details

Table 2-2. Grouping of Known Abdominal Diseases by Symptoms

Pain/Vomiting/No rigidity	**Pain/Vomiting/Distension**	**Pain/(+/– vomiting)**
Acute pancreatitis	Bowel obstruction	Acute diverticulitis
Diabetic ketoacidosis	Cecal volvulus	Mesenteric ischemia
Incarcerated hernia	Sigmoid volvulus	Myocardial infarction*
		Ovarian torsion
		Testicular torsion
Pain/Shock	**Pain/Shock Rigidity**	**Distention/(+/– Pain)**
Abdominal sepsis	Perforated appendix	Elderly with bowel obstruction/volvulus
Aortic dissection	Perforated ulcer	
Hemorrhagic pancreatitis	Ruptured diverticulum	
Leaking/ruptured AAA	Ruptured esophagus	
Mesenteric ischemia (late)	Spontaneous splenic rupture	
Myocardial infarction*		
Ruptured ectopic pregnancy		

Abbreviation: AAA, abdominal aortic aneurysm.
These symptoms and etiologic groupings are a guideline and not intended to be a rule.
*The symptoms of myocardial ischemia are variable.

Table 2-3. Differential Diagnosis by Abdominal Pain Location, Patient's Perspective

Diffuse pain
Aortic Aneurysm
Aortic dissection
Appendicitis (early)
Bowel obstruction
Gastroenteritis
Mesenteric ischemia
Metabolic disorder
Pancreatitis
Perforated bowel
Peritonitis (of any cause)
Sickle cell crisis

Right upper quadrant pain	**Left upper quadrant pain**
Appendicitis	Gastric ulcer
Biliary colic	Gastritis
Cholecystitis	Herpes zoster
Hepatitis	Myocardial ischemia
Hepatic abscess	Pancreatitis
Hepatic congestion	Pneumonia (LLL)
Herpes zoster	Splenic rupture/distension
Myocardial ischemia	Splenic infarction
Perforated duodenum	
Pneumonia (RLL)	

Right lower quadrant pain	**Left lower quadrant pain**
Aortic aneuyrsm	Aortic aneurysm
Appendicitis	Diverticulitis (sigmoid)
Crohn disease (terminal ileitis)	Ectopic pregnancy
Diverticulitis (Cecal)	Endometriosis
Ectopic pregnancy	Inguinal hernia
Endometriosis	Mittelschmerz
Inguinal hernia	Ovarian cyst (ruptured)
Meckel diverticulum	Ovarian torsion
Mittelschmerz	Pelvic inflammatory disease
Ovarian cyst (ruptured)	Psoas abscess
Ovarian torsion	Regional enteritis
Pelvic inflammatory disease	Testicular torsion
Psoas abscess	Ureteral calculi
Regional enteritis	
Testicular torsion	
Ureteral calculi	

regarding the appropriate use of laboratory tests in the evaluation of patients with acute abdominal pain, see Chapter 4. The essential items are: urinalysis (assessment for urinary tract infection, hematuria); electrolytes (prolonged vomiting can cause hypokalemia, contraction alkalosis, and azotemia); BUN and creatinine (important measures of hydration status and renal function); and CBC (as a marker of infection or blood loss). In adults and children, a single white blood cell count cannot exclude surgical disease.[35] The prothrombin time is a quick, easy screen for liver dysfunction. Serum lipase should be checked in patients with suspected pancreatitis.[36,37]

No serum marker confirms acute mesenteric ischemia.[38–41] Urinalysis is indicated for most patients with abdominal pain. Urine HCG is mandatory in women of childbearing capacity. Cervical cultures for chlamydia and gonorrhea should be obtained if pelvic infection is suspected.

Radiologic Testing

Radiologic testing does not take the place of a conscientious history and physical examination. For details regarding the appropriate use of radiologic tests in the evaluation of patients with acute abdominal pain, see Chapter 5. The most important test is an immediate, portable upright chest x-ray in patients with suspected perforation—although up to 20% of patients with perforation will not demonstrate free air.[34] An acute abdominal series (flat/erect abdomen or decubitus film) may demonstrate air/fluid levels, dilated loops of bowel, vascular calcifications, urinary stones, or free air. In the absence of suspected perforation or obstruction, plain abdominal films have limited usefulness.[42] The appropriate use of abdominal CT improves diagnosis and reduces the use of hospital resources.[43–49] Ultrasound, while strongly operator dependent, is the preferred modality for the evaluation of biliary tract disease.[50,51] An electrocardiogram (ECG) should be considered in all patients with upper abdominal pain, especially if the patient is more than 40 years of age.[52]

ARE THERE SPECIAL CONDITIONS (RISK FACTORS) THAT WOULD MAKE IT DIFFICULT TO IDENTIFY THE CRITICAL ILLNESS OR KNOWN DISEASE PROCESS?

A number of conditions camouflage critical illness in patients with acute abdominal pain. High risk groups include: patients with cognitive impairment secondary to dementia, intoxication, psychosis, mental retardation, or autism; patients who cannot communicate effectively (infants and preverbal children, patients with aphasia, patients with language barriers); patients in whom physical or laboratory findings may be minimal (the elderly) or obscured (paraplegics); and patients who are immune suppressed by disease (HIV) or medication (chemotherapy, steroids, tumor necrosis factor inhibitors). Typhlitis, for example, a condition that mimics appendicitis, is seen almost exclusively in immunocompromised patients. See Chapter 3 for a diagnostic approach.

PATIENT DISPOSITION

If the patient's diagnosis is still uncertain, the emergency physician should consider uncommon or systemic causes of abdominal pain. A consultation with general surgery, GYN, or GI may be indicated. Ideally, a brief period of emergency department observation (6 to 8 hours) may be necessary, with repeated abdominal exams by the same physician. Special consideration should be given to admitting all high-risk patients with acute abdominal pain, including children, the elderly, patients with spinal cord injuries or paralysis, and patients on steroids or immunosuppressives. Patients who are not sick and who have an unclear diagnosis can usually be discharged to follow up with their primary care provider within 24 hours.

Discharge instructions should address diet (clear liquids only, push fluids, no fatty foods, no acidic foods); medications (antacids, analgesics, avoid narcotics); and clearly defined follow-up plans (whom to see and when). It is imperative to communicate clearly with the patient and the patient's family. They should understand that the diagnosis is uncertain, and they should know which symptoms warrant a return to the emergency department (increased/different pain, fever, vomiting, syncope, bleeding).[53,54]

ELDERLY PATIENTS WITH ACUTE ABDOMINAL PAIN

Elderly patients with abdominal pain present a special challenge for emergency physicians. As a group, they have more serious illness and more surgical disease than do younger patients with abdominal pain.[2,55] Their symptoms tend to be mild and vague; their presentations late and atypical.[2,15,40,56,57] In one prospective study of patients with endoscopically proven peptic ulcer disease, 30% of elderly patients had no history of abdominal pain.[58] The overall mortality for elderly patients with acute abdominal pain is 14 to 34%.[59,60] The risk is much higher in patients over the age of 80 years,[60] and doubles if the diagnosis is incorrect at the time of admission.[60,61] Assessment of the elderly patient with abdominal pain may be limited by a decrease in the patient's cognitive status secondary to previous cerebrovascular accidents or dementia. Poor hearing and decreased vision may impair the patient's ability to give an adequate history. Underreporting of symptoms is common in the elderly, perhaps due to the perception among patients and family members that pain is a "normal" part of aging.[62,63] Fear of invasive treatments, hospitalization, and loss of independence contribute to underreporting. In addition, patients often ascribe their GI symptoms to medication effects or to the physiology of increased age. Gastric motility and emptying do not decrease in healthy, unmedicated elderly persons.[64]

Numerous studies have demonstrated that surgical emergencies are more common in the elderly than in any other patient population.[2,15,55] Surgical disease is consistently more advanced at the time of diagnosis; half of the elderly patients with appendicitis have had symptoms for more than 72 hours.[15] Complications are much more common: perforated viscus, gangrenous gallbladder, necrotizing pancreatitis, strangulated hernia, and infarcted bowel.[65] While certain variables have been associated with poor outcome (age greater than 84 years, bandemia, free air) and others with the need for surgery (hypotension, abnormal bowel sounds, massively dilated loops of bowel, extreme leukocytosis), the absence of these variables does not preclude significant disease.[66] Fever is not a reliable marker for surgical disease in the elderly,[14,50] who may be hypothermic in the presence of serious abdominal infection.[57] White blood cell count has a low predictive value for surgical disease in the elderly.[14,50] Bandemia should be considered worrisome. Computed tomography scanning has been shown to alter clinical decision making for elderly patients with abdominal pain.[49]

Cholecystitis is the most common surgical entity in elderly patients with abdominal pain,[67] followed by small bowel obstruction, perforated viscus, appendicitis, and large bowel obstruction (Table 2-4). The incidence of peptic ulcer disease is rising among elderly patients.[64] Viral gastroenteritis is uncommon among the elderly, but diarrhea occurs in 35% of patients with mesenteric ischemia.[38] Any acute abdominal pain should be considered important in an elderly patient. In one study of patients more than 80 years of age with acute abdominal pain, 86% required admission; the in-hospital mortality was 17% for patients who did not need surgery and 34% for patients who did.[60] **Clinical suspicion rather than hard data should guide the decision regarding admission of elderly patients with acute abdominal pain. No single test can distinguish among patients who should be admitted and patients who can be safely discharged.[66] A liberal admission policy is strongly advocated when the diagnosis is in doubt or follow-up is uncertain.**

PEDIATRIC PATIENTS WITH ACUTE ABDOMINAL PAIN

The evaluation of acute abdominal pain in pediatric patients differs from that of adults in several critical respects. The likely etiologies of abdominal pain in children differ based on age as well as gender (Table 2-5). While the etiology of pediatric abdominal illness is usually medical rather than surgical, there are several life-threatening abdominal conditions that occur almost exclusively in pediatric patients and for which immediate recognition and surgical consultation are imperative (midgut malrotation, necrotizing enterocolitis [NEC], intussusception). It can be very difficult to assess the degree of physiologic compromise in small children, especially infants; recognition of shock requires an extremely high index of suspicion. Age-related limitations of language and cognition constrain the patient's ability to give a useful history; children often have trouble localizing pain and relating the chronology of their symptoms.[68] Symptoms reported by parents or caregivers may also be nonspecific: lethargy, irritability, poor feeding, or fever. Moreover, pediatric patients (similar to elderly patients) may be pain free despite serious abdominal disease.[69] Nonabdominal disease (pharyngitis, diabetic ketoacidosis, adrenal crisis, vaso-occlusive sickle cell crisis) may also present with GI complaints. Emergency physicians must understand appropriate developmental milestones, know the range of normal vital signs by age,

Table 2-4. Common Causes of Abdominal Pain in the Elderly

Infectious/Inflammatory	Obstructive	Vascular
Cholecystitis	Small bowel obstruction	Abdominal aortic
Diverticulitis	(adhesions, cancer, hernia)	aneurysm
Pancreatitis	Large bowel obstruction	Mesenteric ischemia/
Peptic ulcer disease	(cancer)	infarction
	Volvulus (sigmoid, cecal)	Myocardial ischemia

Table 2-5. Differential Diagnosis of Abdominal Pain in Children by Age Group

Infant	Younger Child	Adolescent
Appendicitis	Appendicitis	Appendicitis
Colic	Constipation	Cholecystitis
Constipation	Diabetic ketoacidosis	Diabetic ketoacidosis
Gastroenteritis	Drug toxicity/overdose	Drug toxicity/overdose
Hirschsprung disease	Esophagitis	Epididymitis
Incarcerated hernia	Gastroenteritis	Esophagitis
Intussusception	Henoch-Schönlein purpura	Gastritis
Malrotation with midgut volvulus	Hepatitis	Gastroenteritis
Necrotizing enterocolitis	Incarcerated hernia	Hemolytic-uremic syndrome
Peritonitis (any etiology)	Inflammatory bowel disease	Inflammatory bowel disease
Pneumonia (lower lobe)	Intussusception	Mittelschmertz
Pyloric stenosis	Meckel diverticulum	Pancreatitis
Trauma (consider abuse)	Mesenteric adenitis	Pelvic inflammatory disease
	Peptic ulcer disease	Peritonitis (any etiology)
	Peritonitis (any etiology)	Sickle cell crisis
	Pneumonia (lower lobe)	Testicular torsion
	Psychosocial	Trauma (consider abuse)
	Sickle cell crisis	Urinary tract infection
	Streptococcal pharyngitis	
	Testicular torsion	
	Trauma (consider abuse)	
	Urinary tract infection	

and be able to estimate patient weight for fluid and medication administration. Judicious use of IV narcotics in pediatric patients with acute abdominal pain does not affect the ability to detect surgical disease.[70] Special care must be given to the emotional needs of pediatric patients and their parents. **The importance of a thorough physical examination in children with acute abdominal pain cannot be overemphasized.**

REFERENCES

1. McCaif LF, Burt CW. National Hospital Ambulatory Medical Care Survey: 2003 Emergency Department Summary. Advanced Data from Vital Health Statistics. No. 358; Hyattsville, MD: National Center for Health Statistics, 2005.
2. Brewer RJ, Golden GT, Hitch DC, et al. Abdominal pain: An analysis of 1,000 consecutive cases in a university hospital emergency room. *Am J Surg.* 1976;131:219.
3. Nagurney JT, Brown DF, Chang Y, et al. Use of diagnostic testing in the emergency department for patients presenting with non-traumatic abdominal pain. *J Emerg Med.* 2003; 25:363.
4. Selbst SM, Friedman MJ, Singh SB. Epidemiology and etiology of malpractice lawsuits involving children in u.s. emergency departments and urgent care centers. *Pediatr Emerg Care.* 2005;21:165.
5. Karcz A, Korn R, Burke MC, et al. Malpractice claims against emergency physicians in Massachusetts: 1975–1993. *Am J Emerg Med.* 1996;14:341.
6. Trautlein JJ, Lambert RJ, Miller J. Malpractice in the emergency department—review of 200 cases. *Ann Emerg Med.* 1984;13:709.
7. Fink S. Rectal examination and appendicitis malpractice claims. *South Medical J.* 1995;88:1279.
8. Kern KA. Medical malpractice involving colon and rectal disease: A 20-year Rreview of United States civil court litigation. *Dis Colon Rectum.* 1993;36:531.
9. Hasdai D, Holmes DR Jr, Califf RM, et al. Carcinogenic shock complicating acute myocardial infarction: Predictors of death. *Am Heart J.* 1999;138:21.
10. Gong MN, Thompson BT, Williams P, et al. Clinical predictors of and mortality in acute respiratory distress syndrome: Potential role of red cell transfusion. *Crit Care Med.* 2005; 33:1191.
11. Inayet N, Amoateng-Adjepong Y, Upadya A, et al. Risks for developing critical illness with GI Hemorrhage. *Chest.* 2000;188:473.

12. Zimmerman JE, Kraus WA, Sun X, et al. Severity stratification and outcome prediction for multisystem organ failure and dysfunction. *World J Surg.* 1996;20:401.

13. Jones AE, Stiell IG, Nesbitt LP, et al. Nontraumatic out-of-hospital hypotension predicts inhospital mortality. *Ann Emerg Med.* 2004;43:106.

14. Parker JS, Vukov LF, Wollan PC. Abdominal pain in the elderly: Use of temperature and laboratory testing to screen for surgical disease. *Fam Med.* 1996;28:193.

15. Hui TT, Major KM, Airtal I, et al. Outcome of elderly patients with appendicitis. *Arch Surg.* 2002;137:995.

16. Castle SC, Norman DC, Yeh M, et al. Fever response in elderly nursing home residents: Are the older truly colder? *J Am Geriatr.* 1992;39:853.

17. Kroesen S, Widener AF, Nesler P. Serious bacterial infections in patients with rheumatoid arthritis under anti-TNF-therapy. *Rheumatology.* 2003;42:617.

18. Whitney TM, Macho JR, Russell TR, et al. Appendicitis in acquired immunodeficiency syndrome. *Am J Surg.* 1992; 164:467.

19. Yen K, Karpas A, Pinkerton HJ, et al. Interexaminer reliability in physical examination of pediatric patients with abdominal pain. *Arch Pediatr Adolesc Med.* 2005;159:373.

20. Pines J, Uscher Pines L, Hall A, et al. The interrater variation of ED abdominal examination findings in patients with acute abdominal pain. *Am J Emerg Med.* 2005;23:483.

21. Paulson EK, Kalady MF, Pappas TN. Clinical practice: Suspected appendicitis. *N Engl J Med.* 2003;348:236.

22. Lederle FA, Simel DL. Does this patient have abdominal aortic aneurysm? *JAMA.* 1999;281:77.

23. Fink HA, Lederle FA, Roth CS, et al. The accuracy of physical examination to detect abdominal aortic aneurysm. *Arch Intern Med.* 2000;160:833.

24. Tayal VS, Graf CD, Gibbs MA. Prospective study of accuracy and outcome of emergency ultrasound for abdominal aortic aneurysm over two years. *Acad Emerg Med.* 2003; 10:867.

25. Walker A, Brenchly J, Sloan JP, et al. Ultrasound by emergency physicians to detect abdominal aortic aneurysms: A U.K. case series. *Emerg Med J.* 2004;21:257.

26. Kuhn M, Bonnin RLL, Davey MJ, et al. Emergency department ultrasound scanning for abdominal aortic aneurysm: Accessible, accurate, and advantageous. *Ann Emerg Med.* 2000;36:219.

27. Knaut AL, Kendall JL, Patten R, et al. Ultrasonographic measurement of aortic diameter by emergency physicians approximates results obtained by computer tomography. *J Emerg Med.* 2005;28:119.

28. Wagner JM, McKinney WP, Carpenter JL. Does this patient have appendicitis? *JAMA.* 1996;276:1589.

29. Dart RG, Kaplan B, Varallis K. Predictive value of history and physical examination in patients with suspected ectopic pregnancy. *Ann Emerg Med.* 1999;33:283.

30. Wolfe JM, Smithline HA, Phipen S, et al. Does morphine change the physical examination in patients with acute appendicitis? *Am J Emerg Med.* 2004;22:280.

31. Thomas SH, Silen W. Effect on diagnostic efficiency of analgesia for undifferentiated abdominal pain. *Br J Surg.* 2003;90:5.

32. Brownfield E. AHRQ. Use of analgesics in the acute abdomen. Available at http://www.ahrq.gov/clinic/ ptsaftey/ chapter37a.htm. Accessed September 28, 2007.

33. Pace S, Burke TF. Intravenous morphine for early pain relief in patients with acute abdominal pain. *Acad Emerg Med.* 1996;3:1086.

34. Silen W. Cope's *Early Diagnosis of the Acute Abdomen.* 21st ed. New York: Oxford University Press; 2005.

35. Mackway-Jones K. Towards evidence based emergency medicine: Best bets from the Manchester Royal Infirmary. *Emerg Med J.* 2002;19:428.

36. Steinberg W, Tenner S. Acute pancreatitis. *N Engl J Med.* 1994;330:1198.

37. Vissers RJ, Abu-Laban RB, McHugh DF. Amylase and lipase in the emergency department evaluation of acute pancreatitis. *J Emerg Med.* 1999;17:1027.

38. Park WM, Gloviczki P, Cherry KJ, et al. Contemporary management of acute mesenteric ischemia: Factors associated with survival. *J Vasc Surg.* 2002;35:445.

39. American Gastroenterological Association. AGA technical review on intestinal ischemia. *Gastroenterology.* 2000; 118:954.

40. Hendrickson M, Naparst TR. Abdominal surgical emergencies in the elderly. *Emerg Med Clin N Am.* 2003;21:937.

41. Yasuhara H. Acute mesenteric ischemia: The challenge of gastroenterology. *Surg Today.* 2005;35:185.

42. Stower MJ, Amar SS, Mikulin T, et al. Evaluation of the plain abdominal x-ray in the acute abdomen. *J R Soc Med.* 1985;78:630.

43. Rao PM, Rhea JT, Novelline RA, et al. Effect of computed tomography of the appendix on treatment of patients and use of hospital resources. *N Engl J Med.* 1998;338:141.

44. Rao PM, Feltmati CM, Rhea JT, et al. Helical computed tomography in differentiating appendicitis and acute gynecologic conditions. *Obstet Gynecol.* 1999;93:417.

45. Rosen MP, Sands DZ, Longmaid HE, et al. Impact of abdominal CT on the management of patients presenting to the emergency department with acute abdominal pain. *Am J Roentgenol.* 2000;174:1391.

46. Christopher FL, Lane MJ, Ward JA, et al. Unenhanced helical CT scanning of the abdomen and pelvis changes disposition of patients presenting to the emergency department with possible acute appendicitis. *J Emerg Med.* 2002;23:1.

47. Tsushima Y, Yamada S, Aoki J, et al. Effect of contrast enhanced computed tomography on diagnosis and management of acute abdomen in adults. *Clin Radiol.* 2002;57:507.

48. Rhea JT, Halpern EF, Ptak T, et al. The status of appendicial CT in an urban medical center 5 years after its introduction: Experience with 753 patients. *AJR Am J Roentgenol.* 2005;184:1802.

49. Esses D, Birnbaum A, Bijur P, et al. Ability of CT to alter decision making in elderly patients with abdominal pain. *Am J Emerg Med.* 2004;22:270.

50. Parker LJ, Vukov LF, Wollan PC. Emergency department evaluation of geriatric patients with acute cholecystitis. *Acad Emerg Med.* 1997;4:51.

51. Bree RL, Ralls PW, Balfe DM, et al. Evaluation of patients with acute right upper quadrant pain. American College of Radiology. ACR Appropriateness Criteria. *Radiology.* 2000; 215(Suppl):153.

52. Pope JH, Aufderheide TP, Ruthazer R, et al. Missed diagnosis of acute cardiac ischemia in the emergency department. *N Engl J Med.* 2000;342:1163.

53. Kamin RA, Nowicki TA, Courtney DS, et al. Pearls and pitfalls in the emergency department evaluation of abdominal pain. *Emerg Med Clin N Am.* 2003;21:61.

54. American College of Emergency Physicians Clinical Policy: critical issues for the initial evaluation and management of patients presenting with a chief complaint of nontraumatic abdominal pain. *Ann Emerg Med.* 2000; 36:406.

55. Bugliosi TF, Meloy TD, Vukov LF. Acute abdominal pain in the elderly. *Ann Emerg Med.* 1990;19:1383.

56. Horattas MC, Guyton DP, Wu D. A reappraisal of appendicitis in the elderly. *Am J Surg.* 1990;160:291.

57. Cooper GS, Shlaes DM, Salata RA. Intraabdominal infection: Differences in presentation and outcome between younger patients and the elderly. *Clin Infect Dis.* 1994;19:146.

58. Hilton D, Iman N, Burke GJ, et al. Absence of abdominal pain in older persons with endoscopic ulcers: A prospective study. *Am J Gastroenterol.* 2001;96:380.

59. Bender JS, Busuito MJ, Graham C, et al. Small bowel obstruction in the elderly. *Am Surg.* 1989;55:385.

60. van Geloven AAW, Biesheuvel TH, Luitse JSK, et al. Hospital admissions of patients aged over 80 with acute abdominal complaints. *Eur J Surg.* 2000;166:866.

61. Fenyo G. Acute abdominal disease in the elderly: Experience from two series in Stockholm. *Am J Surg.* 1982;143:751.

62. Ferrell BA. Pain management in elderly people. *J Am Geriatr Soc.* 1991;39:64.

63. Barucha AE, Camilleri M. Functional abdominal pain in the elderly. *Gastroenterol Clin N Am.* 2001;30:517.

64. Borum ML. Peptic ulcer disease in the elderly. *Clin Geriatr Med.* 1999;15:457.

65. Flum DR, Morris A, Koepsell T, et al. Has misdiagnosis of appendicitis decreased over time? *JAMA.* 2001;286:1748.

66. Marco CA, Schoenfeld CN, Keyl PM, et al. Abdominal pain in geriatric emergency patients: Variables associated with adverse outcomes. *Acad Emerg Med.* 1998;5:1163.

67. de Dombal FT. Acute abdominal pain in the elderly. *J Clin Gastroenterol.* 1994;19:331.

68. Anders JF, Powell EC. Urgency of evaluation and outcome of acute ovarian torsion in pediatric patients. *Arch Pediatr Adolesc Med.* 2005;159:532.

69. Mader TJ, McHugh TP. Acute pancreatitis in children. *Pediatr Emerg Care.* 1992;8:157.

70. Kim MK, Strait RT, Sato TT, et al. A randomized clinical trial of analgesia in children with acute abdominal pain. *Acad Emerg Med.* 2002;9:281.

3

Abdominal Pain in Special Populations

Henderson D. McGinnis
David M. Cline

HIGH YIELD FACTS

- The most important determinant of the human immunodeficiency virus positive (HIV+) patient's course when presenting with abdominal pain is the CD4 count.
- The three most common nonobstetric causes of surgical disease in pregnant patients presenting with acute abdominal pain are, in decreasing frequency: appendicitis, cholecystitis, and bowel obstruction.
- The most common symptom of an acute abdomen in a spinal cord injury patient is autonomic dysreflexia (84%), which is experienced by the patient as increased spasticity of limbs, sphincters or adjacent abdominal muscles, or abnormal sweating.

Patients presenting with atypical symptoms or unique diseases deserve special mention. The presentation and differential diagnosis of pediatric and elderly patients are discussed in Chapter 2. Sickle cell patients are discussed in Chapter 45. Readers should refer to those chapters for discussion of differential diagnoses in those patient groups. Classic presentations of abdominal emergencies can be altered by the patient's immunologic state as well as changes in the patient's physiology, such as pregnancy or spinal cord injury.

PATIENTS WITH ALTERED IMMUNOLOGIC FUNCTION

Epidemiology

Patients with altered immunologic function can be divided into two basic groups that affect management:

(1) mild/moderate immunologic dysfunction, and (2) severe immunologic compromise. The first group has altered presentations yet similar surgical pathology compared to the general population while the second group requires a greatly expanded differential diagnosis listing to include opportunistic infections and their complications. Abdominal pain necessitating medical evaluation is common in patients with HIV infection, affecting 12% to 45% of patients.[1] In patients hospitalized for hematologic malignancies the incidence of neutropenic enterocolitis (typhlitis) is 5.3%, while the incidence of severe, life-threatening infections may be as high as 28.5%.[2,3]

Mild to Moderate Immunologic Dysfunction

Patients in this group include those with malignancies (but not on chemotherapy), the elderly, the malnourished, diabetics, anergic patients, uremic patients, and patients with acquired immunodeficiency syndrome (AIDS) but CD4 counts are over 200/mm.[3] The primary problem in this group is delayed or atypical presentations of common surgical diseases. However, these patients have similar differential diagnoses compared to the general population.

Highly active antiretroviral therapy (HAART) has dramatically changed the course of patients with AIDS. Patients who are maintained on HAART and have CD4 counts over 200/mm^3 are much less likely to have opportunistic infections and the ensuing complications as described below. Comparing data from the 1980s to a recent study illustrates this point. The overwhelming majority of HIV+ patients presenting with abdominal pain detailed in a study published in 1986 had AIDS related infections or complicaitons.[1] In contrast, a retrospective study of 108 cases of HIV+ patients with abdominal pain presenting to the emergency department published in 2001 found the diagnosis of AIDS-related opportunistic infection in only 7% of patients[4] (Table 3-1). This percentage is down from 65% of cases in the pre-HAART era.[1,5] In the HAART era, surgery was found to be necessary in 8% of patients, with only 1% having complications of AIDS related opportunistic infections.[4]

Severe Immunologic Compromise

Patients in this group are likely to present with opportunistic infections and the ensuing complications as a cause of abdominal pain. The differential and workup must include viruses, mycobacteria, parasites, and fungi. Patients in this group include AIDS patients with CD4 counts less than 200/mm^3 transplant patients, patients

Table 3-1. Causes of Abdominal Pain in HIV+ Patients[4]

Cause	Percentage
Nonspecific abdominal pain	19%
Gastroenteritis/diarrhea	14%
Gastritis/peptic ulcer disease	9%
Urinary tract infection	6%
Pancreatitis	5%
Appendicitis	5%
Disseminated mycobacterium	4%
Other AIDS-related opportunistic infection	3%

Abbreviations: HIV+, human immunodeficiency virus positive; AIDS, acquired immunodeficiency syndrome.

actively undergoing chemotherapy for malignancy, neutropenic patients, or any patient with an active disease process that has lead to opportunistic infection in the past. Patients in this group are at risk for severe sepsis with opportunistic infection, unique surgical diseases and complications, such as bowel perforation secondary to cytomegalovirus, or neutropenic enterocolitis. A case series of AIDS patients taken to emergency surgery in the pre-HAART era found bowel perforation in 61%, of which 46% was due to cytomegalovirus (CMV);[6] mortality was 46% of patients. The most common preoperative diagnoses in the modern era is perforated viscus, bowel obstruction, intraabdominal abscess, and hemorrhage. In contrast to the pre-HAART era, the most common finding at surgery for suspected perforated viscus is lymphoma or disseminated mycobacterial disease, with CMV related perforation found much less commonly.[7] Some antiviral medications are known to cause pancreatitis (didanosine) and some lead to ureterolithiasis (indavir). Antiretroviral medications may also cause abdominal pain associated with lactic acidosis.

Neutropenic enterocolitis (previously termed typhlitis, the ileocecal syndrome, or necrotizing enterocolitis) has emerged as the most common cause of the acute abdomen in the neutropenic cancer patient.[2,3] It is a direct complication of profound neutropenia from chemotherapy, aplastic anemia, cyclic neutropenia, or from end-stage AIDS.

Clinical Features

The most common associated symptoms of patients with HIV presenting with abdominal pain include nausea and vomiting (58%), diarrhea (32%), and fever (21%).[4] Approximately 11% are sent for computed tomography

(CT).[4] CD4 counts less than $200/mm^3$ are associated with disseminated mycobacterium and other AIDS related pathology.[6] Weight loss is also associated with AIDS related pathology at laparotomy.[7]

The most important determinant of the HIV+ patient's course is the CD4 count. The mean survival of patients found to have non-Hodgkin lymphoma or disseminated mycobacterial disease is 6 months or less. Toxic megacolon has been associated with CMV opportunistic infections or *Clostridium difficile* colitis. Approximately 50% of HIV patients are infected with hepatitis B or C; cirrhosis follows if hepatitis is not controlled. Hepatic opportunistic disease is seen with CD4 counts less than $100/mm^3$, which includes CMV and fungal infections. Splenomegaly is a common physical finding and is usually caused by CMV, *Mycobacterium tuberculosis, Mycobacterium avium intracellulare (MAI)*, or *Pneumocystis carinii*.

Symptoms of neutropenic enterocolitis include fever, nausea, vomiting, abdominal distention, diarrhea (frequently bloody), with pain localizing to the right lower quadrant mimicking appendicitis. Presentations with hypotension and other signs of sepsis are common.

Diagnosis and Differential

In HIV+ patients with normal CD4 counts, typical differential tables for abdominal pain apply (Table 3-1). In the event of CD4 counts below $200/mm^3$ opportunistic infections and potentially perforation associated with CMV disease, MAI, or non-Hodgkin lymphoma should be considered (Table 3-2). Splenic abscess can the pre-

Table 3-2. Differential Diagnosis of Abdominal Pain in AIDS Patients with Severe Immunocompromise

Bowel perforation due to CMV, lymphoma, Kaposi sarcoma, or MIA
Cholecystitis, including CMV associated acalculous disease
Perforated diverticulitis
Splenic abscess, infarction, or rupture
Appendicitis
Pancreatitis with or without hemorrhage
Bowel obstruction secondary to adhesions or volvulus
Traumatic rectal perforation
Intraabdominal abscess
Lymphoma with hemorrhage
Toxic megacolon

Abbreviations: CMV, cytomegalovirus; MIA, *Mycobacterium avium intracellulare*; AIDS, acquired immunodeficiency syndrome.

senting symptom of atypical infections in the AIDS patient due to atypical mycobacterium, tuberculosis, and *P. carinii*.

Lactic acidosis can be a serious complication of antiretroviral treatment and is more common in woman. Nonspecific symptoms such as nausea, vomiting, and abdominal pain are the most common complaints. The patient may have a mildly elevated lactate with no symptoms or may appear toxic. It is thought that the lactic acidosis is caused by mitochondrial toxicity.

Contrast CT scan is an important diagnostic tool to determine pathology and potentially avoid surgery in the immunocompromised patient. Findings of neutropenic enterocolitis on CT scan include a thickened colonic wall >4 mm with decreased attenuation of contrast due to necrosis or edema, and/or extraluminal fluid collection in the area of the cecum.[2] Ultrasound (US) may also demonstrate increased cecal wall thickness. Blood cultures may show enteric pathogens and/or fungemia.

Differential diagnosis of patients with suspected neutropenic enterocolitis includes acute appendicitis, pseudomembranous colitis (which can be excluded by *C. difficile* toxin assay and/or sigmoidoscopy), hepatic veno-occlusive disease, paralytic ileus, bowel obstruction, obstructed hernia, and intussception.[8]

Emergency Department Management

In general, patients presenting with immunocompromise and abdominal pain are best managed medically. The more severe the immunocompromise, the greater the mortality with surgery, which is chiefly due to associated sepsis. Conversely, HIV+ patients on HAART therapy with CD4 counts above 200/mm^3 should not have surgery delayed if it is indicated because these patients can be expected to have a near normal course with surgery.

Treatment of suspected or documented neutropenic enterocolitis includes fluid resuscitation, broad spectrum antibiotic treatment, and bowel rest to give the patient time for neutropenia to reverse itself. Antibiotic section includes monotherapy with cefepime, ceftazidime, or a carbapenem or combined therapy with an antipseudomonal beta-lactam antibiotic in combination with an aminoglycoside as empiric therapy.[2,9] Piperacillin-tazobactam is another choice.[10] Surgery is reserved for cases of documented or suspected perforation.

Because prognosis is poor in severely immunocompromised patients taken to surgery, conservative therapy should be considered first. After negative CT, careful serial abdominal examination should be used to follow the patient.[11] Medical management of the AIDS patient with severe abdominal pain and suspected infection includes fluid resuscitation and broad spectrum antibiotic treatment, with consideration to opportunistic organisms such as atypical mycobacterium, tuberculosis, fungi, and *P. carinii*. Lactic acidosis associated with retroviral therapy is treated with aggressive administration of fluids.

ABDOMINAL PAIN IN THE PREGNANT FEMALE

Ectopic pregnancy is the most important diagnosis to be ruled out in pregnant female patients presenting to the emergency department with abdominal pain. After this has been excluded, a number of diagnoses should be considered.

Epidemiology

Approximately 0.2 to 1% of pregnant patients require nonobstetric general surgery.[12] The incidence of appendicitis is 0.4 to 1.4 per 1000 pregnancies, and is the most common nonobstetric surgical emergency in pregnant patients.[13] Rupture of the appendix occurs 2 to 3 times more commonly in pregnancy due to delays in diagnosis and operation. Perforated appendicitis is the number 1 surgical cause of fetal loss during pregnancy. Causes of abdominal pain in the pregnant patient are listed in Table 3-3.

Table 3-3. Differential Diagnosis of Pregnant Patients with Abdominal Pain

Ectopic pregnancy
Placental abruption
Appendicitis
Cholecystitis
Pancreatitis
Intussusception
Pyelonephritis
Round ligament syndrome
Renal colic, hydronephrosis
HELLP syndrome
Spontaneous abortion
Ovarian torsion
Uterine fibroid degeneration
Ovarian cysts or tumors
Intraabdominal abscess
Rectus muscle abscess
Crohn disease
Intestinal obstruction
Splenic artery aneurysm
Hepatic adenoma rupture

Abbreviation: HELLP, hemolysis, elevated liver enzymes, low platelets.

Pathophysiology

During pregnancy a number of physiologic changes take place that complicate the diagnosis of surgical disease. There is increased cardiac output and heart rate accompanied by physiologic anemia and leukocytosis, increased gastric acidity with decreased gastric motility, and increased minute ventilation accompanied by decreased functional residual capacity. The enlarging uterus causes displacement of the intraperitoneal organs and pressure on the inferior vena cava leads to decreased venous return. The stretching of the abdominal wall and compression of the viscera results in diminished response to peritoneal irritation and altered or referred pain perception. This changes and makes more difficult the localization of pain.

Clinical Features

After the first trimester, the appendix is gradually displaced above the McBurney point, with horizontal rotation of its base. The upward displacement occurs until the eighth month of gestation when more than 90% of appendices lie above the iliac crest, and 80% rotate upward and toward the right subcostal area.[13,14] However, the most consistent clinical symptom of appendicitis in pregnant woman is vague right lower quadrant abdominal pain, regardless of gestational age.[14] Fever with appendicitis is less common during pregnancy (25%) and leukocytosis is difficult to interpret. The laxity of the abdominal musculature makes rebound tenderness less reliable, but is found in 70% of pregnant patients with appendicitis.[13]

Biliary tract disease is the second most common surgical disease presenting during pregnancy. Pregnancy predisposes to gallstone formation, occurring in approximately 7% of nulliparous woman but 19% of woman with two or more pregnancies.[15] Symptoms are similar to nonpregnant patients. Invasive procedures are well tolerated, especially if surgery is during the second trimester. Pancreatitis in pregnant patients is usually secondary to biliary tract disease. Pancreatitis occurs more frequently in the third trimester and the postpartum period. Signs and symptoms are similar to nonpregnant patients.

Intestinal obstruction is the third most common nonobstetrical reason for laparotomy during pregnancy, complicating 1 in 1500 to 3000 pregnancies. As in the general population, it is most commonly seen in association with adhesions. Its incidence increases as pregnancy progresses.

Splenic artery aneurysms are rare, but are more common in pregnant woman. It is often asymptomatic until rupture, which frequently results in shock or unexplained death. Rupture occurs more frequently during the third trimester and often during labor.

Hepatic adenoma rupture is more common during pregnancy. Most patients can be treated conservatively with frequent US monitoring of the fetus and the mother.

Crohn disease relapses during pregnancy occur more frequently in the first trimester. Abscess formation is more difficult to control during pregnancy, and there is a higher risk of free perforation. Therefore, patients with a history of Crohn disease presenting with peritoneal signs should undergo diagnostic testing without delay and when indicated, exploration.

Diagnosis and Differential

The differential diagnosis of abdominal pain in pregnancy is listed in Table 3-3.[16] Leukocytosis is normal in pregnancy and therefore is less helpful in the differentiation of surgical disease. When HELLP syndrome (hemolysis, elevated liver enzyme levels, and a low platelet count) is suspected, complete blood count to assess platelets, and liver function tests should be obtained. Otherwise, indications for and interpretation of laboratory testing in the pregnant patient is similar to the nonpregnant patient.

The estimated dose of radiation from a plain film of the abdomen is 250 mrad, while the dose of radiation to the fetus from a CT scan of the abdomen is 3000 mrad. Radiation exposure should be kept to a minimum, shielding the fetus whenever possible if radiographs are taken.

Ultrasound is the diagnostic imaging modality of choice and can be used to assess for appendicitis, free fluid or blood accumulations, ovarian torsion, ovarian cysts, degenerating fibroids, pancreatitis, urolithiasis, or biliary tract disease. When considering the diagnosis of ectopic pregnancy, transvaginal US should be considered (see Chapter 32). If the diagnosis cannot be confirmed by US, magnetic resonance imaging should be considered, as well as laparoscopy. In selected cases, where the risk of a missed diagnosis outweighs the risk of radiation to the fetus, CT scanning may be performed. Finally, exploratory laparotomy may be considered in cases where peritonitis is evident but the diagnosis remains unclear.

Emergency Department Care and Disposition

After the diagnosis of surgical disease is made in the pregnant patient, management is similar to the nonpregnant patient with a few selected differences. Affects on the fetus should be considered whenever the choice of pharmacologic agent is being made. Tocolytics should be reserved for patients who are having active contractions and not given prophylactically. See the appropriate chapters in this book for the management of selected surgical or medical conditions.

ABDOMINAL EMERGENCIES IN PATIENTS WITH SPINAL CORD INJURY

Epidemiology

In the past, acute abdominal conditions have been found to be a cause of death in 10% of spinal-cord-injury patients.[17,18] Perforated viscus with peritonitis and sepsis is reported as the most common cause of these deaths.

Pathophysiology

Normal somatic sensation to the abdominal wall originates from T7 through T12 or L1. Patients with complete cord injuries above T7 will have no abdominal wall sensation. Painful stimuli from the abdominal viscera reach the spinal cord through thoracic sympathetic, splanchnic, hypogastric, or pelvic nerves. The sympathetic outflow to most of the viscera comes from T5 or below. Patients with injuries above the level of T6 are referred to as having "high" cord lesions. Patients with complete high cord lesions may have no perception of pain. Chronic constipation is common in spinal cord injury patients and many of these patients will have chronic abdominal distension.

Clinical Features

Patients with high cord lesions presenting with an acute abdomen may experience no pain, while patients with lower lesions may have pain, but be unable to localize the pain because of loss of sensation to the abdominal wall. The most common symptom of an acute abdomen in spinal-cord-injury patients is autonomic dysreflexia (84%), which is experienced by the patient as increased spasticity of limbs, sphincters, or adjacent abdominal muscles and/or abnormal sweating.[19] Any change from normal function should alert the clinician to the possibility of peritoneal irritation.[19] In addition to increased spasticity, symptoms include abdominal pain (35%), abdominal distension (35%), fever (15%), shock (8%), and vomiting (8%).[19,20] Other symptoms include pain referred to the shoulder or scapula, change in bowel habits, headache, elevated blood pressure, or simply the feeling that "something is wrong."

Diagnosis and Differential

Peptic ulcer disease with or without perforation is the most common early surgical disease post-spinal cord injury, followed by intestinal obstruction.[17] As time progresses, all surgical disease should be considered, but according to one case series, biliary disease is more common than in the general population.[20] Urinary tract infections, often in association with urinary catheters, are common, but the presence of pyuria does not rule out surgical disease as the cause of a patient's acute presentation.

Leukocytosis should not be relied on to predict acute abdomen in spinal cord injured patients as it is found in as few as 33% of patients.[20] Diagnostic imaging is particularly helpful in the assessment of the acute abdomen in spinal cord injured patients. Use of ultrasound or CT scanning can improve the diagnostic accuracy to 77%.[17] When considering surgical disease, the differential should remain broad as the patient's ability to localize pain is so limited. The most important part of the nonsurgical differential is unsuspected life threatening infections.

Emergency Department Care and Disposition

If the diagnosis remains unclear and the patient has signs of acute disease, the patient should be admitted to the hospital until serious pathology can be reasonably ruled excluded. Infections, whether intraabdominal or otherwise, should be aggressively treated with indicated antibiotics (see appropriate chapters in this book for antibiotic choice and indications). Fluid resuscitation should be undertaken. Once the diagnosis is in hand, a guide to further management can be found in the appropriate titled chapters following this one.

Pitfalls

- Failure to verify an intrauterine pregnancy to rule out ectopic pregnancy as you are considering other causes of abdominal pain in the pregnant patient.

- Failure to consider atypical causes of infections in immunocompromised patients as a cause of abdominal pain.

- Failure to recognize the atypical symptoms of the acute abdomen in spinal cord injury patients.

- Attributing abdominal pain to urinary tract infection in the spinal cord patient before more serious causes have been ruled out.

REFERENCES

1. Barone JE, Gingold BS, Arvantits ML, et al. Abdominal pain in patients with acquired immune deficiency syndrome *Ann Surg.* 1986:204:219.
2. Gorschlüter M, Mey U, Strehl J, et al. Neutropenic enterocolitis in adults: Systematic analysis of evidence quality *Eur J of Haematol.* 2005;75;1.
3. Micozzi A, Caton Ic, Monaco M, et al. High incidence of infectious gastrointestinal complications observed in patients with acute myeloid leukemia receiving intensive chemotherapy for first induction of remission. *Supp Care Cancer.* 2005;4:294.
4. Yoshida D, Caruso JM. Abdominal pain in the HIV patient. *J Emerg Med.* 2002;23:111.
5. Parente F, Cernuschi M, Antin S, et al. Severe abdominal pain in patients with AIDS: Frequency, clinical aspects, causes, and outcome. *Scand J Gastroenterol.* 1994;29:511.
6. Wilson SE, Robinson G, Williams RA, et al. Acquired immune deficiency syndrome: Indications for abdominal surgery, pathology, and outcome. *Ann Surg.* 1989; 210:428.
7. Chambers AJ, Lord RSA. Incidence of acquired immune deficiency syndrome (AIDS) related disorders at laparotomy in patients with AIDS. *Br J Surg.* 2001;88:294.
8. Pandey M, Mathew A, Geetha N, et al. Acute abdomen in patients receiving chemotherapy. *Indian J Cancer.* 2001; 38:68.
9. Hughes WT, Armstrong D, Bodey GP, et al. 2002 guidelines for the use of antimicrobial agents in neutropenic patients with cancer. *Clin Infect Dis.* 2002;34:730.
10. Gorschluter M, Hahn C, Fixson A, et al. Piperacillin-tazobactam is more effective than ceftriaxone plus gentamicin in febrile neutropenic patients with hematologic malignancies: a randomized comparison. *Support Care Cancer.* 2003;11:362.
11. Scott-Conner CEH, Fabrega AJ. Gastrointestinal problems in the immunocompromised host. *Surg Endosc.* 1996; 10:959.
12. Malangoni MA. Gastrointestinal surgery and pregnancy. *Gastroenterol Clin North Am.* 2003;32:181.
13. Tamir IL, Bongard FS, Klein SR. Acute appendicitis in the pregnant patient. *Am J Surg.* 1990;160:571.
14. Mourad J, Elliot JP, Erickson L, et al. Appendicitis in pregnancy; new information that contradicts long-held clinical beliefs. *Am J Obstet Gynecol.* 2000;182:1027.
15. Gilat T, Konikoff F. Pregnancy and the biliary tract. *Can J Gastroenterol.* 2000;14:55D.
16. Parangi S, Levine D, Henry A, et al. Surgical gastrointestinal disorders during pregnancy. *Am J Surg.* 2007;193:223.
17. Neumayer LA, Bull DA, Mohr JD, et al. The acutely affected abdomen in paraplegic spinal cord injury patients. *Ann Surg.* 1990;212:561.
18. Sheridan R. Diagnosis of the cuate abdomen in neurologically stable spinal cord injured patients. *J Clin Gastroenterol.* 1992;15:325.
19. Strauther GR, Longo WE, Vergo KS, et al. Appendicitis in patient with previous spinal cord injury *Am J Surg.* 1999; 178:403.
20. Miller BJ, Geraghty TJ, Wong CH, et al. Outcome of the acute abdomen in patients with spinal cord injury. *ANZ J Surg.* 2001;71:407.

4

Utility and Limitations of Laboratory Studies

Michael T. Fitch

HIGH YIELD FACTS

- Laboratory studies in the absence of appropriate clinical suspicion are of limited use.
- History and clinical findings should guide the use of laboratory studies.
- White blood cell (WBC) count may be useful in conjunction with other clinical parameters in the diagnosis of appendicitis but is controversial and should not be relied on as an isolated laboratory test.
- Laboratory studies alone cannot rule out acute cholecystitis.
- Lipase should be used instead of amylase in the diagnosis of pancreatitis.
- Urinalysis with microscopy can help with diagnosis of urinary tract infections (UTIs).

INTRODUCTION

Laboratory investigations are a common component of the emergency department (ED) evaluation of patients with acute abdominal pain. These tests can be a valuable component of the patient's clinical evaluation and may help with diagnosis and treatment planning. As with all ancillary testing, it is important for physicians to understand the diagnostic limitations of these studies in order to appropriately interpret their results for patient care. Overreliance on laboratory values can lead to diagnostic error, especially if such studies are used without appropriate clinical suspicion or physical findings. If "routine" laboratory testing is ordered on all patients with abdominal pain, the diagnostic performance of these studies will be less useful than when the same studies are ordered in a population of patients with specific suspected disease processes. Therefore, judicious use of testing is appropriate to maximize this important

diagnostic modality, and there are published clinical guidelines that may help clinicians in determining which tests are most appropriate for various clinical situations.[1]

Screening Laboratory Testing

When considering the use of "screening tests" in a patient presenting with acute abdominal pain, there are some basic concepts that can be learned from studies of asymptomatic patients. Preoperative testing is one area of medicine that has examined the concept of routine laboratory testing as screening for potentially unsuspected medical conditions. Critical analysis of this practice in a comprehensive review of patients being considered for elective surgical procedures demonstrates that the likelihood of an abnormal test in the absence of disease goes up with each additional test that is ordered on a population of patients, and that most laboratory studies do not meet the criteria to perform as a screening test for asymptomatic patients.[2]

While not directly comparable to a population of patients presenting to the ED with acute abdominal pain, the general concept of test performance in the absence of clinical suspicion and adequate pretest probability does apply to our decision to order laboratory testing. In some institutions, ED protocols automatically generate orders for laboratory studies in all patients with abdominal pain.[3] Ordering labs prior to history and physical examination may lead to testing of patients whose pretest probability for specific disease entities is not high enough for the subsequent results to be of clinical value in decision-making. Even in the setting of acute medical admissions to the hospital, some authors suggest that the routine use of emergency laboratory testing does not significantly impact patient management in the majority of patients.[4] In this study of acute medical admissions, only 17% of all tests performed on patients admitted to the hospital were abnormal, and of these few abnormalities, only one-third were found to be helpful for diagnostic purposes. Electrolytes and BUN serum testing were only abnormal 7% of the time, and these results were rarely helpful with diagnosis or treatment.[4]

Emergency department patients who present with acute abdominal pain also may not benefit from unstructured laboratory testing. Few studies have specifically looked at the question of the diagnostic utility of laboratory testing in the absence of other tests (such as radiologic imaging). One prospective study of ED patients with nontraumatic abdominal pain attempted to determine the utility and diagnostic value of laboratory and radiology testing in the ED.[3] Results suggested that the most likely diagnosis and change in disposition occurred in more than one-third of the patients. However, the majority of this benefit came from imaging studies, as no laboratory test alone changed disposition or diagnosis in greater than 16% of patients.

Laboratory Testing in Acute Abdominal Pain

The WBC count of a complete blood count (CBC) is one laboratory test that has been studied in acute abdominal pain. Despite anecdotal evidence, the literature suggests that CBC results are nonspecific and do not perform well as a screening test in acute abdominal pain.[5] In a review of 1000 cases of abdominal pain in the ED, 56% of patients with intestinal obstruction and 43% of the patients with gastroenteritis had increased WBC counts, while 31% of patients with no specific discharge diagnosis also had leukocytosis.[6] Such nonspecific findings are supported by other studies that suggest the WBC fails to discriminate degrees of intraabdominal inflammation,[7] and that CBC results only rarely change patient management or diagnosis.[8]

The published studies that examine the use of specific laboratory tests for nonspecific abdominal pain suggest that this is not an efficient or accurate way to evaluate patients with this complaint. The positive and negative predictive values of a diagnostic test will change with the prevalence of a disease in the population being studied, and thus indiscriminate use of any laboratory test will decrease its reliability for diagnosing or ruling out specific disease entities. In addition, there are no studies in ED patients that demonstrate useful sensitivity or specificity for the "routine" use of CBC, electrolyte panels, liver function tests, amylase, lipase, or urinalysis in acute abdominal pain.

Directed use of laboratory studies to answer specific clinical questions is most appropriate to maximize the information obtained from this type of testing. The focused use of laboratory studies is recommended based on patient history and physical exam findings, as laboratory data may help to confirm a diagnosis that is suggested by clinical exam. Table 4-1 lists a number of laboratory tests that may be considered after a history and physical exam are completed in the setting of the appropriate suspicion based on clinical impression. This table is not intended to be an exhaustive list of all possibilities, and the reader is encouraged to consult additional resources such as the position statement published by a national committee that may provide

Table 4-1. Suggested Laboratory Studies for Goal-directed Clinical Testing in Acute Abdominal Pain

Laboratory Test	Clinical Suspicion
Amylase	Pancreatitis (if lipase not available)
Lipase	Pancreatitis
Beta-HCG	Pregnancy Ectopic or molar pregnancy
Coagulation studies (PT/PTT)	GI bleeding End-stage liver disease Coagulopathy
Electrolytes	Dehydration Endocrine or metabolic disorder
Glucose	Diabetic ketoacidosis Pancreatitis
Gonococcal/Chlamydia testing	Cervicitis/urethritis Pelvic inflammatory disease
Hemoglobin	GI bleeding
Lactate	Mesenteric ischemia
Liver function tests	Cholecystitis Cholelithiasis Hepatitis
Platelets	GI bleeding Coagulopathy
Renal function tests	Dehydration Renal insufficiency Acute renal failure
Urinalysis	Urinary tract infection Pyelonephritis Nephrolithiasis

Abbreviations: GI, gastrointestinal; PT, prothrombin time; PTT, Partial thromboplastin time; HCG, human chorionic gonadotrophin.

additional guidance for a structured approach to diagnosis and ancillary testing.[1] Furthermore, additional information on the utility of diagnostic tests specific to diseases can be found in the appropriate individual chapters in this book. The remainder of this chapter will discuss a few representative clinical entities from Table 4-1 and the laboratory studies that may be used when considering these diagnoses.

White Blood Cell Count and Acute Appendicitis

Laboratory testing has long been a traditional component of the evaluation of patients with abdominal pain who are being considered for a diagnosis of acute appendicitis. Complex scoring systems have been devised to predict the risk of appendicitis, and many of these include the WBC count as a component of the score.[9–11] A retrospective study utilizing a scoring system with 305 patients suggests high sensitivity (93%) but poor specificity (38%) for leukocytosis.[9] However, when the WBC count is evaluated in isolation (without the use of a scoring system) it appears to be of limited usefulness in the diagnosis of individual patients, as 50% of patients without appendicitis may have elevated WBC counts and 13% of those with appendicitis may have normal WBC counts.[11]

The limited utility of this single test is further demonstrated in a retrospective analysis of 359 patients where 21% of patients with appendicitis had normal WBC counts; there was a similar distribution of WBC counts in those individuals with and without appendicitis.[12] Despite these limitations, several prospective studies argue that an increased WBC count may add confidence to a clinical diagnosis already established and should be included in the diagnostic workup,[13, 14] but do point out that 19% of patients with appendicitis had a normal WBC count.[14] The available evidence suggests that WBC count may be useful as a component of a large number of clinical variables to consider in patients with appendicitis and should not be relied on as an isolated laboratory test. For a discussion of the comprehensive approach to appendicitis, see Chapter 9.

Liver Function Tests and Acute Cholecystitis

When evaluating patients with right upper quadrant abdominal pain, acute cholecystitis is one disease process that carries significant morbidity and mortality that must be considered. While elevated liver enzymes may be diagnostic for a clinical entity such as hepatitis, the diagnosis of acute cholecystitis involves a combination of clinical, laboratory, and radiographic findings. This sometimes difficult diagnosis is examined extensively in a systematic review that includes 17 previous studies of the diagnostic workup of cholecystitis.[15] This analysis of the literature finds that no single clinical or laboratory finding has a negative likelihood ratio low enough to rule out acute cholecystitis. The most helpful findings that contributed to the diagnosis of acute cholecystitis were elevations of bilirubin, AST, and alkaline phosphatase. However, elevation of any one of these has only 70% sensitivity and 42% specificity, while elevation of all three has poor sensitivity (34%) with only moderate specificity (80%). Leukocytosis, as an independent variable, had only 63% sensitivity and 57% specificity. Overall, this diagnosis can be supported with laboratory testing but also requires clinical impression and radiologic imaging and cannot be confirmed or excluded with laboratory testing alone. (See Chapter 22, for more information about the diagnosis and treatment of biliary disease.)

Amylase or Lipase to Diagnose Pancreatitis

Amylase and lipase are two serum laboratory tests that are often ordered when clinical findings suggest pancreatitis as a possible diagnosis.[16] Amylase levels in the serum typically increase in 2 to 12 hours, peak in 12 to 72 hours, and normalize in 5 days. Lipase is more specific for acute pancreatitis and increases in 4 to 8 hours, peaks at 24 hours, and normalizes in 8 to 14 days. Clinical history and physical finding are important, as the diagnosis of pancreatitis is sometimes made in the absence of enzyme elevation, with up to 20% of patients with pancreatitis having normal amylase levels while comparatively few patients have normal lipase levels.[17,18]

Lipase has been shown in multiple studies to have superior sensitivity and specificity to amylase,[17–21] and several authors have suggested that ordering both enzymes is redundant and not helpful for diagnosis.[19, 21] The sensitivity and specificity of both of these laboratory studies are dependent on the threshold values selected for diagnosis. Amylase levels 3 times the upper limit of normal have a sensitivity of 90% and a specificity of 75%, while lipase levels of twice the upper limit of normal are equally sensitive with increased specificity of 80 to 99%.[21] A recent retrospective study of 10,931 mostly ED patients demonstrated a lipase sensitivity of 90% with 93% specificity using a cutoff value of 208 U/L with a higher diagnostic accuracy than amylase levels.[18] These studies support the recent suggestion to replace the use of amylase levels with lipase for the diagnosis of acute pancreatitis with no benefit to ordering both tests. (See Chapter 23, for further discussion of the diagnosis and treatment of acute pancreatitis.)

Urinalysis for Urinary Tract Infection

Urinary tract infection (UTI) and pyelonephritis are diagnosed in as many as 7% of patients who present with acute abdominal pain to the ED.[6] Urinalysis (UA), urine microscopy, and urine culture are commonly used laboratory tests when clinical suspicion for such infections exists. Interpretation of these results in the ED can be

Table 4-2. Test Performance Summaries for Urinalysis[26–29, 31–33]

Urinalysis component	Sensitivity	Specificity	PPV	NPV
Leukocyte esterase	68–91%	41–87%	3–56%	82–99%
Nitrite	0–59%	8–98%	0–83%	70–99%
Leukesterase OR Nitrite	87–92%	9–84%	2–77%	79–88%
Leukesterase AND Nitrite	38%	91–100%	0–100%	56–99%
Pyuria	34–96%	47–89%	43–64%	74–95%
Bacteriuria	33–63%	72–100%	60%	74%

Abbreviations: PPV, positive predictive value; NPV, negative predictive value

challenging, as culture results are not available immediately, and quality of specimen collection technique may influence UA and microscopy. A number of studies have attempted to determine whether clean-catch techniques are adequate or whether catheterized specimens are necessary for proper test interpretation in female patients where vaginal contamination may influence UA. Using culture results as the gold-standard, a prospective ED study demonstrated that in the nonmenstruating female patient clean-catch results are not significantly different from catheterization results.[22] For menstruating female patients, catheterization does reduce differences when comparing clean-catch and catheter specimens.[23] Studies of clean-catch techniques have found that holding the labia apart during urine collection is more important than midstream catch or perineal cleaning.[24] Clinicians should consider these aspects when making decisions about the optimal collection technique for urine studies in the ED.

No single urine test available in the ED has adequate sensitivity and specificity to be used alone for the diagnosis of UTI.[25] Table 4-2 illustrates some of the broad ranges of sensitivity, specificity, positive predictive value, and negative predictive value from some of the most commonly used portions of UA and microscopy. Note that none of these tests in isolation has adequate test characteristics to confidently diagnose or rule out urinary infection. However, combinations of leukocyte esterase and nitrites have been shown to have good sensitivity (87 to 92% for leukocytes esterase or nitrites) and good specificity (91 to 100% for leukocyte esterase AND nitrites). This has led some studies to suggest that UA alone is sufficient and that microscopy does not add to diagnostic accuracy.[26] However, other studies have suggested that microscopy plays an important role in evaluating for urine infection.[27] Since a negative UA with a negative microscopy rarely grows positive urine cultures,[28] a number of studies have recommended a combination approach to urine studies by combining leukocyte esterase, nitrites, and microscopy to maximize the sensitivity and specificity.[28–30]

Rational Use of Laboratory Testing in Patients with Abdominal Pain

Clinicians should be aware of the utility and limitations of laboratory testing when applied to patients in the ED who present with acute abdominal pain. Use of history and physical examination findings to guide judicious use of laboratory tests will lead to more meaningful results that can be helpful for diagnosis and treatment decisions. The examples discussed in this chapter and the detailed discussions of specific disease processes throughout this book will help clinicians to understand the circumstances in which ancillary laboratory testing can help in the diagnosis of patients with abdominal pain.

Pitfalls

- Do not rely on laboratory information alone for diagnosis.
- Avoid laboratory tests for diseases that are not suspected clinically.
- Understand the diagnostic limitations of laboratory studies.

REFERENCES

1. ACEP. Clinical policy for the initial approach to patients presenting with a chief complaint of nontraumatic acute abdominal pain. American College of Emergency Physicians. *Ann Emerg Med.* 1994;23:906.
2. Smetana GW, Macpherson DS. The case against routine preoperative laboratory testing. *Med Clin North Am.* 2003;87:7.
3. Nagurney JT, Brown DF, Chang Y, et al. Use of diagnostic testing in the emergency department for patients presenting with non-traumatic abdominal pain. *J Emerg Med.* 2003; 25:363.

4. Sandler G. Do emergency tests help in the management of acute medical admissions? *Br Med J (Clin Res Ed)*. 1984;289:973.

5. Young GP. CBC or not CBC? That is the question. *Ann Emerg Med*. 1986;15:367.

6. Brewer BJ, Golden GT, Hitch DC, et al. Abdominal pain; An analysis of 1,000 consecutive cases in a university hospital emergency room. *Am J Surg*. 1976;131:219.

7. Blennerhassett L, Hall JL, Hall JC. White blood cell counts in patients undergoing abdominal surgery. *Aust N Z J Surg*. 1996;66:369.

8. Silver BE, Patterson JW, Kulick M, et al. Effect of CBC results on ED management of women with lower abdominal pain. *Am J Emerg Med*. 1995;13:304.

9. Alvarado A. A practical score for the early diagnosis of acute appendicitis. *Ann Emerg Med*. 1986;15:557.

10. Malik AA, Wani NA. Continuing diagnostic challenge of acute appendicitis: Evaluation through modified Alvarado score. *Aust N Z J Surg*. 1998;68:504.

11. Ramirez JM, Deus J. Practical score to aid decision making in doubtful cases of appendicitis. *Br J Surg*. 1994; 81:680.

12. Nase HW, Kovalcik PJ, Cross GH. The diagnosis of appendicitis. *Am Surg*. 1980;46:504.

13. Andersson RE, Hugander AP, Ghazi SH, et al. Diagnostic value of disease history, clinical presentation, and inflammatory parameters of appendicitis. *World J Surg*. 1999;23:133.

14. Lyons D, Waldron R, Ryan T, et al. An evaluation of the clinical value of the leucocyte count and sequential counts in suspected acute appendicitis. *Br J Clin Pract*. 1987; 41:794.

15. Trowbridge RL, Rutkowski NK, Shojania KG. Does this patient have acute cholecystitis? *JAMA*. 2003;289:80.

16. Frank B, Gottlieb K. Amylase normal, lipase elevated: is it pancreatitis? A case series and review of the literature. *Am J Gastroenterol*. 1999;94:463.

17. Orebaugh SL. Normal amylase levels in the presentation of acute pancreatitis. *Am J Emerg Med*. 1994;12:21.

18. Smith RC, Southwell-Keely J, Chesher D. Should serum pancreatic lipase replace serum amylase as a biomarker of acute pancreatitis? *ANZ J Surg*. 2005;75:399.

19. Chase CW, Barker DE, Russell WL, et al. Serum amylase and lipase in the evaluation of acute abdominal pain. *Am Surg*. 1996;62:1028.

20. Corsetti JP, Cox C, Schulz TJ, et al. Combined serum amylase and lipase determinations for diagnosis of suspected acute pancreatitis. *Clin Chem*. 1993;39:2495.

21. Vissers RJ, Abu-Laban RB, McHugh DF. Amylase and lipase in the emergency department evaluation of acute pancreatitis. *J Emerg Med*. 1999;17:1027.

22. Walter FG, Knopp RK. Urine sampling in ambulatory women: Midstream clean-catch versus catheterization. *Ann Emerg Med*. 1989;18:166.

23. Guss DA, Dunford JV, Griffith LD, et al. Clean-catch versus straight-catheter urinalysis results in women. *Am J Emerg Med*. 1985;3:369.

24. Baerheim A, Digranes A, Hunskaar S. Evaluation of urine sampling technique: Bacterial contamination of samples from women students. *Br J Gen Pract*.1992;42:241.

25. Leman P. Validity of urinalysis and microscopy for detecting urinary tract infection in the emergency department. *Eur J Emerg Med*. 2002;9:141.

26. Lammers RL, Gibson S, Kovacs D, et al. Comparison of test characteristics of urine dipstick and urinalysis at various test cutoff points. *Ann Emerg Med*. 2001;38:505.

27. Semeniuk H, Church D. Evaluation of the leukocyte esterase and nitrite urine dipstick screening tests for detection of bacteriuria in women with suspected uncomplicated urinary tract infections. *J Clin Microbiol*. 1999; 37:3051.

28. Smith P, Morris A, Reller LB. Predicting urine culture results by dipstick testing and phase contrast microscopy. *Pathology*. 2003;35:161.

29. Al-Daghistani HI, Abdel-Dayem M. Diagnostic value of various urine tests in the Jordanian population with urinary tract infection. *Clin Chem Lab Med*. 2002;40:1048.

30. Van Nostrand JD, Junkins AD, Bartholdi RK. Poor predictive ability of urinalysis and microscopic examination to detect urinary tract infection. *Am J Clin Pathol*. 2000; 113:709.

31. Lifshitz E, Kramer L. Outpatient urine culture: Does collection technique matter? *Arch Intern Med*. 2000; 160:2537.

32. Leman P. Validity of urinalysis and microscopy for detecting urinary tract infection in the emergency department. *Eur Journal of Emerg Med*. 2002;9:141.

33. Sultana RV, Zalstein S, Cameron P, et al. Dipstick urinalysis and the accuracy of the clinical diagnosis of urinary tract infection. *J Emerg Med*. 2001;20:13.

5

The Role of Imaging in Evaluating Emergency Patients with Abdominal Pain

Lawrence M. Lewis

THE ROLE OF IMAGING IN EVALUATING EMERGENCY PATIENTS WITH ABDOMINAL PAIN

This chapter reviews the advantages and disadvantages of various imaging modalities in patients with abdominal pain and is not intended to teach the interpretation of radiographic/ultrasonic images. It is becoming increasingly important for emergency physicians to become more familiar with interpreting ultrasound (US) and computed tomography (CT) imaging, and there are several references which can be helpful in learning this skill.[1–3] Characteristic images specific to individual diagnostic entities can be found throughout this book in their corresponding chapters.

INTRODUCTION

Abdominal pain comprised the single largest symptom-related cause for visiting an emergency department (ED) in 2003 (6.7% of all visits) accounting for approximately 7.5 million ED visits that year.[4] This complaint is common among all age groups and both genders, although the diagnostic probabilities and prognostic implications differ.

The etiology of abdominal pain varies significantly between younger and older adults, with younger adults having a higher percentage of "undifferentiated abdominal pain" and a higher incidence of appendicitis and seniors having higher rates of cholecystitis, bowel obstruction, and diverticulitis.[5,6]

The surgical rate for seniors with acute abdominal pain is approximately 25%.[7,8] Mortality for seniors (with or without surgical intervention) rises sharply with age, being well under 1% for those under 50 years and increasing to 7% for patients aged 80 or more.[5] It is for these reasons that diagnostic imaging has become an important tool in our armamentarium in the evaluation of the older patient with acute abdominal pain. Recommended imaging strategies differ based on age and other factors.

Computed tomography utilization in the United States has more than doubled for inpatients between 1996 and 2002.[9] This growing reliance on sophisticated imaging is evident in our evaluation of patients in the ED with acute nontraumatic abdominal pain. A multicenter study of seniors with nontraumatic abdominal pain showed that academic EDs were using CT in their diagnostic evaluation in over one-third of such patients.[8] An update of that study showed a 9% absolute increase in CT utilization between 2002 and 2004 in the ED evaluation of seniors with abdominal pain.[10]

The increasing need to improve throughput in the ED requires consideration of more than just the sensitivity and specificity of various diagnostic and imaging tests. We present recommendations for diagnostic imaging in the evaluation of abdominal pain, focusing on CT and US, and discuss cost and time efficiencies. This chapter briefly discusses nuclear imaging and magnetic resonance imaging (MRI), particularly where these modalities show superiority or promising potential.

GENERAL IMAGING RECOMMENDATIONS

There are costs and delays (as well as other risks, particularly for CT) associated with imaging; these must be weighed against the potential benefit. There is direct[11,12] and indirect[13] evidence that the two groups in whom the cost and delays associated with radiologic imaging outweigh the benefits: Those are (1) patients in whom there is a high index of suspicion for the need for prompt surgical intervention (unstable, obvious peritonitis) and (2) those in whom there is high confidence of a nonsurgical diagnosis based on history, physical examination, and/or other laboratory tests yielding a low index of suspicion of serious abdominal pathology.[10]

Thus diagnostic imaging is reserved for patients who are stable, do not have obvious signs of peritonitis, do not have a well substantiated diagnosis based on initial evaluation, and are felt to be at high enough risk that further testing is required to help exclude potentially serious pathology. The one caveat is that bedside ultrasonography can be performed in some centers quickly and give additional information that may facilitate the care of the unstable or critically ill patient. Upon consultation, following initial evaluation and stabilization, surgical specialists may request imaging to facilitate the surgical approach or to specify the involvement of surgical subspecialists. However, emergency physicians should not feel the need to obtain imaging studies prior to consultation, in cases where the need for surgery or surgical consultation is obvious from the history and physical examination.

PATIENT POPULATION SUBGROUPS

Imaging recommendations will vary based on patient age, gender, and other special circumstances such as pregnancy. A general rule is that radiation exposure should be more strongly considered as a relative contraindication in younger patients and particularly in pregnant patients.

Pediatric Patients

The risk of radiation exposure is cumulative throughout life. Therefore younger patients are at increased risk of developing a malignancy as a result of ionizing radiation than are older patients. The risk of developing a cancer from a single abdominal CT has been estimated to be as high as 1 in 2000.[14] Thus we need to have heightened awareness of the risk involved with abdominal CT, particularly in younger patients, and weigh it against the purported benefits.

Appendicitis continues to be the most common cause of surgical abdominal pain in children, although it is unlikely to occur in children less than 5 years of age.[15] There have been a number of studies looking at the usefulness of US or CT in diagnosing appendicitis in the pediatric age group. The sensitivity of US for detecting appendicitis ranges from about 50%[16] to 90%[17] averaging above 80% in most studies.[18–22] Because specificity for US has been high (88% to 99%)[23] a number of authors suggest first performing US in patients with equivocal findings for appendicitis. If the US is positive, no further testing is required. Unfortunately a negative US does not rule out appendicitis (with the exception of a clearly visualized normal appendix).[23] Therefore a negative or equivocal US should be followed up by CT for patients with a reasonably high index of suspicion for acute appendicitis.[23] There is debate as to the need for intravenous and/or rectal contrast enhanced CT, with protocols being institution specific. Finally, there have been reports of using criteria to risk-stratify children for selective diagnostic imaging strategies.[24,25]

Pregnancy

There are obvious concerns regarding the use of ionizing radiation in pregnant patients. Ionizing radiation can be measured in several ways. The amount of radioactivity a substance emits is measured in curies (Ci) the International System of units (SI) equivalent is the Becquerel (Bq). Biologic effects are based on the amount of radiation that is absorbed by tissue. Total absorbed doses are modified for any radiation exposure by time, shielding, and distance. Absorbed doses are measured in rads (SI equivalent is the gray [Gy]). A third method for measuring radiation exposure is the dose equivalent (measured in rem or sievert). For diagnostic radiographs the dose equivalent is essentially the same as the absorbed dose.[26] It is estimated that an abdominal/pelvic CT using multidetector technology exposes the fetus to approximately 30 milligray (mGy).[27] Absorbed doses less than 50 mGy are felt to be associated with no increased risk of spontaneous abortion, malignancies, or congenital malformations compared to those seen in persons exposed only to background radiation.[28] Taking the prudent approach, the American College of Radiology (ACR) Appropriateness Criteria for imaging strongly recommends the use of US for diagnostic imaging in this patient population in lieu of CT, regardless of the location of pain. Obviously, there will be exceptions, most notably in patients with multiple traumas, who may require imaging to determine the extent of intraabdominal injury.

Geriatrics

Older patients have the most to gain and sustain the least malignancy risk from CT imaging. They often present atypically,[29] have a much higher rate of surgical disease,[30,31] and have a number of potential life-threatening conditions that can be excluded with a high level of certainty using CT.[31] Because of their older age, the risk of radiation induced malignancy is also lower. Likely as a result of these considerations, this patient population has been shown to have a high rate of CT utilization for the complaint of abdominal pain.[8]

Human Immunodeficiency Virus Patients

Patients with HIV and abdominal pain constitute a distinct patient population with a significantly increased risk of serious abdominal pathology, including acquired immunodeficiency syndrome associated opportunistic infections (AIDS-OI), often requiring imaging for diagnosis. Several authors suggest the liberal use of CT scanning in AIDS patients with abdominal pain,[32,33] despite no prospective studies evaluating its use in this patient population.

Although a number of previous studies suggest a high (40% to 65%) rate of AIDS-OI,[34,35] a fairly recent study from San Francisco suggested that only a small percentage (10%) of all AIDS patients that present to the ED with abdominal pain will actually have an AIDS-OI or require surgery (8%).[36] Their findings may reflect the increased use of highly active antiretroviral therapy (HAART) in the San Francisco population. The rate of abdominal CT in this group was low (11%). However, 75% of the CTs were diagnostic. The admission rate for the HIV patients (37%) was twice that of non-HIV patients, and there is some question as to whether increased use of CT might have helped reduce the admission rate.

IMAGING RECOMMENDATIONS SPECIFIC TO PAIN LOCATION

The American College of Radiology has published imaging guidelines that are location specific.[37] They also have published guidelines for patients with diffuse abdominal pain and fever. The evidence for these recommendations will be reviewed and evaluated.

Diffuse Pain and Fever

The recommendations for immunocompetent patients with fever and diffuse abdominal pain suggest that CT has a "preeminent role in the evaluation of [these] patients," with two reports finding CT superior to clinical evaluation for diagnosis.[38,39] Despite several referenced examples in the paper where CT outperformed plain films, and the statement that "[plain films] offer no incremental information if CT is performed" the appropriateness rating for CT with oral and intravenous (IV) contrast and that for plain films are an identical 8 with the highest rating being 9. Computed tomography without contrast has a rating of 6. We believe the evidence supports using CT in this setting, unless there are contraindications or overriding considerations; even without contrast, CT outperforms plain films in the identification of serious pathology.

In the setting of fever and abdominal pain in the HIV patient, CT with oral, IV, and occasionally rectal contrast is considered the first procedure of choice for the majority of potential pathological conditions.[32,40,41]. Despite this statement the appropriateness rating of CT with contrast and that of plain films are an identical 8 out of 9. Biliary US is also rated an 8 but the only supportive statement for this regards the evaluation of HIV-related cholangitis. We believe the evidence supports the use of CT with contrast in the setting of fever and abdominal pain in an HIV patient, unless there are contraindications or overriding considerations.

Right Lower Quadrant

Evaluation of acute right lower quadrant pain focuses mainly on the diagnosis of appendicitis.[42] The ACR authors suggest that most patients with acute appendicitis can be diagnosed clinically. However, a number of recent articles suggest that the use of CT in patients with suspected appendicitis would improve care by reducing unnecessary surgery and decreasing overall hospital resource utilization.[43,44] The ACR statement suggesting that graded compression sonography be used as the initial screening test to exclude appendicitis in children, young women, and pregnant patients seems prudent and is supported by the literature cited above.

Left Lower Quadrant

Evaluation of left lower quadrant pain focuses mainly on the diagnosis of acute sigmoid diverticulitis, although there are a number of other etiologies of left lower quadrant pain, including ureteral calculi, hernias, ischemic colitis, inflammatory or infectious colitis, ovarian or testicular pathology, colonic malignancy, and genitourinary infections. Computed tomography is reported to have sensitivity ranging from 79% to 98% for sigmoid diverticulitis, and the ACR recommendation is to use CT as the primary imaging test in the evaluation of patients with left lower quadrant pain. One exception is in young women where sonography is recommended initially, since it is at least as good at diagnosing ovarian pathology, has fair sensitivity at diagnosing diverticulitis, and does not involve ionizing radiation.

Right Upper Quadrant

Evaluation of right upper quadrant pain focuses on the diagnosis of acute cholecystitis and recommends the use of US as the primary imaging modality (appropriateness rating of 8). Cholescintigraphy is recommended in patients with a normal US when there is a high index of suspicion of acute cholecystitis. Interestingly, CT and plain films have the same appropriateness score (4) for patients with fever, elevated WBC, and a positive Murphy sign. This score increases to 6 in patients in whom an US of the gallbladder is normal. There is no justification given for the appropriateness scores of CT and US. There have been no prospective studies comparing US to CT in acute cholecystitis; however, one retrospective study did show superior sensitivity of US to CT for diagnosing acute cholecystitis.[45] Newer generation multidetector scanners may improve the sensitivity of CT in this condition.

IMAGING RECOMMENDATIONS SPECIFIC TO SUSPECTED DIAGNOSIS

Imaging recommendations based on clinical diagnosis is problematic for the physician who is first attempting to diagnose the patient. However, this system offers an advantage when there is a single diagnostic possibility that far outweighs the others (e.g., rule out appendicitis). A recent study confirmed that emergency physicians order CT for older patients with abdominal pain more often to rule out potentially serious disease than for any other reason.[10] Thus, it is reasonable to evaluate the usefulness of various imaging modalities for the top diagnoses that emergency physicians want to exclude.

Appendicitis

We have previously discussed diagnostic imaging in suspected appendicitis. Several studies suggest that US is superior to clinical judgment in diagnosing acute appendicitis.[46,47] One review article evaluating both US and CT in suspected appendicitis found sensitivities for US and CT of 73% to 100% and 87% to 100%, respectively.[48] Specificities were also similar (86% to 98% for US and 83% to 97% for CT). This reported sensitivity and specificity for US is similar to the 85% sensitivity and 92% specificity reported in a large metaanalysis.[49] The reported sensitivity for CT improved to 97% to 100% with oral and rectal contrast and a focused appendiceal technique.[48] Others have found CT to be generally superior to US for the evaluation of acute appendicitis.[16] The literature suggests that CT is more accurate and less equivocal than is US for ruling out appendicitis (particularly in obese patients) and should be considered in any older patient with suspected appendicitis who is stable and without obvious peritonitis.[50] The use of screening US in children, adolescents, pregnant patients, and young adults is recommended (see "Pediatric Patients" section).

Renal Disease

The use of noncontrast CT for evaluating renal colic has been well studied and has been shown to have a sensitivity for detecting ureteral calculi of 95% or better with a similar specificity.[51,52] This is significantly higher than plain radiography (sensitivity about 50% to 60%)[53] or US, which ranges in sensitivity from 19%[54] to 93%,[55] with most reported studies showing sensitivity in the 6% to 70% range. However, the use of repeated CTs in frequent stone formers is problematic due to cumulative radiation exposure. Because of this, some authors suggest using US and KUB first, and only using CT in patients where these two modalities were negative or equivocal.[53,56,57]

Imaging serves several purposes: (1) It helps rule out other potentially serious conditions that can mimic ureteral calculi, for example, aortic dissection/aneurysm, or appendicitis; (2) It can give an indication of the degree of obstruction; and (3) It can accurately determine the

size and location of the stone, thereby allowing assessment of the likelihood of spontaneous passage. The main reason to use CT acutely would be to exclude serious alternative diagnoses. Patients with signs and symptoms of renal colic with a previous history of stones and a low suspicion of other potentially serious disease do not require CT imaging urgently. If you choose to treat empirically, and the stone does not pass or the pain does not resolve within 3 to 5 days, the patient will require imaging to confirm the diagnosis and determine size and location of stone, and degree of obstruction. A noncontrast study will not give information regarding the functioning of the kidney.

The diagnosis of pyelonephritis is usually made based on clinical and laboratory findings. However, in cases where the diagnosis is in doubt or where there is a suspicion of complicated pyelonephritis (unresolved fever after several days of antibiotics, diabetes mellitus) CT and US are both able to confirm the diagnosis and demonstrate anatomical abnormalities which may lead to alterations in management.[58,59]

Gallbladder Disease

Ultrasound is considered the test of choice for evaluating patients with suspected gallbladder disease (ACR). Whereas US has over 90% sensitivity for detecting gallstones, CT has a sensitivity around 70% to 75%.[60] Moreover, US has been shown to be superior to CT for diagnosing cholecystitis.[45] However, in many centers CT is more readily available, particularly after hours, than is US. The newer generation scanners may have improved sensitivity for cholecystitis, although this has not been demonstrated in comparative studies to date. Computed tomography scan, of course, can evaluate other organs including the liver, kidneys, and pancreas, all of which may lead to right upper quadrant pain.

Computed tomography is more sensitive for the rare condition of acalculous cholecystitis than is US.[61] Recent advances in technology and reformatting have improved CT sensitivity for choledolithiasis and biliary tract obstruction and can identify significant complications of gallbladder disease such as ascending cholangitis and perforation.[34] For suspected uncomplicated cholecystitis (stable patient without peritonitis), US should be the imaging procedure of choice whenever available. Patients with a negative CT but who show signs and symptoms highly suggestive of gallbladder disease should have either US or other diagnostic tests such as cholescintigraphy or MR cholangiopancreatography performed (see section on "Other Imaging Modalities").

Bowel Obstruction

Small bowel obstruction is responsible for about 15% of surgical admissions in patients with acute abdominal conditions.[62] The diagnosis of bowel obstruction can be made clinically when the classic presentation of abdominal distension, crampy abdominal pain, nausea, and vomiting are present particularly in a patient who is not passing stool or gas per rectum. Confirmation can be accomplished with plain radiography. However, about a third to a fourth of small bowel obstructions may be missed with the traditional obstructive series.[63,64] Several previous studies from before the era of multidetector row scanners had comparable sensitivity for plain radiography and CT to detect bowel obstruction.[63,64] These and other studies showed a much higher sensitivity for both modalities for complete obstruction than for partial obstruction.[65,66] Other studies show a high sensitivity of CT (over 90%) to detect high-grade obstruction[67] as well as partial obstruction.[68] Furthermore, CT allows the determination of the cause and location of obstruction,[63,64] and is quite good at detecting closed loop obstruction and accompanying ischemia.[54,68,69] Both conditions require urgent surgical intervention. A recent systematic review showed an aggregate sensitivity of 92% for CT to detect complete obstruction and an 83% sensitivity to detect ischemia (strangulation).[33]

The disadvantage to CT is increased radiation and the frequent use of contrast (both PO and IV). Before choosing a specific imaging test, one should consider the culture at her or his institution. Which test is faster to obtain? The use of IV/PO contrast with CT is associated with significant delays.[70] However, at institutions where IV/PO contrast is not mandatory, CT may be as quick to obtain as an obstructive series. Particularly, if surgeons at your institution usually want a CT even if the obstructive series is positive, then it makes sense to perform the more sensitive and specific test initially.

Although not commonly considered in adults, US has been shown to be at least as sensitive as plain radiography for detecting bowel obstruction and can be performed at the bedside.[71,72] Dilated, fluid-filled small bowel loops often with an edematous wall are the hallmarks of obstruction. In early or incomplete obstruction, hyperperistalsis with a to-and-fro motion of the bowel contents may be observed during real-time imaging. Ultrasound is also at least as good as plain films in detecting pneumoperitoneum.[73]

Diverticulitis

Computed tomography is very sensitive for diverticulitis (79%–98%).[37,74] It also can help distinguish this from other possible causes of left lower quadrant pain. But does every older patient with left lower quadrant pain and mild tenderness require a CT? There are patients with mild symptoms, previous episodes, and perhaps a low grade fever and mild or no elevation in their white blood cell count. Clinical judgment is obviously required, but many practitioners would empirically treat such a patient as long as they had reasonable confidence in patient compliance and follow up.

The use of US for diverticulitis has also been studied and sensitivity is reported to be in the 84% to 90% range.[47,57,75,76] This is a reasonable alternative and is the preferred imaging procedure in younger or pregnant patients. However, at least one study showed US to be significantly less sensitive in detecting abscesses,[77] and the CT detection of abscess in patients with diverticulitis suggests a high risk of failure from nonoperative management.[19]

Mesenteric Ischemia

Acute mesenteric ischemia is an uncommon cause (1%) of abdominal pain but is associated with a high mortality rate that increases significantly with delay in diagnosis.[78,79] Thus, it is important to diagnose this condition quickly prior to mesenteric infarction.

Mesenteric ischemia may be due to arterial occlusion (either thrombotic or embolic), venous obstruction, or nonocclusive conditions (arterial spasm). It also may result from strangulation of the blood supply such as occurs in intestinal obstruction. The sensitivity of various imaging modalities will differ for each of the underlying etiologies.

Arterial Occlusion (Celiac, Superior Mesenteric, or Inferior Mesenteric Artery)

Based on earlier studies showing a sensitivity of less than 70% for detecting acute mesenteric ischemia,[80–82] particularly when due to arterial occlusion, the American Gastroenterological Association (AGA) in their 2000 review on intestinal ischemia recommended selective mesenteric angiography as the "gold standard" for diagnosing this condition.[83] A report using multidetector row scanners and biphasic CT with CT mesenteric angiography achieved a sensitivity of 96% and a specificity of 94% among 62 patients with suspected mesenteric ischemia.[84] However, unless specifically ordered, CT angiography is not routinely performed. We have found routine CT to have a sensitivity of less than 80% for mesenteric/colonic ischemia.[85] If mesenteric ischemia is suspected, a discussion with the radiologist will help to ensure performance of the optimum study.

Plain x-ray has low sensitivity for detecting mesenteric ischemia in the early stages, although an abnormal plain film (usually showing ileus) suggests a poor prognosis.[79] Duplex sonography has relatively low sensitivity for detecting mesenteric ischemia but a high specificity, allowing its use to rule in the disease.[74] In centers where rapid bedside duplex sonography is available, a positive US/Doppler scan may allow the patient to move expeditiously to surgery or perhaps percutaneous endovascular stenting.[86]

Venous Occlusion (Mesenteric Venous Thrombosis)

Patients with suspected mesenteric venous occlusion (hypercoagulable state, recurrent thrombophlebitis, or venous thrombosis) were an exception to the AGA recommendation for selective angiography. It was suggested that a contrast-enhanced CT be the initial diagnostic study in these patients.[83] An earlier, fairly large series suggests the high sensitivity of CT in mesenteric venous thrombosis (MVT).[87]

Nonocclusive Mesenteric Ischemia

This condition is usually found in critically ill, hospitalized patients with low cardiac output on vasopressors. However, it can present in the ED and might be considered in patients with abdominal pain who have taken cocaine or other vasoactive drugs, and it has also been associated with digitalis, furosemide, and ergotamine. The AGA recommends angiography when this condition is suspected, both for diagnostic and therapeutic reasons.[83]

Strangulation

Strangulation of the blood supply to the bowel may result from vovulus or other causes of closed loop obstruction. These conditions are diagnosed readily with CT (see bowel obstruction above). Computed tomography has better than 80% sensitivity for detecting accompanying ischemia.[33]

Cancer (Space Occupying Lesions)

Computed tomography and US are both capable of detecting intraabdominal masses. The selection of imaging in patients in whom an intraabdominal mass or cancer is suspected depends on several factors. Ultrasound, if readily available, may be faster and less expensive and will not expose the patient to radiation or contrast.

However, in the Unites States, older patients with suspected mass lesions usually undergo contrast-enhanced CT. The use of CT may better demonstrate the relationship of the mass to the great vessels and other important anatomic areas. The success of CT to detect various cancers before they are symptomatic and prior to other screening tests has lead to its use as a screening tool, though the cost-effectiveness of this approach is questionable.[9]

Gastroesophageal Disease

The spectrum of gastroesophageal disease includes gastritis, peptic ulcer disease, and esophagitis. These conditions are usually diagnosed clinically, perhaps with follow-up using endoscopy or contrast studies. Plain radiography, CT, or US is not routinely used, although CT has been shown to be capable of diagnosing ulcer disease.[88]

Ovarian Disease

Ultrasound has been the test of choice for diseases of the ovary. It is safe, sensitive, and well tolerated and can be performed at the bedside. The addition of color flow Doppler has extended its usefulness in helping differentiate benign from malignant disease.[89] A few studies have shown that CT or MR offer some advantages, particularly in malignant disease.[90,91] For suspected ovarian pathology, the initial imaging procedure should be US, whenever available. This may be followed by other imaging modalities when necessary.

Nonspecific Abdominal Pain

Unfortunately, many patients present with a history and physical examination that does not allow the physician to collapse the differential diagnosis into one or two possible diagnoses. In the past several years, a number of articles have been published that look at the utility of CT in aiding triage and in diagnosing patients with undifferentiated abdominal pain[92–98] with several studies focusing on older adults.[8,99,100] Studies that have compared CT to plain radiographs have shown a significant advantage of abdominal CT in patients with nontraumatic abdominal pain.[96,97,100] Furthermore, the use of CT has been shown to alter diagnosis in 37% to 45% of patients, and significantly alters disposition decisions (admit/discharge/surgery) in about a quarter of patients.[92,94,99,101] The disposition changes often resulted in a net decrease in hospital admissions.[94,99] Other studies have shown that "early" CT (within 24 hours of admission) may reduce overall hospital stay and may even reduce mortality among patients admitted to a surgical service for acute abdominal pain.[102]

We need to temper the overall optimism of these studies with several caveats: First, the above studies that look at the usefulness of CT all had selection bias. Almost two thirds of patients who presented during the study periods did not have a CT performed. Therefore, the patients who underwent CT are a selected group and who are more likely to have significant pathology. Even among an older population, nearly half of patients with abdominal pain did not have serious disease[8,100] with only about a quarter having surgical disease.[8,103] Thus, clinical judgment is necessary. The majority of patients, particularly those in lower-risk populations (younger patients with few comorbidities, who also have increased relative contraindications, i.e., radiation exposure) should be evaluated carefully before considering CT scanning.

Another important caveat is that CT is not 100% sensitive. A negative CT does not rule out "badness." A few of the above studies suggest that the most common pathology missed is gallbladder disease,[8,98] but reports on sensitivity for early bowel obstruction[65] or mesenteric/colonic ischemia[82,85] are also sobering (fails to detect approximately 20% of cases). Patients with severe pain, especially with other supporting evidence for serious pathology, should not be discharged based on a negative CT. Nor is CT 100% specific, with specificities averaging about 90% for acute suspected appendicitis.[48] Diagnostic accuracy will often depend on the specific technique used. Above, we have discussed the use of arterial phase imaging when considering mesenteric ischemia. There is no unanimity on the use of oral or IV contrast for abdominal CT, and opinion will vary depending on your clinical setting (institution specific) and the clinical condition being considered (diagnosis specific). Oral contrast conservatively adds 60 to 90 minutes to the time to complete a scan.[104] Intravenous contrast will often dictate a serum creatinine result prior to the study. Because patient populations and the radiologist's technical expertise vary between institutions, clinicians should prospectively determine imagining strategies, as well as outline contrast protocols, that facilitate patient management at their institution. Agreement between clinicians and radiologists should exist for strategies that are diagnosis specific (i.e., small bowel obstruction) as well as chief complaint specific (i.e., right lower quadrant pain).

Finally, besides the obvious radiation exposure and the expense and time required for obtaining an abdominal CT, this procedure is often performed with IV iodinated contrast, which is an allergy risk and a potential nephrotoxin and has been associated with intractable acidosis in patients on metformin. There are a number of conditions that increase the risk of adverse events as a consequence of administering IV iodinated contrast material, some of which are not well recognized.[105] Anaphylactoid reactions are increased among patients with a history of asthma, hay fever, certain food allergies, or drug allergies.[106] There is increased risk of nephrotoxicity in diabetic patients,[34] reports of severe hypertensive crisis in patients with pheochromocytoma,[107] and a significant increase in overall adverse events in patients with cardiac disease.[108] Thus, it is important to discuss clinical findings and diagnostic questions with radiology colleagues, in order to select the optimum diagnostic imaging for any given clinical situation.

OTHER IMAGING MODALITIES

There are other imaging procedures, besides plain radiography, US, and CT, which are occasionally used to evaluate the patient with abdominal pain. These procedures are usually not as available as the aforementioned work horses of radiology, but they occasionally can be very helpful in those patients who appear ill but in whom the diagnostic workup has been negative, or in patients in whom some of the above tests may be relatively contraindicated.

Magnetic Resonance Imaging

Magnetic resonance imaging has been used for a variety of abdominal imaging procedures. Although MR provides good anatomical detail with high intrinsic soft-tissue contrast, it is usually not easily available and has been reserved mostly for patients in whom CT is contraindicated and in whom US is not diagnostic. This applies in particular to pregnant patients with abdominal/pelvic pain where it has been shown to be very sensitive.[77] Magnetic resonance imaging has also been shown to be very useful in imaging aortic disease as well[109] and should be strongly considered for any patient with a potential abdominal emergency in whom ionizing radiation or iodinated contrast media is contraindicated.[110]

Magnetic resonance imaging is currently the diagnostic test of choice for imaging the pancreatic and biliary tree, and MR cholangiopancreatography is considered diagnostically equivalent to endoscopic retrograde cholangiopancreatography for pancreatic and biliary ductal disease.[111]

Cholescintigraphy

Cholescintigraphy is an imaging technique used to assess hepatocytic function, gallbladder function, and cystic duct/biliary duct patency. There is a role for cholescintigraphy in patients with suspected cholecystitis in whom US is nondiagnostic. One study showed significantly higher sensitivity for diagnosing acute cholecystitis using the hepatobiliary ^{99m}Tc-iminodiacetic acid (HIDA) scan than US,[112] whereas others have shown comparable sensitivity with decreased specificity for HIDA scans compared to US.[113] It appears that HIDA scans are more sensitive than US for acute acalculous cholecystitis.[114]

Technetium Scans

Technetium labeled sulfur colloid (^{99m}Tc-sulfur colloid) and technetium labeled red blood cell (^{99m}Tc-RBC) scans are often used to determine the source of gastrointestinal bleeding. The superiority of ^{99m}Tc-sulfur colloid scans over angiography for localizing GI bleeds was demonstrated more than two decades ago.[115] Although there is theoretical advantage to the longer half-life of tagged RBCs, if scanning time is limited to one hour, the ^{99m}Tc-sulfur colloid is as sensitive at localizing the site of bleeding as ^{99m}Tc-RBC scan and is simpler and lower cost.[116]

CONCLUSION

The evaluation of patients with abdominal pain is one of the great challenges in emergency medicine. Today, we have an array of imaging modalities that can be extremely helpful in rapidly and accurately diagnosing these patients. Thirty years after Fenyo reported missed diagnosis rates that ranged from 30% for acute appendicitis and acute pancreatitis to 62% for acute diverticulitis,[117] a multicenter study showed an overall missed diagnosis rate of less than 20% for patients presenting to the ED with abdominal pain.[100] This marked improvement, in large part, is due to advances in diagnostic imaging. However, the optimal and most efficient use of diagnostic imaging requires that we perform a good history and physical examination, consider other appropriate diagnostic tests, and confer with our radiology colleagues to determine the most appropriate imaging study and technique.

REFERENCES

1. Ma OJ, Mateer JR. *Emergency Ultrasound*. New York, NY: McGraw-Hill; 2003.
2. Lee JKT, Sagel SS, Stanley RJ, et al. *Computed Body Tomography with MRI Correlation*. 3rd ed. Philadelphia, PA: Lippincott; 1998.
3. Schwartz DT, Reisdorff E. *Emergency Radiology*. New York, NY: McGraw-Hill; 2000.
4. McCaig LF, Burt CS. National Hospital Ambulatory Medical Care Survey: 2003 Emergency Department Summary. Hyattsville, Maryland: National Center for Health Statistics: Department of Health and Human Services & Centers for Disease Control and Prevention; 2005.
5. Telfer S, Fenyo G, Holt PR, et al. Acute abdominal pain in patients over 50 years of age. *Scand J Gastroenterol Suppl.* 1998;144:47.
6. de Dombal FT. Acute abdominal pain in the elderly. *J Clin Gastroenterol.* 1994;19:331.
7. Ha HK, Kim JS, Lee MS, et al. Differentiation of simple and strangulated small-bowel obstructions: usefulness of known CT criteria. *Radiology.* 1997;204:507.
8. Hustey FM, Meldon SW, Banet GA, et al.. The use of abdominal computed tomography in older ED patients with acute abdominal pain. *Am J Emerg Med.* 2005;23:259.
9. Beinfeld MT, Gazelle GS. Diagnostic imaging costs: are they driving up the costs of hospital care? *Radiology.* 2005;235:934.
10. Lewis LM, Klippel AP, Bavolek RA, et al. Quantifying the usefulness of CT in evaluating seniors with abdominal pain. *Eur J Radiol.* 2007;61:290.
11. Henriksson AE, Bergqvist D. Spontaneous pancreatic bleeding. *World J Surg.* 2003;27:187.
12. Safran DB, Pilati D, Folz E, Oller D. Is appendiceal CT scan overused for evaluating patients with right lower quadrant pain? *Am J Emerg Med.* 2001;19:199.
13. Colucciello S. Assessing abdominal pain in adults: A rational, cost-effective, and evidence-based strategy. *Emerg Med Pract.* 1999;1:1.
14. Jacob K, Steel JR. X-ray dose training: are we exposed to enough? A reply to Dr McCoubrie's letter published in Vol. 60, No. 6 (2005) on p. 730. *Clin Radiol.* 2005;60:936.
15. Graham JM, Pokorny WJ, Harberg FJ. Acute appendicitis in preschool age children. *Am J Surg.* 1980;139:247.
16. Garcia Pena BM, Mandl KD, Kraus SJ, et al. Ultrasonography and limited computed tomography in the diagnosis and management of appendicitis in children. *JAMA.* 1999;282:1041.
17. Hahn HB, Hoepner FU, Kalle T, et al. Sonography of acute appendicitis in children: 7 years experience. *Pediatr Radiol.* 1998;28:147.
18. Dilley A, Wesson D, Munden M, et al. The impact of ultrasound examinations on the management of children with suspected appendicitis: a 3-year analysis. *J Pediatr Surg.* 2001;36:303.
19. Kaiser S, Frenckner B, Jorulf HK. Suspected appendicitis in children: US and CT—a prospective randomized study. *Radiology.* 2002;223:633.
20. Lessin MS, Chan M, Catallozzi M, et al. Selective use of ultrasonography for acute appendicitis in children. *Am J Surg.* 1999;177:193.
21. Ramachandran P, Sivit CJ, Newman KD, et al. Ultrasonography as an adjunct in the diagnosis of acute appendicitis: a 4-year experience. *J Pediatr Surg.* 1996; 31:164.

22. Sivit CJ, Applegate KE, Stallion A, et al. Imaging evaluation of suspected appendicitis in a pediatric population: effectiveness of sonography versus CT. *Am J Roentgenol.* 2000;175:977.

23. Taylor GA. Suspected appendicitis in children: in search of the single best diagnostic test. *Radiology.* 2004;231:293.

24. Garcia Pena BM, Cook EF, Mandl KD. Selective imaging strategies for the diagnosis of appendicitis in children. *Pediatrics.* 2004;113:24.

25. Samuel M. Pediatric appendicitis score. *J Pediatr Surg.* 2002;37:877.

26. Ratnapalan S, Bona N, Chandra K, et al. Physicians' perceptions of teratogenic risk associated with radiography and CT during early pregnancy. *Am J Roentgenol.* 2004;182:1107.

27. Parry RA, Glaze SA, Archer BR. The AAPM/RSNA physics tutorial for residents: Typical patient radiation doses in diagnostic radiology. *Radiographics.* 1999;19:1289.

28. Council on Radiation: *Medical Radiation Exposure of Pregnant and Potentially Pregnant Women: Report Number 54* National Council on Radiation Protection and Measurement, Washington DC, 1977.

29. Cooper GS, Shlaes DM, Salata RA. Intraabdominal infection: Differences in presentation and outcome between younger patients and the elderly. *Clin Infect Dis.* 1994;19:146.

30. Bugliosi TF, Meloy TD, Vukov LF. Acute abdominal pain in the elderly. *Ann Emerg Med.* 1990;19:1383.

31. Hendrickson M, Naparst TR. Abdominal surgical emergencies in the elderly. *Emerg Med Clin North Am.* 2003;21:937.

32. Kuhlman JE, Fishman EK. Acute abdomen in AIDS: CT diagnosis and triage. *Radiographics.* 1990;10:621.

33. Slaven EM, Lopez F, Weintraub SL, et al. The AIDS patient with abdominal pain: a new challenge for the emergency physician. *Emerg Med Clin North Am.* 2003;21:987.

34. Baron RL, Tublin ME, Peterson MS. Imaging the spectrum of biliary tract disease. *Radiol Clin North Am.* 2002; 40:1325.

35. Parente F, Cernuschi M, Antinori S, et al. Severe abdominal pain in patients with AIDS: frequency, clinical aspects, causes, and outcome. *Scand J Gastroenterol.* 1994;29:511.

36. Yoshida D, Caruso JM. Abdominal pain in HIV infected patient. *J Emerg Med.* 2002;23:111.

37. Balfe DM, Levine MS, Ralls PW, et al. Evaluation of left lower quadrant pain. American College of Radiology. ACR Appropriateness Criteria. *Radiology.* 2000;215:167.

38. Siewert B, Raptopoulos V, Mueller MF, et al. Impact of CT on diagnosis and management of acute abdomen in patients initially treated without surgery. *Am J Roentgenol.* 1997;168:173.

39. Taourel P, Baron MP, Pradel J, et al. Acute abdomen of unknown origin: impact of CT on diagnosis and management. *Gastrointest Radiol.* 1992;17:287.

40. Merine DS, Fishman EK, Jones B, et al. Right lower quadrant pain in the immunocompromised patient: CT findings in 10 cases. *Am J Roentgenol.* 1987;149:1177.

41. Wyatt SH, Fishman EK. The acute abdomen in individuals with AIDS. *Radiol Clin North Am.* 1994;32:1023.

42. Bree RL, Ralls PW, Balfe DM, et al. Evaluation of patients with acute right upper quadrant pain. American College of Radiology. ACR Appropriateness Criteria. *Radiology.* 2000;215:153.

43. Berger MY, van der Velden JJ, Lijmer JG, et al, Abdominal symptoms: do they predict gallstones? A systematic review. *Scand J Gastroenterol.* 2000;35:70.

44. Rao PM, Rhea JT, Novelline RA, et al. Helical CT technique for the diagnosis of appendicitis: prospective evaluation of a focused appendix CT examination. *Radiology.* 1997;202:139.

45. Harvey RT, Miller WT, Jr. Acute biliary disease: initial CT and follow-up US versus initial US and follow-up CT. *Radiology.* 1999;213:831.

46. Chen SC, Wang HP, Hsu HY, et al. Accuracy of ED sonography in the diagnosis of acute appendicitis. *Am J Emerg Med.* 2000;18:449.

47. Zielke A, Hasse C, Nies C, et al. Prospective evaluation of ultrasonography in acute colonic diverticulitis. *Br J Surg.* 1997;84:385.

48. Rothrock SG, Pagane J. Acute appendicitis in children: emergency department diagnosis and management. *Ann Emerg Med.* 2000;36:39.

49. Berger RG, Boxwala A. Multimedia medical case authorship and simulator program. *Medinfo.* 1995;8:1693.

50. Keyzer C, Zalcman M, De Maertelaer V, et al. Comparison of US and unenhanced multi-detector row CT in patients suspected of having acute appendicitis. *Radiology.* 2005;236:527.

51. Jackman SV, Jarrett TW. A comparison of noncontrast computerized tomography with excretory urography in the assessment of acute flank pain. *J Urol.* 1999;162:1707.

52. Homer JA, Davies-Payne DL, Peddinti BS. Randomized prospective comparison of non-contrast enhanced helical computed tomography and intravenous urography in the diagnosis of acute ureteric colic. *Australas Radiol.* 2001; 45:285.

53. Kobayashi T, Nishizawa K, Watanabe J, et al. Clinical characteristics of ureteral calculi detected by nonenhanced computerized tomography after unclear results of plain radiography and ultrasonography. *J Urol.* 2003; 170:799.

54. Obuz F, Terzi C, Sokmen S, et al. The efficacy of helical CT in the diagnosis of small bowel obstruction. *Eur J Radiol.* 2003;48:299.

55. Patlas M, Farkas A, Fisher D, et al. Ultrasound vs CT for the detection of ureteric stones in patients with renal colic. *Br J Radiol.* 2001;74:901.

56. Shokeir AA. Renal colic: new concepts related to pathophysiology, diagnosis and treatment. *Curr Opin Urol.* 2002;12:263.

57. Ripolles T, Agramunt M, Martinez MJ, et al. The role of ultrasound in the diagnosis, management and evolutive prognosis of acute left-sided colonic diverticulitis: a review of 208 patients. *Eur Radiol.* 2003;13:2587.

58. Britt H, Bridges-Webb C, Sayer GP, et al. The diagnostic difficulties of abdominal pain. *Aust Fam Physician*. 1994; 23:375.

59. Kawashima A, Sandler CM, Goldman SM. Current roles and controversies in the imaging evaluation of acute renal infection. *World J Urol*. 1998;16:9.

60. Memel DS, Balfe DM, Semelka RC. The biliary tract. In Lee JKT, Sagel SS, Stanley RJ, Heiken JP, eds. *Computed Body Tomography with MRI Correlation*. 3rd ed. Philadelphia, PA: Lippincott; 1998: 779.

61. Paulson EK. Acute cholecystitis: CT findings. *Semin Ultrasound CT MR*. 2000;21:56.

62. Welch JP. General consideration and mortality in bowel obstruction. In: Welch JP, ed. *Bowel obstruction: differential diagnosis and clinical management*. Philadelphia, PA: W.B. Saunders;1990:59.

63. Maglinte DD, Gage SN, Harmon BH, et al. Obstruction of the small intestine: accuracy and role of CT in diagnosis. *Radiology*. 1993;188:61.

64. Maglinte DD, Reyes BL, Harmon BH, et al. Reliability and role of plain film radiography and CT in the diagnosis of small-bowel obstruction. *Am J Roentgenol*. 1996;167:1451.

65. Burkill G, Bell J, Healy J. Small bowel obstruction: the role of computed tomography in its diagnosis and management with reference to other imaging modalities. *Eur Radiol*. 2001;11:1405.

66. Burkill GJ, Bell JR, Healy JC. The utility of computed tomography in acute small bowel obstruction. *Clin Radiol*. 2001;56:350.

67. Daneshmand S, Hedley CG, Stain SC. The utility and reliability of computed tomography scan in the diagnosis of small bowel obstruction. *Am Surg*. 1999;65:922.

68. Frager D, Baer JW, Medwid SW, et al. Detection of intestinal ischemia in patients with acute small-bowel obstruction due to adhesions or hernia: efficacy of CT. *Am J Roentgenol*. 1996;166:67.

69. Maglinte DD, Heitkamp DE, Howard TJ, et al. Current concepts in imaging of small bowel obstruction. *Radiol Clin North Am*. 2003;41:263.

70. Huynh LN, Coughlin BF, Wolfe J, et al. Patient encounter time intervals in the evaluation of emergency department patients requiring abdominopelvic CT: oral contrast versus no contrast. *Emerg Radiol*. 2004;10:310.

71. Musoke F, Kawooya MG, Kiguli-Malwadde E. Comparison between sonographic and plain radiography in the diagnosis of small bowel obstruction at Mulago Hospital, Uganda. *East Afr Med J*. 2003;80:540.

72. Chavhan GB, Masrani S, Thakkar H, et al. Sonography in the diagnosis of pediatric gastrointestinal obstruction. *J Clin Ultrasound*. 2004;32:190.

73. Brooks SE, Mullins CD, Guo C, et al. Resource utilization for patients undergoing hysterectomy with or without lymph node dissection for endometrial cancer. *Gynecol Oncol*. 2002;85:242.

74. Werner A, Diehl SJ, Farag-Soliman M, et al. Multi-slice spiral CT in routine diagnosis of suspected acute left-sided colonic diverticulitis: a prospective study of 120 patients. *Eur Radiol*. 2003;13:2596.

75. Zielke A, Hasse C, Bandorski T, et al. Diagnostic ultrasound of acute colonic diverticulitis by surgical residents. *Surg Endosc*. 1997;11:1194.

76. Chou YH, Chiou HJ, Tiu CM, et al. Sonography of acute right side colonic diverticulitis. *Am J Surg*. 2001;181:122.

77. Birchard KR, Brown MA, Hyslop et al. MRI of acute abdominal and pelvic pain in pregnant patients. *Am J Roentgenol*. 2005;184:452.

78. Levy PJ, Krausz MM, Manny J. Acute mesenteric ischemia: improved results—a retrospective analysis of ninety-two patients. *Surgery*. 1990;107:372.

79. Ritz JP, Runkel N, Berger G, et al. Prognostic factors in mesenteric infarct. *Zentralbl Chir*. 1997;122:332.

80. Alpern M. Walter Stanley Stiles. 15 June 1901–15 December 1985. *Biogr Mem Fellows R Soc*. 1988;34:815.

81. Smerud MJ, Johnson CD, Stephens DH. Diagnosis of bowel infarction: a comparison of plain films and CT scans in 23 cases. *Am J Roentgenol*. 1990;154:99.

82. Taourel PG, Deneuville M, Pradel JA, et al. Acute mesenteric ischemia: diagnosis with contrast-enhanced CT. *Radiology*. 1996;199:632.

83. Brandt LJ, Boley SJ. AGA technical review on intestinal ischemia. American Gastrointestinal Association. *Gastroenterology*. 2000;118:954.

84. Kirkpatrick ID, Kroeker MA, Greenberg HM. Biphasic CT with mesenteric CT angiography in the evaluation of acute mesenteric ischemia: initial experience. *Radiology*. 2003;229:91.

85. Boyko AT, Ullery BS, Bhalla S, et al. LM. Sensitivity of computed tomography to detect mesenteric ischemia/ infarction. *Acad. Emerg Med*. 2002;9:378.

86. Sharafuddin MJ, Olson CH, Sun S, et al. Endovascular treatment of celiac and mesenteric arteries stenoses: applications and results. *J Vasc Surg*. 2003;38:692.

87. Rhee RY, Gloviczki P, Mendonca CT, et al. Mesenteric venous thrombosis: still a lethal disease in the 1990s. *J Vasc Surg*. 1994;20:688.

88. Pun E, Firkin A. Computed tomography and complicated peptic ulcer disease. *Australas Radiol*. 2004;48:516.

89. Guerriero S, Ajossa S, Garau N, et al. Ultrasonography and color Doppler-based triage for adnexal masses to provide the most appropriate surgical approach. *Am J Obstet Gynecol*. 2005;192:401.

90. Mitchell DG, Mintz MC, Spritzer CE, et al. Adnexal masses: MR imaging observations at 1.5 T, with US and CT correlation. *Radiology*. 1987;162:319.

91. Tempany CM, Zou KH, Silverman SG, et al. Staging of advanced ovarian cancer: comparison of imaging modalities—report from the Radiological Diagnostic Oncology Group. *Radiology*. 2000;215:761.

92. Tsushima Y, Yamada S, Aoki J, et al. Effect of contrast-enhanced computed tomography on diagnosis and management of acute abdomen in adults. *Clin Radiol*. 2002; 57:507.

93. Marincek B. Nontraumatic abdominal emergencies: acute abdominal pain: diagnostic strategies. *Eur Radiol.* 2002; 12:2136.

94. Rosen MP, Siewert B, Sands DZ, et al. Value of abdominal CT in the emergency department for patients with abdominal pain. *Eur Radiol.* 2003;13:418.

95. Mindelzun RE, Jeffrey RB. Unenhanced helical CT for evaluating acute abdominal pain: a little more cost, a lot more information. *Radiology.*1997;205:43.

96. Nagurney JT, Brown DF, Novelline RA, et al. Plain abdominal radiographs and abdominal CT scans for nontraumatic abdominal pain—added value? *Am J Emerg Med.* 1999;17:668.

97. Nagurney JT, Brown DF, Chang Y, et al. Use of diagnostic testing in the emergency department for patients presenting with non-traumatic abdominal pain. *J Emerg Med.* 2003;25:363.

98. Brown DF, Fischer RH, Novelline RA, et al. The role of abdominal computed tomography scanning in patients with non-traumatic abdominal symptoms. *Eur J Emerg Med.* 2002;9:330.

99. Esses D, Birnbaum A, Bijur P, et al. Ability of CT to alter decision making in elderly patients with acute abdominal pain. *Am J Emerg Med.* 2004;22:270.

100. Lewis LM, Banet GA, Blanda M, et al. Etiology and clinical course of abdominal pain in senior patients: a prospective, multicenter study. *J Gerontol A Biol Sci Med Sci.* 2005;60:1071.

101. Nagurney JT, Sane S, Brown DF, et al. Physician certainty in the diagnosis of abdominal pain. *Acad Emerg Med.* 2003;10:563.

102. Ng CS, Watson CJ, Palmer CR, et al. Evaluation of early abdominopelvic computed tomography in patients with acute abdominal pain of unknown cause: prospective randomised study. *BMJ.* 2002;325:1387.

103. Marco CA, Schoenfeld CN, Keyl PM, et al. Abdominal pain in geriatric emergency patients: variables associated with adverse outcomes. *Acad Emerg Med.* 1998;5:1163.

104. Cartmell S, Huynh K, Lin A, et al. Quantitative microcomputed tomography analysis of mineralization within three-dimensional scaffolds in vitro. *J Biomed Mater Res A.* 2004;69:97.

105. Konen E, Konen O, Katz M, et al. Are referring clinicians aware of patients at risk from intravenous injection of iodinated contrast media? *Clin Radiol.* 2002;57:132.

106. Wilson MS, Ellis H, Menzies D, et al. A review of the management of small bowel obstruction. *Ann R Coll Surg Engl.* 1999;81:320.

107. Raisanen J, Shapiro B, Glazer GM, et al. Plasma catecholamines in pheochromocytoma: effect of urographic contrast media. *Am J Roentgenol.* 1984;143:43.

108. Katayama H, Yamaguchi K, Kozuka T, et al. Adverse reactions to ionic and nonionic contrast media. A report from the Japanese Committee on the Safety of Contrast Media. *Radiology.* 1990;175:621.

109. Bhalla S, Menias CO, Heiken JP. CT of acute abdominal aortic disorders. *Radiol Clin North Am.* 2003;41:1153.

110. Pedrosa I, Rofsky NM. MR imaging in abdominal emergencies. *Radiol Clin North Am.* 2003;41:1243.

111. Barish MA, Yucel EK, Ferrucci JT. Magnetic resonance cholangiopancreatography. *N Engl J Med.* 1999; 341:258.

112. Alobaidi M, Gupta R, Jafri SZ, et al. Current trends in imaging evaluation of acute cholecystitis. *Emerg Radiol.* 2004;10:256.

113. Johnson H, Jr., Cooper B. The value of HIDA scans in the initial evaluation of patients for cholecystitis. *J Natl Med Assoc.* 1995;87:27.

114. Puc MM, Tran HS, Wry PW, et al. Ultrasound is not a useful screening tool for acute acalculous cholecystitis in critically ill trauma patients. *Am Surg.* 2002;68:65.

115. Alavi A, Ring EJ. Localization of gastrointestinal bleeding: superiority of 99mTc sulfur colloid compared with angiography. *Am J Roentgenol.* 1981;137:741.

116. Ponzo F, Zhuang H, Liu FM, et al. Tc-99m sulfur colloid and Tc-99m tagged red blood cell methods are comparable for detecting lower gastrointestinal bleeding in clinical practice. *Clin Nucl Med.* 2002;27:405.

117. Fenyo G. Diagnostic problems of acute abdominal diseases in the aged. *Acta Chir Scand.* 1974;140:396.

6

Vomiting

David M. Cline

HIGH YIELD FACTS

- The differential diagnosis of vomiting is voluminous and the clinician should consult the differential tables in this chapter (Tables 6-1 through 6-3) when in doubt of the cause.
- Clinicians frequently fail to consider causes of vomiting due to etiologies originating from outside of the abdomen (Table 6-2).

Vomiting is a forceful expulsion of gastric contents through the mouth, which is facilitated by a series of motor and autonomic responses. Nausea is an unpleasant feeling that one is about to imminently vomit. Vomiting differs from retching and regurgitation. Retching is the term used to describe the labored, rhythmic respiratory activity, and abdominal musculature contractions that frequently precede vomiting. Retching in the absence of vomiting does not result in the oral expulsion of gastric contents. Regurgitation is the effortless movement of gastric contents into the mouth without the characteristic motor and autonomic changes that occurs with vomiting. Regurgitation is a common and more benign manifestation of many disorders that may proceed to vomiting.

EPIDEMIOLOGY

The epidemiology of vomiting can be divided into major group headings, which facilitate the clinician's pursuit of the diagnosis and the treatment likely to be the most effective. Conditions associated with vomiting are listed in Tables 6-1 through 6-3. Clinicians are advised to keep their differential diagnoses broad when first approaching the patient with vomiting as the causes are numerous with great variability in prognosis and indicated management of the underlying disorder. Conditions associated with vomiting significantly affect patients with lost time from work and restricted activities.[1] A study in the United States that assessed the financial burden of gastrointestinal (GI) illness associated with vomiting found costs exceeding \$3.4 billion for food-borne and non-food-borne gastroenteritis.[2] Lost productivity due to acute enteric infections in 1980 was reported to be \$21.8 billion.[3] Vomiting is the eighth most common reason to visit the emergency department.[4]

PATHOPHYSIOLOGY

Vomiting is a complex and highly coordinated reflex activity that involves multiple organ systems including the GI tract, the central nervous system, and the vestibular system. Three stages of vomiting exist: nausea, retching, and emesis.[5] The central emetic mechanism was identified as being located in the medulla and was published in 1952.[6] The nausea stage is characterized by an unpleasant feeling accompanied by hypersalivation and tachycardia (or bradycardia in some patients) with or without diaphoresis. Retching occurs as the pylorus muscles contract while the fundus of the stomach relaxes. This process moves the gastric contents up to the cardiac portion of the stomach. Emesis occurs as the abdominal wall muscles contract simultaneously with the pylorus muscles and thus propel the food and gastric secretions from the stomach up and out through the esophagus and mouth. Individuals with intact function of the epiglottis rarely sustain aspiration. The acid content of the gastric secretions produces a burning sensation and a foul taste in the mouth. The odor of the gastric contents may exacerbate the feeling of nausea experienced by the patient.

Repeated episodes of vomiting can lead to metabolic alkalosis, hypokalemia, but more commonly, hypovolemia. Forceful vomiting can injure the esophageal mucosa, leading to a Mallory-Weiss tear, or more significantly, an esophageal perforation, (Boerhaave syndrome).

CLINICAL FEATURES

Because the differential diagnosis of vomiting is broad, taking into account acute and chronic presentations of neurologic, ophthalmologic, vestibular, endocrine, respiratory, cardiac, GI, gynecologic, testicular, urinary, vascular, and immune systems, the clinical symptoms that accompany vomiting will vary widely. Historical variables pertinent to the severity and nature of vomiting include frequency, duration, volume (these first three give an index of potential dehydration); contents (blood, food, or mucus); color (blood or bile); odor (acidic, feculent); persistence; and symptom free periods of the vomiting. The accompanying symptoms, before, during, and after the vomiting episodes are most helpful in focusing in on the diagnosis.

Table 6-1. Gastrointestinal/Abdominal Conditions Associated with Vomiting

Cyclic vomiting syndrome

Esophageal disorders
Esophageal foreign body
Esophagitis
Gastroesophageal reflux disease

Functional gastrointestinal disorders
Constipation
Gastroparesis
Chronic intestinal pseudoobstruction
Nonulcer dyspepsia
Irritable bowel syndrome

Gynecological disorders
Pelvic inflammatory disease
Ovarian torsion
Tubo-ovarian abscess

Infectious causes
Gastroenteritis
Hepatitis
Spontaneous bacterial peritonitis
Intraabdominal abscess
Urinary tract infection

Kidney disorders
Renal colic
Nephrolithiasis
Renal tubular acidosis
Uremia

Mechanical obstruction
Gastric outlet obstruction
Pyloric stenosis
Hernia (multiple types)
Intussusception
Large bowel obstruction
Volvulus
Midgut rotation
Small bowel obstruction

Organic gastrointestinal disorders
Crohn disease
Cholecystitis
Hepatitis
Mesenteric ischemia
Pancreatitis
Peptic ulcer disease

Testicular disorders
Testicular torsion

Table 6-2. Extraabdominal Conditions Associated with Vomiting

Central nervous system disorders
Increased intracranial pressure
Malignancy
Hemorrhage
Infarction
Abscess
Meningitis
Congenital malformation
Hydrocephalus
Pseudotumor cerebri
Migraine
Seizure disorders

Endocrinologic and metabolic disorders
Acute intermittent porphyria
Addison disease
Diabetic ketoacidosis
Hyperparathyroidism
Hypoparathyroidism
Hyperthyroidism
Inborn errors of metabolism
Pregnancy

Infections (nonabdominal)
Otitis media
Meningitis
Pneumonia, cough associated
Reye syndrome
Sepsis
Other infections

Labyrinthine disorders
Labyrinthitis
Meniere disease
Tumors

Psychiatric disease and stimuli
Anorexia nervosa
Anxiety disorders
Bulimia nervosa
Depression
Pain
Psychogenic vomiting

Toxic ingestions
Alcohol
Insecticides
Mushrooms
Nicotine
Heavy metals

(Continued)

Table 6-2. Extraabdominal Conditions Associated with Vomiting (Continued)

Toxic ingestions
Digoxin
Salicylate
Isonazid

Miscellaneous acute conditions
Acute cardiac disease
Acute cardiac ischemia
Congestive heart failure
Glaucoma
Poisoning/overdose
Radiation therapy

Table 6-3. Medications Associated with Vomiting

Cancer Therapy
Chemotherapy

Analgesics
Aspirin
Auranofin
Nonsteroidal anti-inflammatory drugs

Antiasthmatics
Theophylline

Anticonvulsants

Antimicrobial Drugs
Acyclovir
Antituberculous drugs
Erthryomycin
Sulfonamides
Tetracycline

Antiparkinsonian drugs

CNS-active drugs

Colchicine

Cardiovascular medications
Digoxin
Antiarrhythmics
Antihypertensives
Beta Blockers
Calcium channel antagonists
Diuretics

Ethanol

Gastrointestinal medications
Sulfasalazine
Azathioprine

Hormonal preparations/therapies
Oral hypoglycemic agents
Oral contraceptives

Narcotics

Nicotine

Vitamins in excess

Sudden onset of severe headache with vomiting should alert clinicians to the possibility of subarachnoid hemorrhage. Increased intracranial pressure from any cause can produce vomiting, frequently without any preceding nausea. Headache, fever, and neck pain may represent meningitis, while migraine is the most frequent cause of patients presenting to the emergency department complaining of headache associated with vomiting. Vestibular symptoms (vertigo with or without nystagmus) and vomiting may represent labyrinthitis but may also represent cerebellar stroke. Eye pain associated with vomiting may represent glaucoma. Vomiting associated with tachycardia, diaphoresis, and elevated blood pressure may represent hyperthyroidism (but these symptoms may accompany the marked nausea that occurs in some patients who vomit).

Vomiting that occurs exclusively after cough points to the respiratory system. Asthma will sometimes be accompanied by vomiting. Certain respiratory infections have more GI symptoms, such as Legionnaires' disease.

Chest pain accompanied by vomiting should caution the clinician to the possibility of myocardial ischemia, but may represent an acute esophageal rupture (Boerhaave syndrome). Congestive heart failure may be accompanied by vomiting due in part to congestion of the liver.

Gastrointestinal causes of vomiting are indeed the most frequent, but clinicians should avoid quickly focusing on gastroenteritis (especially in the absence of diarrhea) or gastritis as the cause until more serious conditions have been considered. Inability to pass flatus or abdominal distension should point to the possibility of intestinal obstruction. Abdominal pain that is relieved by vomiting may represent delayed gastric emptying from diabetic gastropareses or gastric outlet obstruction due to contraction from ulcer disease.

Pregnancy should be the first thought in a vomiting women who is of childbearing potential (including women with a history of tubal ligation, who are at risk for ectopic pregnancy). Severe, persistent vomiting with pregnancy is clinically diagnosed as hyperemesis gravidarum and is generally associated with a 5% weight loss and ketonuria, with or without electrolyte abnormalities. Vomiting with vaginal discharge or pain with intercourse may be associated with pelvic inflammatory disease or tubo-ovarian abscess. Sudden onset of one-sided, lower abdominal pain could represent ovarian torsion. Testicular pain or tenderness associated with vomiting could represent testicular torsion. Urinary tract infection, especially pyelonephritis, may be accompanied with vomiting and may predict the need for inpatient treatment.

Historical clues point to the need for a detailed physical exam of identified systems of interest; however, all patients with vomiting need a complete abdominal exam. First consider the vital signs that will help to predict the need for fluid resuscitation. It is important to realize that normal vital signs do not rule out a life threatening emergency. Orthostatic hypotension has long been used to assess for the presence of hypovolemia or hemorrhage, but other pathophysiologic mechanisms may explain orthostatic changes, such as acute alcohol intoxication.[7] Positive criteria are a 20-point increase in pulse, or a 20-point fall in blood pressure when going from a supine position to standing. The inability to maintain an erect posture due to the feeling of impending syncope is also considered positive. Abnormal pupillary size and response to light may herald herniation of the brain in an unconscious patient who is vomiting; protecting the patient's airway with intubation may be required. Patients with epistaxis may become nauseated and vomit blood they have swallowed and accumulated in the stomach; evidence of a bleeding point may be noted on close inspection of the nares.

Patients who are vomiting in response to respiratory disease may have abnormal breath sounds, or simply be prompted to cough and experience nausea in response to the deep breathing necessary for thorough auscultation of the lungs. Patients with right-sided heart failure, and significant congestion of the liver, can be expected to have jugular venous distension.

In neonates, bilious vomiting should clue the clinician into malrotation (Chapter 35), while projectile vomiting increases the likelihood of pyloric stenosis (Chapter 39).

The abdominal examination is vitally important in the evaluation of the vomiting patient. Starting with observation, a distended abdomen may be the only physical sign of bowel obstruction in elderly patients. While vomiting alone can cause minor epigastric tenderness, marked tenderness of the epigastric region in association with pain should clue the clinician into the possibility of perforated viscous as a cause or consequence of repeated episodes of vomiting. High-pitched bowel sounds may be a sign of bowel obstruction (Chapter 13), but their absence does not rule out obstruction.

Localized abdominal tenderness will help to focus the differential (see Chapter 2 for differential diagnosis stratified by abdominal quadrant). Rebound tenderness and or guarding should increase the suspicion for surgical disease. Pelvic examination is essential in women with significant abdominal pain. In mean, examination of the testes will help to identify testicular torsion. A rectal examination is essential in patients complaining of vomiting blood to check stool for blood, or when bowel obstruction is being considered to identify fecal impaction as a cause of vomiting (Chapter 8). Recurrent episodes of abdominal pain associated with rectal blood in children should point to the diagnosis to intussusception. While a positive Murphy sign will increase the index of suspicion for acute cholecystitis, a sonographic Murphy sign is more specific (Chapter 22).

Neurologic examination is essential when cerebral causes of vomiting are suspected. Consider neurologic examination in all patients complaining of vomiting associated with headache or any neurologic symptom or sign.

In patients presenting with vomiting and vertigo, the Hallpike test is used to aid the diagnosis of benign positional vertigo. The patient should be positioned first in the seated position with the head rotated 45° to one side. The patient is then assisted to a supine position with the head hanging over the edge of the bed an additional 30° to 45°. Patients with benign positional vertigo will exhibit a latent and short-lived nystagmus with the rapid component toward the affected ear while complaining of vertigo. The patient is then returned to the sitting position and the other side is tested. Psychiatric assessment should be made in patients suspected of these disorders (Table 6-2); bulimia may produce life-threatening hypokalemia.

Specific Disorders

The majority of disorders associated with vomiting are discussed in the designated chapters of this book. The etiologies below are exclusive to this chapter.

Cyclic Vomiting Syndrome

Cyclic vomiting syndrome (CVS) is characterized by recurrent episodes of vomiting lasting hours to days with complete resolution of symptoms between episodes. The cause is not known, but patients have been found to have autonomic dysfunction with positive tilt testing.[8] The patients typically have discrete severe nausea, vomiting, lethargy, and abdominal pain. The disorder is similar to migraine headache as patients frequently have antecedent auras, headache, and photophobia.[9] It is more common in childhood, and childhood CVS may evolve into common migraine in later life. The diagnosis is made clinically, but care should be taken to rule out acute pathology before this chronic diagnosis is made. Treatment includes behavioral modification to avoid identified triggers, prophylactic migraine therapy (beta blockers), and abortive migraine therapy (triptans) with reported success rates of 40% to 90%.[10] Tricyclic antidepressants have been studied in this setting and provided a 93% success rate with decreased symptoms, and 26% of patients had full remission.[11]

Diabetic Gastroparesis

Diabetic gastroparesis is characterized by delayed gastric emptying in the absence of mechanical obstruction of the stomach.[12] The most common symptoms include postprandial fullness, nausea, vomiting, and bloating.[13] Patients commonly have several manifestations of diabetes including autonomic neuropathy, nephropathy, and retinopathy, although it may occur in the absence of these associated disorders.[12] Barium swallow may be helpful in ruling out gastric outlet obstruction. In general, food retained in the stomach after a 12-hour fast is suggestive of gastroparesis. Treatment includes metoclopramide 10 mg as required as well as dimenhydrinate 50 mg as needed.[12] Other medications that may be of help include domperidone 10 mg to 20 mg three times daily before meals, with or without erythromycin 40 mg to 250 mg three times daily before meals.[12] Prochlorperazine 25 mg is also used for nausea.

Gastric Outlet Obstruction

Gastric outlet obstruction is most commonly caused by chronic peptic ulceration with pyloric stenosis or by a malignancy of the prepyloric gastric antrum. Patients typically vomit partially digested food several hours after eating. Gastric decompression with a nasogastric tube will help initially with symptoms and reveal the typical gastric contents. The diagnosis can be confirmed with saline load test, or barium swallow; however, barium may make endoscopy difficult. Treatment with endoscopic balloon dilatation of the pylorus and a course of endoscopic dilation is successful in 50% of patients with peptic ulcer diseases. Malignancy is treated surgically, but symptomatic relief can be accomplished endoscopically with expandable stents in poor surgical candidates.

Mallory-Weiss Syndrome

Mallory-Weiss syndrome is characterized by bloody vomitus that follows a bout of forceful retching and nonbloody vomiting. The lesion is typically a 1 cm to 4 cm tear in the mucosa and submucosa. The majority occur in the stomach, with the remainder of the gastroesophageal junction. The bleeding is usually mild and self limited. Rarely, bleeding becomes severe; 3% of deaths from GI bleeds are reported to be caused by Mallory-Weiss tears. Treatment is supportive with bowel rest.

Boerhaave Syndrome

Boerhaave syndrome is characterized by perforation of the three layers of the esophagus due to forceful retching or vomiting. The overlying pleura is ruptured yielding free passage of esophageal contents into the mediastinum and thorax. This disorder is a surgical emergency. Mortality is as high as 50% if surgery is not performed within the first 24 hours.

DIAGNOSIS AND DIFFERENTIAL

The differential diagnosis of vomiting can be aided by reviewing Tables 6-1 to 6-3. New medications are frequently a cause (Table 6-3).

Diagnostic testing in the patient presenting with vomiting will be highly individualized and should be guided by the associated symptoms and signs. The most common cause of idiopathic ketotic hypoglycemia in children is repeated episodes of vomiting associated with dehydration; children with this history should have finger stick glucose checks. Electrolytes are commonly ordered and may aid patient management of dehydration, but are not required on all patients. Repeated episodes of vomiting produce a metabolic alkalosis due to loss of hydrogen ions in the vomitus. The disorder produces a large amount of bicarbonate ion being delivered to the distal tubule of the kidney. Potassium is selected over sodium for concomitant excretion of bicarbonate as volume contraction produces a secondary hyperaldosteronism, resulting in the urinary wasting of potassium and hypokalemia.

Complete blood counts may be indicated in specific circumstances elucidated in other chapters in this book, but given their limitations (Chapter 4), the results will not narrow the differential diagnosis in the vomiting patient. A urine pregnancy test should be considered in all women of childbearing potential presenting with vomiting. A complete metabolic workup (electrolytes, kidney function, ketones, blood, or capillary gas) should be considered in the patient suspected of having diabetic ketoacidosis. Hepatic function should be considered in the patient at risk for hepatic failure (alcoholism, cirrhosis, jaundice, known hepatitis) or in the child suspected of having Reyes syndrome.

The indications for radiographic testing are primarily guided by the severity and acuity of the presentation. Using the differential tables as a starting point (Tables 6-1 and 6-2), the reader is referred to Chapter 5 and the chapters that follow this one for a more detailed discussion of imaging options for specific suspected disease processes.

EMERGENCY DEPARTMENT CARE AND DISPOSITION

The management of disorders that produce vomiting should be directed first to the underlying cause. This chapter presents measures that provide symptomatic relief.

The decision to provide intravenous fluids should be individualized to each patient. An attempt at oral rehydration should be considered. Medications to control vomiting are the sixth most common medication given in U.S. emergency departments.[4] Medications that are used to treat vomiting come from several different classes that should be selected based on the physician's understanding of the underlying pathophysiology in each case (Table 6-4).

The phenothiazines are recommended as first line agents and they have broad indications[14] (Table 6-4). Side effects of the phenothiazines include sedation, extrapyramidal or dystonic reactions, QTc prolongation, neuroleptic malignant syndrome, and seizures. Side effects appear to be more common in the elderly.[15] Many clinicians use promethazine for pregnant patients; however, it is a class C (uncertain safety in pregnancy). Perhaps the most commonly used agent for pregnant patients who vomit is metoclopramide, which is a class B

Table 6-4. Pharmacologic Treatment of Vomiting

Medication Class	Examples	Indications/Uses	Dose
Phenothiazine, dopamine antagonist	Promethazine	Gastroenteritis, metabolic, toxins, medications, migraine	12.5–25 mg IV or PO, every 6 hours, or suppository
Phenothiazine, dopamine antagonist	Prochlorperazine	Gastroenteritis, metabolic, toxins, medications, migraine	5–10 mg IV or PO every 6 hours, 25 mg suppository every 12 hours
Phenothiazine, dopamine antagonist	Chlorpromazine	Metabolic, toxins, medications, migraine	25–50 mg IM or PO
Serotonin 5-HT$_3$ antagonist	Ondansetron	Chemotherapy, postsurgery, migraine, used in children for gastroenteritis[14]	4–8 mg IV or PO, 3 times a day
5-HT$_4$ agonist	Metoclopramide	Gastroparesis functional dyspepsia	10 mg IV or PO, every 6 hours
Butyrophenone dopamine antagonist	Droperidol	2002 FDA black box warning, Metabolic, toxins, medications	0.675–1.25 mg IV or IM
Peripheral antidopaminergic	Domperidone	Gastroparesis functional dyspepsia	10–20 mg 3 to 4 times a day
Antihistamine	Dimenhydrinate	Labyrinth disorders motion sickness	50–100 mg PO, 3 to 4 times a day
Antihistamine	Meclizine	Labyrinth disorders motion sickness	25 mg PO 3 times a day
Motilin agonist	Erythromycin	Gastroparesis	40–250 mg PO 3 times a day
Benzodiazepine	Lorazepam	Anticipatory nausea, chemotherapy	1–2 mg IV, PO, or sublingual
Tricyclic antidepressant	Nortriptyline	Functional vomiting	25–100 mg PO before bedtime
Unknown mechanism	Trimethobenzamide	Gastroenteritis	250 mg IM or PO every 6 hours

Abbreviations: IV, intravenous; IM, intramuscular; PO, oral; FDA, Food and Drug Administration.

(presumed safe based on animal studies). Metoclopramide is also a prokinetic agent, useful in gastroparesis and functional dyspepsia. Metoclopramide is associated with many of the same side effects as the phenothiazines. Ondansetron has been studied in the setting of gastroenteritis presenting to the emergency department and was found to reduce vomiting and facilitate oral rehydration.[16,17] An older study found that children receiving ondansetron had significantly fewer emetic episodes and that more of them did not vomit at all during the initial observation period in the emergency department (87% versus 65%; however, a statistically significant difference was not found during a 48-hour follow-up period).[18] In the ondansetron group, there were fewer admissions and shorter lengths of stay in hospital, but children receiving ondansetron had a higher rate of return visits, for either persistent vomiting or persistent diarrhea, and a higher mean incidence of diarrhea.[18] Ondansetron has found increasing use in the emergency department because of a low side-effect profile. However, ondansetron is associated with increased diarrhea, QTc prolongation, QRS widening, headache, fatigue, and hypersensitivity reaction. In general, pediatricians and emergency physicians commonly prescribe antiemetic agents for children,[19] but their use remains controversial with 1996 guidelines discouraging their use in young children.[20] Droperidol has received a black box warning from the Food and Drug Administration because of an association with dysrhythmias, but this has been challenged.[21] For patients presenting with vomiting associated with vertigo, antihistamines are recommended. Antihistamine side effects include: sedation, dry mouth, constipation, urinary retention, blurred vision, exacerbation of glaucoma, and confusion. Drug therapy for gastroparesis is also listed in Table 6-4. Domperidone may cause gynecomastia and sexual dysfunction. Erythromycin is known for causing gastritis, but is useful for certain patients with gastroparesis because of its prokinetic effects. Use of dexamethasone has been advocated for certain patients treated for vomiting in the emergency department, especially patients with migraine; however, its use for other patient groups requires further study. For additional discussion of pharmacologic management of migraine, see Chapter 43.

PITFALLS

- Missing a life-threatening cause of vomiting because benign abdominal disorders with vomiting are more common.

- Failing to consider the indications and the side-effect profile of an antiemetic before choosing one for use in the acute setting.

REFERENCES

1. Monto AS, Koopman JS. The Tecumseh Study. XI. Occurrence of acute enteric illness in the community. *Am J Epidemiol.* 1980;112:323.
2. Sandler RS, Everhart JE, Donowitz M, et al. The burden of selected digestive diseases in the United States. *Gastroenterology.* 2002;122:1500.
3. Garthright WE, Archer DL, Kvenberg JE. Estimates of incidence and costs of intestinal infectious diseases in the United States. *Public Health Rep.* 1988;103:107.
4. McCaig LF, Nawar EW. National Hospital Ambulatory Medical Care Survey: 2004 Emergency Department Summary. *Adv Data.* 2006;372:1.
5. Lumsden K, Holden WS. The act of vomiting in man. *Gut.* 1969;10:173.
6. Wang SC, Borison HL. A new concept of organization of the central emetic mechanism: recent studies on the sites of action of apomorphine, copper sulphate and cardiac glycosides. *Gastroenterology.* 1952;22:1.
7. Tomaszewski C, Cline DM, Whitley TW, Grant T. Effect of acute alcohol ingestion on orthostatic vital signs. *Ann Emerg Med.* 1995;25:636.
8. Chelimsky TC, Chelimsky GG. Autonomic abnormalities in cyclic vomiting syndrome. *J Pediatr Gastroenterol Nutr.* 2007;44:326.
9. Li BU, Misiewicz L. Cyclic vomiting syndrome: a brain-gut disorder. *Gastroenterol Clin North Am.* 2003;32:997.
10. Sudel B, Li BU. Treatment options for cyclic vomiting syndrome. *Curr Treat Options Gastroenterol.* 2005;8:387.
11. Namin F, Patel J, Lin Z, et al. Clinical, psychiatric and manometric profile of cyclic vomiting syndrome in adults and response to tricyclic therapy. *Neurogastroenterol Motil.* 2007;19:196.
12. Camilleri M. Diabetic gastroparesis. *N Engl J Med.* 2007;356:820.
13. Revicki DA, Rentz AM, Dubois D, et al. Development and validation of a patient-assessed gastroparesis symptom severity measure: the Gastroparesis Cardinal Symptom Index. *Aliment Pharmacol Ther.* 2003;18:141.
14. Hasler WL, Chey WD. Nausea and vomiting. *Gastroenterology.* 2003;125:1860.
15. Sheth HS. Phenothiazine, promethazine adverse events after implementation of a medication shortage interchange. *Ann Pharmacother.* 2005;39:255.
16. Freedman SB, Adler M, Seshadri R, et al. Oral ondansetron for gastroenteritis in a pediatric emergency department. *N Engl J Med.* 2006;354:1698.
17. Stork CM, Brown KM, Reilly TH, et al. Emergency department treatment of viral gastritis using intravenous ondansetron or dexamethasone in children. *Acad Emerg Med.* 2006;13:1027.

18. Ramsook C, Sahagun-Carreon I, Kozinetz CA, et al. A randomized clinical trial comparing oral ondansetron with placebo in children with vomiting from acute gastroenteritis. *Ann Emerg Med.* 2002;39:397.

19. Li ST, DiGiuseppe DL, Christakis DA. Antiemetic use for acute gastroenteritis in children. *Arch Pediatr Adolesc Med.* 2003;157:475.

20. American Academy of Pediatrics, Provisional Committee on Quality Improvement, Subcommittee on Acute Gastroenteritis. Practice parameter; the management of acute gastroenteritis in young children. *Pediatrics.* 1996;97:424.

21. Habib AS, Gan TJ. Food and Drug Administration black box warning on the perioperative use of droperidol: a review of the cases. *Anesth Analg.* 2003;96:1377.

7

Diarrhea

Phillip A. Clement
Kevin J. Corcoran

HIGH YIELD FACTS

- An estimated 85% of cases of diarrhea are of infectious etiology, the remainder are due to noninfectious causes, such as osmotic diarrhea.
- Patients at risk for the greatest morbidity and mortality from diarrheal illnesses include the elderly, infants, and those with significant underlying medical conditions.
- Infectious diarrhea may result in extensive fluid losses and certain invasive pathogens may lead to bacteremia, sepsis, and death.
- Most cases of *Clostridium difficile*-associated diarrhea develop on days 4 to 9 of antibiotic therapy, but may be delayed for as long as 10 weeks.
- Diarrhea may be the presenting symptom of acute abdominal pathology, toxic exposures, endocrine disorders, and other systemic illnesses.

EPIDEMIOLOGY

Diarrhea remains a major health problem worldwide with greater than 4 billion cases each year, resulting in more then 4 million deaths annually.[1,2] The World Health Organization lists diarrhea as a leading cause of death in children less than 5 years of age with an estimated 7000 deaths each day, mostly in developing countries.[1,2] In the United States, children under 5 years of age suffer more than 20 million episodes of diarrhea annually, resulting in 200,000 hospitalizations and more than 300 deaths per year.[1–3] In the adult population of the United States, the estimate is greater than 100 million cases of diarrhea annually.[4] Diarrhea accounts for up to 5% of U.S. emergency department (ED) visits, 1.5% of total hospitalizations, and is second only to the common cold in days lost from work.[4] Patients at risk for the greatest

morbidity and mortality are those at the extremes of age, those with hospital or antibiotic associated diarrhea, and those with comorbidities or immunodeficiencies.

The most common etiology of diarrhea is infectious (Table 7-1), accounting for approximately 85% of cases. While the majority of infectious cases are self-limiting, the potential exists for serious illness, and when combined with susceptible patient populations, may lead to significant morbidity and mortality.

The remaining 15% of cases of diarrhea are due to noninfectious causes (Table 7-2) and if unrecognized, may pose an even greater threat to patient well being and survival. Diarrhea may be the presenting symptom of acute abdominal pathology, endocrine disorders, toxic exposures, central nervous system pathology, inflammatory bowel disease, chemotherapy, radiation therapy, and other systemic illnesses.

PATHOPHYSIOLOGY

Diarrhea can be divided into four major types based on the pathophysiology: osmotic, secretory, inflammatory, and abnormal motility. Osmotic diarrhea occurs due to the ingestion of osmotically active and nonabsorbable substances, which cause the osmotic movement of water into the intestinal lumen. This may result from congenital or acquired causes of malabsorption or maldigestion, resulting in an excess of osmotically active solutes. A more common cause is the ingestion of exogenous agents such as laxatives, dietetic foods containing sorbitol, mannitol, or xylitol, magnesium containing antacids, and certain drugs such as colchicine, cholestyramine, or neomycin. If exogenous agents are the cause, the diarrhea will resolve with fasting.

Secretory diarrhea is the most common mechanism encountered in the acute setting. It results from cytotoxins that produce an increased cellular permeability resulting in the secretion of water and electrolytes into the intestinal lumen. Secretory diarrhea may be induced by enteropathogenic viruses (viral gastroenteritis), bacterial cytotoxins (*Vibrio cholerae*), hormonal hypersecretion, and certain drugs. Stool studies examining electrolyte concentrations and osmolality can help to differentiate between osmotic and secretory diarrhea. However, this is of limited value in the acute setting. With secretory diarrhea, fecal erythrocytes and leukocytes are uncommon, as are extensive systemic symptoms, although significant morbidity and mortality may occur due to fluid loss.

Inflammatory diarrhea is also a commonly encountered mechanism in the acute setting. It results from cellular damage to the intestinal mucosa, leading to the secretion

Table 7-1. Causes of Infectious Diarrhea

Bacterial Inflammatory Diarrhea	Bacterial Secretory Diarrhea	Viral	Parasitic
Salmonella sp.	**Preformed toxins—food poisoning:**	Rotavirus	**Protozoa**
Shigella sp.		Pararotavirus	*Entamoeba histolytica*
Campylobacter sp.	*Staphylococcus aureus*	Norwalk virus	*Entamoeba polecki*
Yersinia enterocolitica	*Bacillus cereus*	Norwalk-like agents	*Giardia lamblia*
Yersinia pseudotuberculosis	*Clostridium botulinum*	Adenovirus	*Cryptosporidium*
Enterohemorrhagic *E. coli* 0157:H7	**Toxins formed after colonization:**	Enteric adenovirus	*Cyclospora*
Enteroinvasive *E. coli*		Coronavirus	*Microsporidia*
Clostridium difficile	*Vibrio cholerae*	Calicivirus	*Enteromonas hominis*
Vibrio parahaemolyticus	*Clostridium perfringens*	Picornavirus	*Isospora belli*
Vibrio vulnificus	*Shigella* sp.	Astrovirus	*Balantidium coli*
Vibrio fluvialis	Enterotoxigenic *E. coli*	Small round viruses	*Blastocystis hominis*
Aeromonas sp.	*Aeromonas hydrophila*	Cytomegalovirus	*Dientamoeba fragilis*
Plesiomonas shigelloides	*Klebsiella pneumoniae*	Hepatitis A-G	*Sarcocystis hominis*
Mycobacterium sp.		Herpes simplex virus	**Helminth**
		HIV enteropathy	*Ascaris lumbricoides*
			Diphyllobothrium latum
			Enterobius vermicularis
			Angiostrongylus costaricense
			Anisakiasis
			Hookworms
			Schistosoma sp.
			Strongyloides stercoralis
			Trichinella spiralis
			Trichuris trichiura
			Taenia sp.

Abbreviation: HIV, human immunodeficiency virus.

of water, electrolytes, blood, mucus, and plasma proteins. This may be caused by invasive bacterial and parasitic pathogens, which produce dysenteric illnesses. Epithelial damage may also occur due to radiation therapy, chemotherapy, autoimmune disorders, hypersensitivity reactions, and inflammatory bowel disease. With inflammatory diarrhea, fecal leukocytes and erythrocytes are typically present, as are systemic symptoms, and affected patients have a greater likelihood of suffering significant illness.

Abnormal motility is a diagnosis of exclusion in the acute setting and is generally seen in patients with chronic diarrhea. Hypomotility may be associated with bacterial overgrowth and results in steatorrhea. Hypermotility decreases contact time between the luminal contents and the absorbing mucosa and thus limits water and electrolyte absorption.

CLINICAL FEATURES

Diarrhea can be defined clinically as a change in the normal pattern of stools with an increased frequency, volume, and fluidity. Many authors have included a requirement of greater then three stools per day. Diarrhea can be further characterized as acute or chronic with acute being of less than 4 weeks duration. The clinical presentation depends on the specific cause and is greatly influenced by the overall state of host defenses. Susceptible patients (the elderly, infants, and the immunosuppressed) tend to experience a more significant course of disease.[4]

The physical examination should focus on the patient's overall health, signs of volume depletion, a toxic appearance, the presence of blood in the stool, or a surgical abdomen. Search for evidence of decreased perfusion such as hypotension, tachycardia, dry mucous membranes,

Table 7-2. Causes of Noninfectious Diarrhea

Gastrointestinal Pathology	Toxins	Toxins	Endocrine Pathology	Systemic Disease—Other
Appendicitis	**Drugs**	**Dietetic foods**	**Hormonal hypersecretion syndromes**	Allergic reactions
Autonomic dysfunction	Antacids	Sorbitol	Zollinger-Ellison syndrome (gastrin)	Alcoholism
Blind loop	Antibiotics	Xylitol	Carcinoid syndrome (serotonin)	Amyloidosis
Bowel obstruction	Antidepressants	Mannitol	Pancreatic cholera (VIP)	Connective tissue disease
Celiac disease	Antiepileptic drugs	**Fish toxins**	Hyperthyroidism (thyroid hormone)	Severe malnutrition
Cholecystitis	Antihypertensives	Scombroid	Medullary carcinoma of the thyroid (calcitonin)	Stevens-Johnson syndrome
Pancreatitis	Antiparkinson drugs	Ciguatera	Somatostatinoma (somatostatin)	Toxic shock syndrome
Hepatitis/Cirrhosis	Caffeine	Tetroton	Systemic mastocytosis (histamine)	Wilson disease
Defects in amino acid transport	Cardiac antiarrhythmics	Echinoderms	**Endocrine disease**	Cystic fibrosis
Diverticular disease	Chemotherapy agents	Neurotoxic shellfish poisoning	Diabetes enteropathy	Hemolytic-uremic syndrome
Familial dysautonomia	Cholesterol-lowering drugs	Paralytic shellfish poisoning	Pancreatic insufficiency	Henoch-Schönlein purpura
Fecal impaction/incontinence	Cholinergic agents	Amnestic shellfish poisoning	Adrenal insufficiency	Lymphoma
Gastrointestinal bleed	Cholinesterase inhibitors	**Plant toxins**	Hypoparathyroidism	Sepsis
Gastrointestinal cancer	Colchicine	Herbal preparations		Gonadal torsion
Hirschsprung disease	Digitalis	Mushrooms—Amanita sp.		Ectopic pregnancy
Inflammatory bowel disease	Diuretics	Pesticides-organophosphates		Otitis media-infants
				Pelvic inflammatory disease
				Tuboovarian abscess
				Pyelonephritis

Intussusception	Fluorouracil	Nicotine
Irritable bowel syndrome	H2-receptor antagonist	Horse chestnut
Ischemic bowel	Lactulose	Rhubarb
Lactose/fructose intolerance	Laxatives/cathartics	Pokeweed
Malabsorption syndromes	Lithium	**Miscellaneous:**
Malrotation	NSAIDs	Carbon monoxide poisoning
Postsurgical/Postvagotomy	Neomycin	Opiate withdrawal
Radiation therapy	Prostaglandins	Ethanol
Short gut syndrome	Quinidine	Heavy metals
Strictures	Ricinoleic acid	Monosodium glutamate
Toxic megacolon	Theophylline	
Tropical sprue	Thyroid hormones	
Volvulus		
Whipple disease		

Abbreviations: NSAIDs, nonsteroidal anti-inflammatory drugs; VIP, vasoactive intestinal peptide.

oliguria, cool pale skin, or altered mentation. In children look for sunken eyes, fontanel depression, poor skin turgor, and a decrease in urinary output. Hypotension and tachycardia are typical responses to volume depletion. However, in young healthy patients, a normal blood pressure and heart rate may be maintained even with significant dehydration. In addition, patients who are taking atrioventricular nodal blockers may not exhibit a typical tachycardic response to volume depletion. Fever is consistent with dysentery, or invasive bacterial and parasitic causes of diarrhea, but could also indicate acute surgical pathology. Fever may or may not be associated with viral and noninvasive bacterial causes of diarrhea or food poisoning. The rectal exam should be used to detect melena, hematochezia, or fecal impaction. Gross blood may indicate gastrointestinal (GI) bleeding, intussusception, ischemic bowel, radiation therapy, or colitis caused by enterohemorrhagic *Escherichia coli* 0157:H7.

DIAGNOSIS AND DIFFERENTIAL

The causes of diarrhea are numerous and the exact etiology is often difficult to determine in the acute setting (Tables 7-1 and 7-2). Although the most common presentation is an infectious, self-limiting gastroenteritis, this diagnosis should be withheld until more serious causes of diarrhea have been considered. The diagnosis of gastroenteritis has been incorrectly applied to processes such as acute appendicitis, carbon monoxide poisoning, opiate withdrawal, and subarachnoid hemorrhage.

A careful history is essential in determining the etiology of diarrhea. The history should clarify the patient's understanding of the term diarrhea as lay definitions vary widely. Ask about the consistency of the stool, watery versus loosely formed, and determine the frequency of stooling. Give special attention to details such as when the diarrhea began in relation to other symptoms, and whether the diarrhea is a major or minor component of the present illness. Crampy abdominal pain after protracted vomiting and copious, watery diarrhea is consistent with gastroenteritis (Table 7-3). In contrast, the onset of abdominal pain followed by nausea and a single loose stool may be suggestive of surgical pathology. Fever, myalgia, cephalgia, and profuse diarrhea are consistent with dysentery (Table 7-4), whereas a sudden severe headache, vomiting, and one loose stool could represent a central nervous system process such as subarachnoid hemorrhage.

Other symptoms associated with the present illness should be reviewed in order of occurrence and severity. Ask about vomiting, fever, abdominal pain, anorexia,

constipation, myalgia, cephalgia, tenesmus, and neurologic symptoms such as paresthesias, weakness, or cranial nerve palsies. Ask about blood or mucous in the stool and inquire about the character of any associated vomitus (bloody or bilious). Differentiate acute (less than 4 weeks) from chronic symptoms.

A dietary history may yield clues as to the cause of diarrhea and should include unusual foods, dairy products, eggs, seafood, unpasteurized, undercooked or poorly prepared foods (Tables 7-3 and 7-4). Ask about common source exposures such as daycare, community outbreaks, recent hospitalizations, or institutional exposures. Inquire about recent travel, especially to developing countries and cruise ships, as well as recent outdoor activities, including backpacking and exposure to new water sources.

An inquiry should be made about the patient's past medical and surgical history, with special attention given to immunocompetency. Ask about a history of malignancies, inflammatory bowel disease, human immunodeficiency virus (HIV), autoimmune disorders, diabetes mellitus, and other endocrine pathology. Ask about recent chemotherapy or radiation therapy, a history of allergic reactions, GI bleeds, and any abdominal surgeries. Ask about a personal or family history of diarrhea, including prior treatment, and whether eating or drinking exacerbates the diarrhea.

The abdominal exam is of particular importance. Significant abdominal pain should prompt the search for causes other than infectious gastroenteritis. Signs and symptoms consistent with surgical pathology include pain that precedes the diarrhea, focal tenderness, and evidence of rebound or peritoneal inflammation. However, diffuse and crampy abdominal pain may occur after protracted vomiting or diarrhea and is consistent with gastroenteritis. In addition, *Campylobacter* sp. and *Yersinia enterocolitica* may mimic appendicitis by causing right lower quadrant pain, anorexia, vomiting, low-grade fever, and an elevated white blood cell count, which may precede the onset of diarrhea by as much as several days. Appendicitis must be ruled out in patients with this presentation.

Early acute abdominal emergencies with diarrhea may be differentiated from infectious causes with serial abdominal exams or in some cases by radiographic imaging such as computed tomography or ultrasonography. Radiographic studies may be of value in patients with a suspected surgical abdomen, and to identify abnormalities such as tumors, obstructions, blind loops, fistulas, and Crohn disease.

Laboratory and other diagnostic tests are of limited value in the acute setting for the majority of cases.

Table 7-3. Diagnosis and Treatment of Gastroenteritis

Infectious Agents	Incubation	Transmision	Diagnostic Features	Adult Therapy
Viral gastroenteritis	12 to 72 hours	Contaminated food or water and from person to person.	Nausea, vomiting and watery diarrhea, mild abdominal cramps, and myalgias. Patients may be afebrile. Epidemics may occur in infants and small children; day care, institutions, and cruse ships. Common in cooler months. Most common causes are Norwalk and Rotovirus.	Symptomatic treatment with oral or intravenous rehydration.
Staphylococcus aureus	1 to 6 hours	Proteinaceous foods which have been previously cooked (chicken, egg, and potato salads, ham, shrimp, and cream filled goods). Infected food handler.	Causes mostly upper GI symptoms, severe nausea and vomiting with only mild diarrhea or abdominal cramps. Patients are usually afebrile. Symptoms develop rapidly and are due to preformed enterotoxins.	Symptomatic treatment with oral or intravenous rehydration. Antibiotics are ineffective against preformed enterotoxins.
Enterotoxigenic *Escherichia coli*	12 to 72 hours	Contaminated water supplies.	Causes a cholerae like illness with profuse watery diarrhea. Infants may be febrile while adults are usually afebrile. Accounts for 30%–70% of travelers diarrhea.	Symptomatic care. For severe cases consider: Ciprofloxacin 500 mg PO BID × 3–5 days.
Vibrio cholerae	12 to 72 hours	Contaminated food or water, person to person. Raw or undercooked seafood (oysters, crabs, and shrimp) most common.	Causes profuse, explosive rice-water diarrhea with vomiting, fever, abdominal cramps, dehydration, lactic acidosis and death if untreated. Caused by enterotoxins which are formed after GI bacterial colonization. Common summer and early fall; Gulf Coast US.	Primary treatment is aggressive fluid resuscitation. Antibiotics may shorten the course of the disease. Consider: Ciprofloxacin 1.0 gram PO × 1-dose. Alternative is Tetracycline or TMP/SMX.
Bacillus cereus	1 to 6 hours	Previously cooked meats, vegetables, dried fruits, fried rice, and powered milk.	Causes mostly upper GI symptoms, an abrupt onset of nausea and vomiting, mild diarrhea. Most patients are afebrile. Symptoms develop rapidly due to preformed enterotoxins.	Symptomatic treatment with oral or intravenous rehydration.

(Continued)

Table 7-3. Diagnosis and Treatment of Gastroenteritis (Continued)

Infectious agents	Incubation	Transmision	Diagnostic features	Adult therapy
Clostridium perfringens	8 to 24 hours	Previously cooked or poorly reheated meats, poultry, and gravy.	Causes mostly lower GI symptoms, abdominal cramps, nausea, watery diarrhea with minimal vomiting. Most patients are afebrile. Caused by enterotoxins formed both before and after GI bacterial colonization.	Symptomatic treatment with oral or intravenous rehydration.
Clostridium botulinum	12 to 36 hours	Home-canned fruits and vegetables and canned commercial fish products.	An uncommon illness causing only mild GI symptoms followed by weakness, muscle incoordination, fatigue, malaise, dry mouth, diplopia, and dysphagia. Respiratory compromise may result from progressive muscle weakness and cranial nerve palsies.	Hospitalization for supportive care including ventilatory support if needed. IGA decontamination should be considered as should the administration of intravenous trivalent antitoxin.
Giardia lamblia	1 to 4 weeks	Contaminated food or water, person to person.	Causes mostly lower GI symptoms, a malabsorptive diarrhea, crampy abdominal pain, bloating, and excessive flatus. Most common intestinal parasite in the US; causes chronic diarrhea. Common in backpackers, travelers, and the elderly.	Treatment is with Metronidazole 250 mg PO TID × 7 days.
Scombroid poisoning	1 to 2 hours	Contaminated scombroid fish (tuna, bonito, and mackerel) or Dolphin fish (mahi-mahi).	Causes flushing of the face, neck and upper trunk, perioral numbness and tingling, dysphagia, headache, and dizziness, with nausea, vomiting, diarrhea, abdominal pain and rarely bronchospasm. Caused by histamine-like substance from contaminated fish.	Antihistamines: diphenhydramine 50 mg IV and H2 receptor antagonist such as cimetidine or ranitidine. Fluid resuscitation and bronchodilators should be used as indicated.
Paralytic shellfish poisoning	0 to 1 hour	Bivalve shellfish (clams, oysters, mussels, and scallops).	May cause nausea, vomiting, diarrhea, abdominal cramps, headache, ataxia, vertigo, paresthesias of face and extremities, cranial nerve palsies, muscle weakness, and paralysis.	Hospitalization for 24 hour observation and supportive care including ventilatory support if needed. IGA decontamination should be considered.

Abbreviations: GI, Gastrointestinal; Mg, milligram; PO, orally; BID, twice a day; TID, three times a day; TMP-SMX, trimethoprim-sulfamethoxazole.

Table 7-4. Diagnosis and Treatment of Dysenteric Enteritis

Infectious Agents	Incubation; Duration	Transmission	Diagnostic Features*	Adult Therapy
Campylobacter sp.	1–7 days; 1 week	Contaminated water (unchlorinated, natural water supplies), contaminated food (unprocessed milk, poultry), animals	Prodrome of fever, myalgias, cephalgia, and abdominal pain followed by diarrhea. Vomiting is minimal. Most common cause of bacterial diarrhea. Occurs primarily in children and young adults during the summer months. May mimic appendicitis. Also called backpackers diarrhea	Ciprofloxacin 500 mg PO, or 400 mg IV, BID × 5 days. Alternative Rx: azithromycin or erythromycin.
Shigella sp.	1–3 days; 4-7 days	Contaminated food, person to person, day care, institutions, poor sanitation	Fever, cephalgia, myalgia, abdominal pain, and diarrhea. Vomiting is minimal. May lead to sepsis and death. Very common in children 1–5 years of age and in institutionalized patients	Ciprofloxacin 500 mg PO, or 400 mg IV, BID × 5 days. Alternative Rx: azithromycin or TMP/SMX.
Salmonella sp.	8–72 hours; 2-5 days	Contaminated water, food (eggs, poultry or milk), animals (chicks, lizards, turtles) and group gatherings	Fever, abdominal pain, headache, myalgia, and diarrhea. Vomiting is minimal. Increased risk of sepsis in the elderly, young, immunocompromised, asplenic, and those with SS disease, HIV, or IVDA	Ciprofloxacin 500 mg PO, or 400 mg IV, BID × 3–7 days. Alternative Rx: azithromycin or ceftriaxone.
Yersinia enterocolitica	1–5 day; 3-12 days	Contaminated water, food (pork or milk), person to person, wild and domestic animals	Low-grade fever, anorexia, vomiting, and abdominal pain which preceding diarrhea. May mimic appendicitis. More common in children and young adults	Usually a self-limiting process. Ciprofloxacin 500 mg PO BID × 3–5 days. Alternative Rx: TMP/SMX.
Enterohemorrhagic E. coli 0157:H7	3–8 days; 5–10 days	Contaminated water or food (raw or undercooked meats, hamburger) person to person, day care, institutions, and poor sanitation	Fever, vomiting, abdominal pain, and grossly bloody diarrhea. May mimic mesenteric ischemia or GI bleed. Childern and the elderly are the most commonly affected. Hemolytic uremic syndrome occurs in 5% of affected patients, 5–20 days post-infection	Antibiotics are not recommended and may increase the risk of complications such as HUS.
Vibrio parahaemolyticus	8–72 hours; 1–2 days	Contaminated water or food (raw or undercooked shellfish)	Low-grade fevers, headaches, abdominal cramps, diarrhea, and nausea with minimal vomiting. More common in the summer months, and in adults	No antibiotic treatment has been proven to be effective although in vitro sensitivity has been shown to the fluoroquinolones and to doxycycline.

(Continued)

Table 7-4. Diagnosis and Treatment of Dysenteric Enteritis (Continued)

Infectious Agents	Incubation; Duration	Transmission	Diagnostic Features*	Adult Therapy
Strongyloides stercoralis	weeks; weeks to months	Soils contaminated with feces, walking bare footed, warm climates (southern US, the tropics), poor sanitation, and institutions	May present with fever, abdominal pain, vomiting, and diarrhea. Cutaneous, pulmonary or CNS symptoms may also develop. Sepsis may occur in the immunocompromised	Thiabendazole 25 mg/kg PO BID × 3–5 days
Aeromonas hydrophilia	1–5 days; 2–10 weeks	Contaminated water	Vomiting, diarrhea, and abdominal cramps, with or without fever. Chronic infection may mimic inflammatory bowel disease. Accounts for 10–15% of cases of pediatric diarrhea. Occurs more commonly in the elderly or the compromised, but the presentation is more severe in children	Ciprofloxacin 500 mg PO BID × 3–7 days. Alternative treatment is TMP/SMX or tetracycline
Clostridium difficile (antibiotic associated)	4 days–10 weeks; weeks	Antibiotic associated, days 4–9 of use, may be delayed for up to 10 weeks, clindamycin, penicillins and cephalosporins most common	Fevers, abdominal pain, and diarrhea. Vomiting is rare. More common in adults but tends to be more severe in children. May cause sepsis especially in the young, the elderly, and the immunocompromised	Discontinue associated antibiotics. Treat with Metronidazole 500 mg PO or IV, TID × 10–14 days. Alternative treatment is with Vancomycin 125 mg PO QID × 10–14 days
Plesiomonas shigelloides	1–2 days; 5–20 days	Uncooked shellfish, raw oysters, travel in Mexico or Asia	Vomiting, severe abdominal cramps, diarrhea, and dehydration. More common in the immunocompromised	Treatment is usually not required. In the immunocom promised treatment is with Ciprofloxicin 500 mg po bid 3–7 days. Alternative Rx: TMP/SMX DS PO BID × 3–7 days
Entamoeba histolytica (amebic dysentery)	1–12 weeks; weeks	Contaminated food or water; poor sanitation, institutionalization, and traveling to developing countries	Abrupt onset of fever, bloody diarrhea, abdominal pain, tenesmus, with vomiting being rare. Chronic illness with malaise, weight loss, bloating, blood streaked diarrhea, and may develop an hepatic abscess	Metronidazole 750mg PO TID × 10 days followed by Iodoquinol 650 mg PO TID × 20 days

* All potential dysenteric illness may have fecal red blood cells and white blood cells on stool smears.

Testing should be considered in patients with a toxic appearance, those who are hemodynamically unstable, those with a suspected noninfectious cause of diarrhea, the very young, the elderly, and immunosuppressed individuals. In addition, testing may be of value in patients with a prolonged course or in those not responding to conservative management.[5,6] Fecal leukocytes and erythrocytes, by stool smear, have long been used to help determine which patients with diarrhea should be treated with empiric antibiotics. However, the presence of fecal cells has never been shown to be a reliable predictor of which patients would benefit from antimicrobial therapy.[7] While fecal leukocytes are common with dysenteric illness (Table 7-4), and are suggestive of an inflammatory diarrhea, they are not specific for a bacterial cause. Fecal cells may result from an inflammatory diarrhea of bacterial, parasitic, or noninfectious causes. In addition, the absence of fecal cells has not been shown to rule out an invasive bacterial enteritis.[7] Furthermore, in an otherwise healthy individual, many cases of bacterial enteritis are self-limiting and may not require antimicrobial therapy. Reliance on guaiac alone is even less reliable as the presence of blood does not always correlate with the presence of fecal leukocytes. Blood without fecal leukocytes may indicate amebiasis, malignancies, bowel ischemia, GI bleeding, fissures, hemorrhoids, or heavy metal poisoning. An assay for *C. difficile* toxin may be of benefit in patients with recent antibiotic use. In addition, testing for *E. coli* 0157:H7 toxin may be considered in endemic areas and in patients with suspected hemolytic-uremic syndrome (HUS).

Routine cultures of the stool for bacteria are of limited value as only 2% have been shown to be positive.[4] However, cultures may be warranted in patients who are febrile, toxic appearing, immunosuppressed, at the extremes of age, experiencing a prolonged course, or in those not responding to conventional treatment. The assessment of stool for ova and parasites, or testing for Giardia antigen, may be considered in patients with chronic diarrhea, a history of travel to developing countries, a history of backpacking, those exposed to poor sanitation, those with exposure to infants in day care centers, and those with HIV infection.[8,9]

INFECTIOUS DIARRHEA

Infectious causes of diarrhea have been estimated to account for 85% of cases and can be divided into viral (60%), bacterial (20%), and parasitic causes (5%) (Table 7-1). The most significant symptoms are seen with bacterial and parasitic pathogens which cause an invasive, inflammatory diarrhea, although any infectious organism may result in morbidity and mortality, especially in susceptible patients. The specific causative agents of infectious diarrhea are rarely identified in the acute setting.

The causes of infections diarrheas are divided by their predilection to cause a dysenteric illness (Tables 7-3 and 7-4). Gastroenteritis is a clinical syndrome that includes nausea, vomiting, and diarrhea. The upper GI symptoms are often more prominent and the diarrhea of variable severity.

Most viral pathogens produce a cytotoxin mediated secretory diarrhea.[10] Viral gastroenteritis is usually self-limiting with mild dehydration and generally requires only supportive care. It is not usually associated with extensive systemic symptoms or significant abdominal pain. Fecal erythrocytes and leukocytes are uncommon. The most frequently identified agents are Norwalk and Rotavirus.[11,12]

Bacterial pathogens may produce either an inflammatory or a secretory diarrhea.[10] Bacterial secretory diarrhea may be caused by cytotoxins that are preformed and rapid acting, as with *Staphylococcus aureus* food poisoning, or by toxins formed after bacterial colonization of the intestinal mucosa, as with *Vibrio cholerae*. Cytotoxin-mediated bacterial gastroenteritis is generally a mild and self-limiting process, clinically similar to viral gastroenteritis. However, fluid losses can be extensive and in susceptible patients may lead to shock and mortality if untreated. Worldwide, *V. cholerae* accounts for a significant number of deaths annually.[13]

Dysentery is an inflammatory diarrhea caused most commonly by bacterial and parasitic pathogens, which invade the intestinal mucosa (Table 7-4). This invasive, inflammatory process typically leads to the presence of blood, mucus, and plasma proteins in the stool. Dysenteric enteritis is typically associated with fever, abdominal pain, anorexia, dehydration, myalgia, cephalgia, and weight loss. Invasive bacterial organisms, most notably *Salmonella* and *Shigella*, may result in bacteremia, sepsis, and death especially in infants, the elderly, and those with significant underlying medical conditions.[14–16]

Inflammatory diarrhea may also be caused by chemotherapy, radiation therapy, hypersensitivity reactions, autoimmune disorders, and inflammatory bowel disease. These disorders may present in a manner similar to that of bacterial dysentery.

Acute amebic dysentery, caused by the parasitic pathogen *Entamoeba histolytica,* may be associated with significant systemic symptoms and may be difficult to distinguish clinically from dysentery of a bacterial cause.[11,17] With an inflammatory enteritis from any cause, stool smears will generally contain both erythrocytes and leukocytes.

Both heterosexual and homosexual contact may be associated with the transmission of amebic dysentery, *Giardia, Salmonella, Shigella,* and *Campylobacter.* Lower GI symptoms may also be caused by sexually transmitted diseases such as *Neisseria gonorrheae, Chlamydia trachomatis,* and herpes simplex. Human immunodeficiency virus-positive and other immunocompromised individuals are subject to infections with Cryptosporidium, cytomegalovirus, and *Mycobacterium avium intracellulare.*[9,11]

Although specific parasitic pathogens are rarely identified in the acute setting, a diagnosis of parasitic enteritis should be considered in patients with a travel history to developing countries, in institutionalized patients, or in the immunocompromised.[8,9] Also consider parasitic causes in patients with a prolonged course and in those not responding to conventional treatment.

NONINFECTIOUS DIARRHEA

Approximately 15% of cases of diarrhea are due to noninfectious causes (Table 7-2) and if not recognized may pose an even greater threat to patient well being and survival. Diarrhea may be a presenting symptom of acute abdominal pathology, endocrine disorders, toxic exposures, central nervous system pathology, chemotherapy, radiation therapy, and other systemic illnesses.

The clinical presentation of patients with noninfectious diarrhea covers a wide range of signs and symptoms and depends primarily on the underlying cause. It is imperative to consider such entities as GI bleeding, mesenteric ischemia, inflammatory bowel disease, acute appendicitis, intussusception, ectopic pregnancy, bowel obstruction, volvulus, diverticular disease, fecal impaction (with overflow diarrhea), and GI tumors. Endocrine pathology, such as diabetic ketoacidosis and adrenal insufficiency, should be considered as well.

The list of toxins that may present with GI symptoms is extensive (Table 7-2). Consider common toxins such as digoxin, salicylates, carbon monoxide, and heavy metals. In addition, consider the ingestion of mushrooms, other plant products, seafood, and fish borne toxins. Ask about occupational exposures, and in farm workers, consider pesticides (organophosphate poisoning) and nicotine poisoning (green tobacco syndrome). If neurologic symptoms exist, consider botulism or shellfish poisoning. Inquire about other medications including, prescription and nonprescription drugs, herbal preparations, and drugs of abuse. Give particular attention to recent antibiotic or laxative use. Consider specific toxidromes, such as cholinergic or sympathomimetic, as well as an evaluation for opiate withdrawal.

ANTIBIOTIC ASSOCIATED DIARRHEA

Diarrhea is a common complication of antimicrobial therapy, occurring in 5% to 25% of patients treated with antibiotics.[18] The diarrhea results from the effects of broad spectrum antibiotics on fecal flora, mitigated by patient host factors. Most cases are self-limiting and improve after withdrawal of the antibiotic and general supportive care. Patients with severe symptoms, and those who appear systemically ill should be evaluated for *C. difficile*-associated diarrhea (CDAD). Clindamycin has been implicated as one of the most common causes of antibiotic associated colitis. Other frequent causes include fluoroquinolones, penicillins, and cephalosporins.[19]

Clostridium difficile is a gram-positive, spore-forming rod that has been implicated in 10% to 20% of antibiotic related cases of diarrhea, and essentially all cases of pseudomembranous colitis.[20] *C. difficile* normally inhabits the colon of only 3% of healthy adults but up to 80% of newborns and infants.[21] Development of CDAD requires several factors including treatment with antimicrobials and colonization by the fecal-oral route. Antimicrobials cause disruption of the normal colonic flora, which facilitates the germination of ingested spores. Other factors that contribute to the development of CDAD include host immunity, patient age, virulence of the *C. difficile* strain, and the timing of antibiotic exposure.[22]

Most cases of CDAD develop on days 4 to 9 of antibiotic therapy, but may be delayed for up to 10 weeks after the completion of therapy.[23,24] *C. difficile* produces two toxins that are responsible for its pathogenesis: Toxin A is primarily an enterotoxin that causes excretion of inflammatory fluid from the intestinal mucosa, while toxin B is cytotoxic in nature.[22] These toxins induce a profound colonic inflammatory response culminating in pseudomembranous colitis with its characteristic raised yellow plaques and pseudomembranes scattered throughout the colorectal mucosa. *C. difficile*-associated diarrhea is a nosocomial infection with *C. difficile* being readily cultured from hospital equipment and patient care areas. It is also acquired by direct contact with hospital workers. Hand washing with soap and water is an important preventive measure, but alcohol-based hand cleaning solutions do not inhibit the transmission of *C. difficile.*[22]

Patients presenting with diarrhea, in the acute setting, should be questioned about recent hospitalizations and antibiotic treatment. A diagnosis of *C. difficile* should be strongly considered in patients with these historical factors. Mild to moderate CDAD is usually accompanied by lower abdominal cramps without other significant systemic symptoms. Patients presenting with moderate

CDAD may have malaise, fever, abdominal distension, crampy abdominal pain, and profuse diarrhea. In 1% to 3% of patients with CDAD, fulminate colitis develops with toxic megacolon, perforation, and death.[21]

Initial evaluation and treatment of patients with CDAD includes supportive care and diagnostic stool studies including enzyme–linked immunosorbent assay (ELISA) to detect toxin A or B. The ELISA assay has a sensitivity of 71% to 94% and a specificity of 92% to 98%.[21] Sigmoidoscopy has also been utilized in the workup of patients with *C. difficile* colitis;however, this must be done with caution to prevent perforation of the inflamed mucosa.

In many cases the diarrhea of CDAD will resolve with withdrawal of the antibiotic and the administration of appropriate resuscitative fluids. Antibiotic treatment directed against *C. difficile* may be required when the diarrhea does not resolve with conservative measures. Early antibiotic treatment should be initiated in older patients, patients with multiple comorbid conditions, and patients who need to be maintained on other antibiotics.

Preferred therapy for *C. difficile* consists of metronidazole 250 mg to 500 mg orally 3 to 4 times a day for 10 to 14 days.[21] Vancomycin 125 mg to 500 mg orally 4 times a day for 10 to 14 days is also an effective, but is reserved for ill patients who do not respond to metronidazole. Intravenous vancomycin is less effective as it does not reach acceptable intraluminal concentrations. Emergent colectomy may be necessary for patients who develop toxic megacolon or colonic perforation. Antimotility and opiate drugs should be avoided as they have been associated with toxic megacolon and may worsen the course of disease.[23]

Symptoms recur in 10% to 30% of patients, despite a high initial response rate to treatment.[23] Symptoms generally reoccur within the first 2 weeks after completion of the initial therapy. Approximately 50% of all recurrent cases are due to reinfection and not to a relapse of the primary infection.[21]

EMERGENCY DEPARTMENT CARE AND DISPOSITION

The evaluation and treatment of patients with diarrhea should begin with a rapid assessment of the severity of the present illness, the extent of volume depletion, and the overall health of the patient, followed by the appropriate resuscitative measures. In unstable patients establish intravenous access and continuous cardiac monitoring, followed by normal saline volume resuscitation. Complete vital signs should be obtained, including blood pressure and pulse rate (with orthostatic changes), pulse oximetry, respiratory rate, and a rectal temperature. Draw blood for electrolytes, a complete blood count, serum lipase, renal and liver function, and a pregnancy test, as indicated. A type and cross-match should be obtained if blood loss is suspected. Search for evidence of sepsis, a surgical abdomen, GI bleeding, toxic exposures, endocrine pathology, or anaphylaxis. Antibiotic use may be indicated in the toxic appearing patient.

The initial treatment for patients with diarrhea, regardless of the cause, consists of supportive care with attention given to the patient's hydration status. Since many cases of diarrhea are self-limiting, this is often the only treatment necessary. Oral rehydration may be used for patients with mild to moderate fluid losses. In pediatric patients give 50 mL to 100 mL per kg of a glucose-electrolyte solution orally given over 4 hours.[3,25] Oral rehydration fluids such as sports drinks, diluted fruit juices, and soft drinks supplemented with soups, broths, or crackers may be sufficient to replace the fluid and sodium losses resulting from acute diarrhea. However, such "clear liquids" may contain excess sugars and insufficient sodium content resulting in an osmotic diarrhea.[3,4] Milk and other lactose containing products should be avoided, as many viral and bacterial pathogens cause a transient lactase deficiency leading to malabsorption and an osmotic diarrhea. Caffeine containing beverages should also be avoided as caffeine increases cyclic adenosine monophosphate (cAMP) levels and may result in a secretory diarrhea. Food intake is encouraged, but foods high in simple sugars should be avoided, due to the tendency to promote an osmotic diarrhea. Foods with a high fat content tend to delay gastric emptying and should also be avoided.[5]

Intravenous fluid resuscitation with normal saline or lactated Ringer solution is the preferred treatment for patients with evidence of more severe dehydration. In pediatric patients, fluid resuscitation should consist of a bolus of 20 mL per kg of normal saline. This may be repeated as needed. As children are particularly susceptible to hypoglycemia after prolonged vomiting, diarrhea, and poor oral intake, a rapid bedside glucose determination should be preformed in ill-appearing pediatric patients.

Patients who appear toxic, those with a suspected invasive enteritis with severe diarrhea, fever, abdominal pain, and other systemic symptoms may require empiric antimicrobial treatment. Antimicrobial choice should be based on knowledge of the common causes of infectious diarrhea and directed against those pathogens most likely to cause harm (Tables 7-3 and 7-4). Ciprofloxacin, 500 mg orally, twice a day, for 3 to 7 days is most commonly given.[26, 27] Alternative treatments include the other fluoroquinolones, azithromycin, or trimethoprim-sulfamethoxazol (TMP-SMZ).[8,9,26,28]

The empiric use of antibiotics in infants and the elderly has been associated with an increased risk of developing HUS. This risk is greatest in patients at the extremes of age, those with more severe illness, those with high volume, grossly bloody diarrhea, and those with entero-hemorrhagic *E. coli* 0157:H7 infections.[29] Hemolytic-uremic syndrome occurs in 5% to 10% of all cases of enterohemorrhagic *E. coli*, and is the most common cause of renal failure in children. Hemolytic-uremic syndrome results in death for 3% to 5% of patients, with 35% experiencing chronic renal failure or other significant sequelae.[30] Although the greatest risk of HUS occurs with enterohemorrhagic *E. coli*, Salmonella, Shigella and Campylobacter have also been implicated.[29] Therefore, empiric antibiotics should not be used in the treatment of infants and the elderly with suspected *E. coli* 0157:H7 and with caution in other infections.[15] Hospital admission, supportive care, and stool studies should be initiated.

Because no broad empiric strategy exists for the treatment of parasitic pathogens, drug therapy is best guided by laboratory analysis. However, if amebic dysentery is of concern (travel history, chronic diarrhea, institutionalized or immunocompromised patients), treatment with metronidazole after stool analysis for ova and parasites should be considered. A second agent, such as iodoquinol, is needed after initial treatment.[17]

Specific treatment for noninfectious diarrhea should be directed toward the suspected cause. Patients with potential surgical pathology require further diagnostic testing such as computed tomography and surgical consultation. Treatment for toxic exposures consists of early decontamination, supportive care, and the administration of specific antidotes if appropriate.

The literature remains divided over the use of anti-motility agents in the treatment of acute enteritis, with bloody diarrhea often being listed as a contraindication. Opiates, loperamide, and diphenoxylate with atropine have been associated with the development of toxic megacolon in patients with ulcerative or antibiotic-associated colitis.[23] In addition, the use of morphine has been associated with Salmonella and Shigella bacteremia.[31] An association has also been noted between the use of antidiarrheal medications and the development of HUS.[29] Therefore, in the acute setting, antimotility agents should be used with caution, if at all, in patients with inflammatory bowel disease, suspected antibiotic-associated colitis, bloody diarrhea, and in patients at the extremes of age. In other patients, antimotility agents may be used, as warranted. The prevention of infectious diarrhea transmission should begin with interruption of the fecal-oral pathway and can be accomplished by adherence to strict hygiene and frequent handwashing.

DISPOSITION

Most patients with diarrhea do not require hospitalization and can be discharged home after careful assessment and symptomatic treatment. Patients with a toxic appearance, severe dehydration, hemodynamic instability, or patients at high risk, should be admitted for supportive treatment, continuous monitoring, and further investigation if the cause is uncertain. Referral to a gastroenterologist may be indicated in the evaluation of chronic diarrhea and for workup beyond the scope of the ED.

PITFALLS

- Many pathologic processes present with GI symptoms and risk being misdiagnosed as gastroenteritis. This includes dysenteric illnesses, acute surgical pathology, toxic exposures, endocrine emergencies, and other systemic illnesses.

- High-risk patients may experience a more significant course of disease, are more susceptible to the effects of fluid losses, and have increased susceptibility to sepsis from invasive bacterial organisms.

- Fecal leukocytes and erythrocytes are not a reliable indicator of which patients require empiric antimicrobial therapy.

- Patients at the extremes of age have an increased risk of developing hemolytic-uremic syndrome when receiving antibiotics or antimotility agents. This risk is greatest in ill-appearing patients with grossly bloody stools.

- In patients with ulcerative colitis or antibiotic-associated colitis, the use of antimotility agents has been associated with the development of toxic megacolon.

REFERENCES

1. Kosek M, Bern C, Guerrant RL. The global burden of diarrhoeal disease, as estimated from studies published between 1992 and 2000. *Bull World Health Organ.* 2003; 81:197.
2. Black RE, Morris SS, Bryce J. When and why are 10 million children dying every year? *Lancet.* 2003;361:2226.
3. King CK, Glass R, Bresee JS, et al. Managing acute gastroenteritis among children: Oral rehydration, maintenance, and nutritional therapy. *MMWR.* 2003;52:1.

4. Dupont HL. Guidelines on acute infectious diarrhea in adults. *Am J Gastroenterol.* 1997;92:1962.

5. Aranda-Michel J, Giannella RA. Acute diarrhea: a practical review. *Am J Med.* 1999;106:670.

6. Manatsathit S, Dupont HL, Farthing M, et al. Guideline for the management of acute diarrhea in adults. *J Gastroenterol Hepatol.* 2002;17:S54.

7. McNeely WS, Dupont HL, Mathewson JJ, et al. Occult blood versus fecal leukocytes in the diagnosis of bacterial diarrhea: a study of U.S. travelers to Mexico and Mexican children. *Am J Trop Med Hyg.* 1996;55:430.

8. Gomi H, Jiang ZD, Adachi JA, et al. In vitro antimicrobial susceptibility testing of bacterial enteropathogens causing traveler's diarrhea in four geographic regions. *Antimicrob Agents Chemother.* 2001;45:212.

9. Oldfield EC. Evaluation of chronic diarrhea in patients with human immunodeficiency virus infection. *Gastroent Disorders.* 2002;2:176.

10. Mathan VI. Diarrheoeal diseases. *Brit Med Bull.* 1998; 54:407.

11. Framm SR, Soave R. Agents of diarrhea. *Med Clin North Am.* 1997;81:427.

12. Hoekstra JH. European Society of Pediatric Gastroenterology, Hepatology and Nutrition Working Group on Acute Diarrhoea: Acute gastroenteritis in industrialized countries: compliance with guidelines for treatment. *J Pediatr Gastroenterol Nutr.* 2001;33:S31.

13. Davidson G, Barnes G, Bass D, et al. Infectious diarrhea in children: working group report of the First world Congress of pediatric gastroenterology, Hepatology, and Nutrition. *J Pediatr Gastroenterol Nutr.* 2002;35:S143.

14. Armon K, Stephenson T, MacFaul R, et al. An evidence and consensus based guideline for acute diarrhea management. *Arch Dis Child.* 2001;85:132.

15. Nazarian LF. A synopsis of the American Academy of Pediatrics' practice parameter on the management of acute gastroenteritis in young children. *Pediatr Rev.* 1997;18:221.

16. Eliason BC, Lewan RB. Gastroenteritis in children: Principles of diagnosis and treatment. *Am Fam Physician.* 1998;58:1769.

17. Fine KD, Schiller LR. AGA technical review on the evaluation and management of chronic diarrhea. *Gastroenterology.* 1999;116:1464.

18. Surawicz CM. Antibiotic-associated diarrhea and pseudomembranous colitis: are they less common with poorly absorbed antimicrobials? *Chemother.* 2005;51:81.

19. Hogenauer C, Hammer HF, Krejs GJ, et al. Mechanisms and management of antibiotic-associated diarrhea. *Clin Infect Dis.* 1998;27:702.

20. Schroeder MS. Clostridium difficile-associated diarrhea. *Am Fam Physician.* 2005;71:921.

21. Mylonakis E, Ryan ET, Calderwood S. Clostridium difficile-associated diarrhea: a review. *Arch Intern Med.* 2001;26:525.

22. Hurley BW, Nguyen CC. The spectrum of pseudomembranous enterolitis and antibiotic-associated diarrhea. *Arch Intern Med.* 2002;162:2177.

23. Cleary RK. Clostridium difficile-associated diarrhea and colitis: clinical manifestations, diagnosis, and treatment. *Dis Colon & Rectum.* 1998;41:1435.

24. Kelly CP, Pothoulakis C, LaMont JT. Clostridium difficile colitis. *N Engl J Med.* 1994;33:257.

25. Duggan C, Lasche J, McCarty M, et al. Oral rehydration solution for acute diarrhea prevents subsequent unscheduled follow-up visits. *Pediatrics.* 1999;104:29.

26. Dryden MS, Gabb RJ, Wright SK. Empirical treatment of severe acute community-acquired gastroenteritis with ciprofloxacin. *Clin Infect Dis.* 1996;22:1019.

27. Daniels NA, MacKinnon L, Bishop R, et al. Vibrio parahaemolyticus infections in the United States, 1973–1998. *J Infect Dis.* 2000;181:1661.

28. Oldfield EC 3rd, Wallace MR. The role of antibiotics in the treatment of infectious diarrhea. *Gastroenterol Clin North Am.* 2001;30:817.

29. Besser RE, Griffin PM, Slutsker L. Escherichia coli O157:H7 gastroenteritis and the hemolytic uremic syndrome: an emerging infectious disease. *Annu Rev Med.* 1999;50:355.

30. Slutsker L, Ries AA, Greene KD, et al. Escherichia coli O157:H7 diarrhea in the United States: clinical and epidemiologic features. *Ann Intern Med.* 1997;126:505.

31. MacFarlane AS, Peng X, Meissler JJ, et al. Morphine increases susceptibility to oral *Salmonella typhimurium* infection. *J Infect Dis.* 2000;181:1350.

8

Constipation

David M. Cline

HIGH YIELD FACTS

- Acute constipation may be the first symptom of colonic cancer.
- The most important management decision on behalf of patients presenting with a complaint of constipation is not what agent to use to relieve the symptoms, but the decision to further investigate with diagnostic testing.
- When a patient presents with constipation accompanied by significant abdominal pain, the clinician should consider bowel obstruction (including volvulus), diverticulitis, and ischemic colitis as potential causes.

EPIDEMIOLOGY

Constipation is a common problem with a prevalence of 12% to 19% in North America.[1] Estimates based on an objective measure (fewer than 3 bowel movements per week) are less than estimates based on patient self reporting. Female to male ratio is 2.2 to 1,[1] and laxative use is more frequent in women. Up to 26% of elderly men and 34% of elderly woman complain of constipation. As much as 75% of elderly patients in nursing homes are given laxatives on a regular basis.

ETIOLOGY

The conditions associated with the complaint of constipation are numerous (Tables 8-1 to 8-3), with inadequate fiber in the diets of symptomatic patients reported as the most common cause.[2] However, in the elderly, constipating medications (Table 8-2) and inadequate caloric intake may be more important causes.[3,4] It has been shown that decreased water intake increases stool firmness, but the evidence for dehydration as a significant cause of constipation is lacking.[5,6] Using a definition of fewer than 3 bowel movements per week,

constipation doubles the risk of colon cancer.[7] Laxative use does not appear to be a marker of similar significance. Prevalence of constipation during pregnancy ranges from 11% to 38%, but a more frequent complaint appears to be the sensation of anal blockage, occurring in 34% to 42% of women. Emergency physicians should pay particular attention to life-threatening conditions that may present with constipation (Table 8-1), the most frequent of which is bowel obstruction. Despite the widespread use of computed tomography (CT) scanning to better identify confusing presentations of bowel obstruction, autopsy studies continue to reveal missed bowel obstruction as an unexpected cause of death.[8]

PATHOPHYSIOLOGY

Constipation results when there is an imbalance between nonpropulsive forces that determine fluid absorption in the large intestine and the propulsive forces that move the fecal material toward the rectum. Colonic transit is affected by the smooth muscle function of the bowel wall regulating motility and the submucosal plexuses regulating absorption, with overall control by the parasympathetic nervous system. Bowel contents affect transit time, especially fiber and water content. Typically only 100 mL per day of ingested fluid or secretions are lost in the stool, and when colonic transit times are prolonged or inadequate fluid is ingested, stool becomes hard and difficult to expel. Elderly patients with idiopathic chronic constipation have prolonged transit times and therefore increased fluid reabsorption. Medications such as narcotics have similar actions. These changes are typically accompanied by decreased rectal sensitivity and decreased rectal reflexes. Ignoring the urge to defecate may also occur in the setting of painful anal lesions or changes in environment. Stool holding promotes fluid absorption and hardened stool. If chronic rectal distension results, motor tone also decreases, which exacerbates the problem.

Normal colonic transit ranges from 18 to 72 hours. Some patients have prolonged times; patients with slow transit constipation have times greater than 72 hours. Slow transit constipation is thought to be due to a disorder of the myenteric plexus. These patients are unlikely to respond to simple treatment measures such as fiber.[9] There are multiple disorders that are grouped as pelvic outlet dysfunction that involve high resting anal canal pressures or failure of anal sphincter relaxation during defecation that impedes the outflow of stool. Rectoceles may result from years of straining and worsen rectal evacuation.

Table 8-1. Acute Causes of Constipation, Clinical Findings and Test Results

	Diagnostic Clues	**Testing***
Anal lesions		
Abscess†	Dull aching pain that persists between bowel movements; palpable with rectal exam	Anoscopy helpful to visualize extent of abscess, pretreat with topical anesthetic
Fissures	Pain with bowel movements, better afterward; visible on rectal exam if tolerated, may bleed	Anoscopy helpful to rule out other pathology, pretreat with topical anesthetic
Hemorrhoids	Pain if thrombosed; external hemorrhoids visible on rectal exam at 2, 5, or 9 o'clock	Anoscopy helpful for internal hemorrhoids, pretreat with topical anesthetic
Herpes	Significant pain; visible on rectal exam	Viral culture, but results not immediate
Bowel disease		
Carcinoma	Family history, weight loss, hematochezia	May have positive stool for occult blood
Diverticulitis (consider perforation)	Tenesmus, left lower quadrant pain, anorexia, fever, diarrhea, symptoms may vary	May have positive stool for occult blood
Inflammatory bowel disease	Tenesmus, bloody diarrhea, anorexia, weight loss, associated arthritis,	May have positive stool for occult blood
Ischemic colitis†	History of cardiovascular disease, pain out of proportion to exam, distension	May have elevated white blood cell count, or elevated lactate; CT scanning
Obstruction, small or large bowel†	Vomiting, abdominal pain and distension (most common symptom in elderly)	Positive obstructive radiography series, or computed tomography
Toxic megacolon†	Inflammatory bowel disease; starts with bloody diarrhea and abdominal pain, followed by fever chills, obstipation, and toxicity	>6 cm dilation on plain film, CT identifies complications
Volvulus, cecal, or sigmoid colon†	Institutionalized patient, mental illness, vomiting, abdominal pain and distension (most common symptom in elderly)	Obstructive radiography series, CT
Dietary habits		
Inadequate fiber intake	History	None
Inadequate fluid intake	History	May have elevated blood urea nitrogen and creatinine levels, or normal values
Medications (Table 8-3)	History	None
Metabolic disorders		
Hypokalemia	Generalized weakness, cramping, hyporeflexia, dysrhythmias,	Low potassium level; U waves and or ST segment depression on ECG
Hypercalcemia	Generalized weakness, cramping, abdominal pain, polyuria and polydipsia	Elevated calcium level
Uremia	Nausea and vomiting, weakness, hypertension, edema	Elevated blood urea nitrogen and creatinine, electrolytes
Hypothyroidism	Fatigue, weakness, cold intolerance, weight gain, dry, scaly skin, nonpitting waxy edema	Thyroid stimulating hormone level
Hypoadrenalism	Weakness, dehydration, hypotension, nausea, weight loss, abdominal pain	Hyponatremia, hypokalemia, hypoglycemia; consider cosyntropin test

(Continued)

Table 8-1. Acute Causes of Constipation, Clinical Findings and Test Results (Continued)

	Diagnostic Clues	**Testing***
Pregnancy (consider ectopic)	Missed menses	Urine pregnancy
Psychosocial change		
Travel	History	None
Depression	History	None
Psychosocial stress	History	None
Immobility	History	None
Toxicologic disorder		
Lead poisoning	Nausea, vomiting, abdominal pain, ataxia,	Anemia, lead level

*Patients deemed to be significantly ill after history and physical exam should have more extensive testing than what was is suggested here.
†Potentially life threatening, if left untreated.
Abbreviations: CT, computed tomography; ECG, electrocardiogram.

Table 8-2. Common Medications Associated with Constipation

Antacids
  Aluminum hydroxide
  Calcium carbonate
Anticholinergics
  Antihistamines
  Tricyclic antidepressants
  Phenothiazines
  Antiparkinsonian agents
  Antispasmodics
Antihypertensives
  ACE-inhibitors
  Calcium-channel blockers
  Clonidine
  Diuretics
Iron
Laxative abuse
Lipid-lowering agents
Narcotics
Nonsteroidal antiinflammatory agents
Phenytoin
Sympathomimetics
  Ephedrine
  Pseudoephedrine
  Terbutaline

Abbreviation: ACE, angiotensin-converting enzyme.

Table 8-3. Chronic Causes of Constipation

Bowel disease
  Irritable bowel syndrome
  Diverticulosis
  Inflammatory bowel disease
  Hirschsprung disease (infants)
  Stricture (colonic)
Debilitated
  Chronic disease
  Institutionalized
Evacuation disorders
  Pelvic outlet dysfunction
  Rectocele
Neurogenic
  Diabetic
  Stroke, dementia
  Multiple sclerosis
  Parkinson disease
  Spinal cord lesions
Pseudo-obstruction (Ogilvie syndrome)
Psychogenic
  Schizophrenia
Slow transit constipation

Obstipation is the absolute inability to pass stool. Fecal impaction is the inability to pass a hard collection of stool and can be regarded as extreme constipation. Risk factors for fecal impaction include physical and mental incapacitation, advanced age, institutionalization, and chronic laxative use. With age, the rectum and anus lose tactile sensitivity, and thus the sensation of fullness in the rectum decreases. Anal lesions that cause pain can inhibit the passage of stool. While stool is retained, ongoing fluid absorption and colonic peristalsis combine to pack stool into a hard bolus that is difficult to pass though the fixed caliber of the anus.

CLINICAL FEATURES

The clinical presentation is highly variable ranging from simple constipation amenable to small changes in diet to life threatening disorders that have a constellation of symptoms that are compatible with constipation: reduced frequency of stooling, abdominal cramping, or pain with defecation. Clues to the diagnosis may be uncovered in the context of the complaint; constipation may be only one of the symptoms that contribute to the total clinical picture. As the use of constipating medications is a common cause of constipation, over-the-counter medication and prescribed medication use should be reviewed in detail. (Patients may recall additional medications after their list has been given to the triage nurse.)

History taking should elicit recent and chronic bowel habits to determine the acute nature of the condition; the frequency of bowel movements should be elicited. Stool description including consistency, caliber, and presence of blood or purulent material should be elicited. Associated symptoms such as pain and vomiting should be determined; simple constipation may be associated with crampy pain, but severe pain and/or vomiting are more frequently associated with ominous conditions. The complaint of pain should be differentiated into abdominal and rectal pain as each has important implications regarding etiology or treatment. History of associated fever, weight loss, poor appetite, diarrhea (which may alternate with constipation), flatulence, and foul smelling feces should be elicited. Systemic symptoms may indicate a systemic process such as hypothyroidism. (See Table 8-1 for symptoms of common causes of acute constipation.)

Abnormal vital signs suggest a serious condition causing constipation. Mild abdominal distension may be noted with simple constipation, but may also be a sign of bowel obstruction; abnormal bowel sounds and signs of peritoneal irritation are more likely associated with serious conditions. In thin patients, stool may be palpable, but should be absent after treatment if this is indeed the cause of a palpable mass.

A rectal exam is an essential part of the evaluation to look for hemorrhoids, rectal fissure, abscess, or fecal impaction. Stool should be checked for blood, as carcinoma must be considered in patients with positive occult blood testing. Decreased tone may be found and be indicative of neurologic disease or long-standing constipation. While the neurologic exam may at first appear superfluous to the complaint, abnormal reflexes may be a clue to an acute electrolyte disorder that ultimately explains the presentation.

DIAGNOSIS AND DIFFERENTIAL

Different causes of constipation are listed in Tables 8-1 through 8-3. The presence of significant abdominal pain should alert the clinician to the possibility of serious conditions such as bowel obstruction including volvulus, diverticulitis, and ischemic colitis. Rectal pain may be associated with fecal impaction, rectal abscess, rectal fissure, or hemorrhoids. Associated bright red blood may accompany these rectal conditions, but may also be associated with malignancy, inflammatory bowel disease, or diverticulitis.

Constipation with intermittent diarrhea may indicate an obstructing colonic lesion such as carcinoma, fecal impaction, or undisclosed rectal foreign body. Alternatively, mixed constipation with diarrhea may be associated with inflammatory bowel disease and irritable bowel syndrome (IBS). Flatulence, bloating, and foul smelling feces may be associated with malabsorption syndrome. Vomiting (especially if recurrent) and inability to pass flatulence is associated with bowel obstruction. Volvulus is more frequent in patients over the age of 80 and in the institutionalized patient. Decreasing caliber of stool could indicate an obstructing carcinoma, while small caliber stool since birth could herald Hirschsprung disease in an infant.

Fecal Impaction

Patients with fecal impaction may have fever or leukocytosis,[10] but the presence of these markers should prompt the physician to consider other more serious conditions such as diverticulitis, urinary tract infection, or pneumonia. Coexistent hemorrhoids are very common with fecal impaction.[10] When fecal impaction is suspected clinically, but the patient has an empty rectal vault, a radiographic investigation for bowel obstruction is warranted, and may verify impaction beyond the reach of the examiner's finger (see below for a discussion for bowel obstruction associated with fecal impaction). Untreated fecal impaction will continue to yield abdominal distension that can limit ventilation, which can lead to tachypnea.[10]

LIFE THREATENING CONDITIONS PRESENTING WITH CONSTIPATION

Emergency physicians should pay particular attention to the life-threatening causes of constipation listed in Table 8-1. These include abscess, bowel obstruction, colon carcinoma, diverticulitis, ischemic bowel, toxic megacolon, and volvulus. While these patients would typically be expected to appear acutely ill, that is not always the case.

The symptoms of abscess are listed in Table 8-1. Deeper abscesses may not be visible on inspection and should be suspected when a patient complains of rectal pain and tenderness, especially when associated with fever. Computed tomography or ultrasound may be required for diagnosis. The symptoms of severe constipation and bowel obstruction (as well as volvulus) can be identical, and therefore, obstruction can be missed, sometimes with fatal results.[8,11] Bowel obstruction and volvulus are discussed in Chapter 13.

Ischemic Large Bowel

There are two clinically distinct presentations of large bowel ischemia that may be associated with a complaint of constipation: bowel obstruction that has progressed to ischemia and ischemic colitis. Unlike small bowel ischemia, colonic ischemia is rarely due to major arterial occlusion. Ischemic colitis typically results from low flow states or small vessel occlusion. Risk factors include hypotension, vascular disease, diabetes mellitus, and vasculitis. Typical symptoms are cramplike abdominal pain, distension, and bloody diarrhea, but may also mimic constipation with overflow diarrhea and hemorrhoid bleeding, or may present without bleeding.[11] Medical management is the mainstay of treatment except when signs of acute abdomen are present, in which case surgery is recommended. All patients suspected of having ischemia in association with obstruction require surgical consultation. Computed tomography has good sensitivity for picking up ischemia in the setting of bowel obstruction, but misses 17% of cases.[12]

Colon Cancer

A retrospective study of 358 patients referred for colonoscopy plus 205 patients referred for flexible sigmoidoscopy who complained of constipation revealed a prevalence of colon cancer of 1.6% and a 14.4% prevalence of adenoma. The authors concluded: "the range of neoplasia in patients with constipation evaluated with lower endoscopy was comparable with what would be expected in asymptomatic subjects undergoing colorectal cancer screening."[13] Indeed, constipation alone is not an indication for urgent colorectal screening for cancer, despite the fact that the incidence of cancer appears to be higher in this group.[7]

Stool that is positive for blood is one of the alarm symptoms that should ultimately prompt a more thorough workup than what would be expected for a stable patient (see Alarm Symptoms below). Outpatient studies to be considered by the primary care physician are elective CT scan, or better, colonoscopy with biopsy of any lesions found. In the stable patient without signs of obstruction, even in the face of weight loss, there is no mandate for CT on an emergent basis. However, patients should have blood counts performed in the emergency department (ED) to help verify clinical stability. The exception is the patient complaining of constipation who is still having bowel movements, with only occult blood positive and who is otherwise stable with follow-up assured.

Toxic Megacolon

Megacolon can occur in association with chronic constipation and may be difficult to distinguish clinically from bowel obstruction or volvulus even after obtaining plain film radiography.[14] Toxic megacolon has defined criteria for the diagnosis using plain film radiography and clinical information. The diagnosis is made by any **three** of the following criteria: (1) fever >101.5°F (>38.6°C), (2) heart rate >120 beats per min, (3) white blood cell count >10.5 × 10^9/L, or (4) anemia; **plus any one** of the following: dehydration, mental status changes, electrolyte disturbances, or hypotension.[15] The majority of patients have a history of inflammatory bowel disease, and present after an episode of exacerbation has started, initially with bloody diarrhea, fevers, chills, and abdominal cramping. The onset of toxic megacolon is variable, but may be present with abdominal distension, obstipation, and reduced bowel sounds accompanied by fever, tachycardia, and hypotension.[16] On plain films, the colon is dilated >6 cm, and dilations of up to 15 cm are not uncommon. Computed tomography scanning is recommended to better define subclinical perforations and abscesses not apparent on physical exam or plain radiography.[17] These patients typically appear ill and require admission for resuscitation including fluids, antibiotics, and surgical consultation.

CHRONIC CONDITIONS CAUSING CONSTIPATION

Chronic conditions associated with constipation are listed in Table 8-4. The management of the patient's constipation would typically begin prior to evaluation in the ED, and care would need to be coordinated by a return visit to the patient's doctor. Pseudo-obstruction or Ogilvie syndrome is discussed in Chapter 13. One condition listed in Table 8-3 deserves further discussion here.

Irritable Bowel Syndrome

Irritable bowel syndrome (IBS) is common; 15% of U.S. adults report symptoms compatible with IBS.[18] Irritable bowel syndrome is more common in women, is the most

Table 8-4. Agents Used in the Treatment of Constipation

ACGCCTF recommended evidenced based treatments for constipation*			
Treatment	**Dose**	**Side Effects/Caution**	**Type/Mechanism**
Polyethylene Glycol plus electrolytes	1 L, in 2 divided doses daily	Nausea, cramping, anal irritation; less luminal electrolyte losses	Hyperosmolar agent, balanced electrolytes
Lactulose	15–30 mL, twice daily	Cramps, flatulence, belching, nausea	Osmotically active nonabsorbable sugars pull fluid into gut
Psyllium	1 tsp TID	Bloating, flatulence	Fiber, increased stool bulk and motility

Other treatments commonly used			
Treatment	**Dose**	**Side Effects/Caution**	**Type/Mechanism**
Polyethylene glycol 3350	17 gm mixed in 240 mls of liquid, and given as 1, or split into 2 doses	Nausea, cramping, anal irritation	Hyperosmolar agent
Bisacodyl	10 mg PO daily	Nausea, cramping	Stimulates secretion and motility of small and large bowel
Magnesium citrate	150–300 mL As needed	Hypermagnesemia can occur in patients with renal failure or in children	Osmotic laxative
Magnesium hydroxide	15–30 mL once or twice daily	Hypermagnesemia can occur in patients with renal failure or in children	Osmotic laxative
Mineral oil	5–15 mL orally	Malabsorption of fat soluble vitamins with chronic use; lipoid pneumonia in debilitated patients	Nonabsorbable oil, acts as anal lubricant
Sorbital	15–30 mL once or twice daily	Cramps, flatulence, belching, nausea	Osmotically active nonabsorbable sugars pull fluid into gut
Senna	187 mg daily	Nausea, cramping, may worsen constipation with chronic use	Stimulant laxative, increases motility of large bowel
Cascara sagrada	325 mg (or 5 mL) daily	Nausea, cramping, may worsen constipation with chronic use	Stimulant laxative, increases motility of large bowel

*For the treatment of chronic constipation.
Abbreviations: ACGCCTF, American College of Gastroenterology Chronic Constipation Task Force; PO, by mouth; TID, three times daily.

frequent disorder seen by gastroenterologists, and accounts for 12% of visits to primary care providers.[19] Many theories have been described, but there remains no pathologic basis for the disease.[20] The diagnosis is made with clinical criteria based on consensus conferences, that is, the Rome criteria. Three symptomatic forms exist forms: pain predominate, diarrhea predominate, and constipation predominate. Treatments for the constipation predominate form include dietary changes, osmotic laxatives, other laxatives, and 5-HT-receptor agonists. Tegaserod was previously recommended for treatment in women, but since has been pulled from the market due to concerns over risk of heart attack or stroke.

DIAGNOSTIC TESTING

In 2005, the American College of Gastroenterology Chronic Constipation Task Force published "An Evidenced-Based Approach to the Management of Chronic Constipation in North America."[23] In the document they comment that no studies examine the utility of laboratory testing for patients who complain of constipation (that is, complete blood count, serum calcium, electrolytes, renal function tests, thyroid function tests, cosyntropin test for adrenal insufficiency, and others). No such document exists for the evaluation of acute constipation. For simple constipation, plain film radiography has not been shown to be helpful, and may be misleading in both adults and children.[24,25] The presence of stool in the large bowel on plain radiography is an expected finding and does not confirm the diagnosis of benign constipation and exclude other more serious conditions. Indeed, all diagnostic testing performed in the ED for the evaluation of constipation should be aimed at the inclusion or exclusion of more serious conditions. Tests to consider include electrolytes, calcium level, renal function tests, complete blood count, and thyroid function tests. If suspecting obstruction, an upright chest and abdomen, and a supine abdomen radiograph may reveal dilated large or small bowel and/or air fluid levels; however, a CT scan of the abdomen and pelvis with oral and intravenous contrast may be needed to rule out more significant pathology or to confirm the presence of obstruction.

Alarm Symptoms

Certain symptoms found in association with constipation warrant a more extensive workup, according to the American College of Gastroenterology Chronic Constipation Task Force.[23] Those symptoms are

(1) hematochezia, anemia, or occult blood in the stool, (2) weight loss greater than 10 pounds, (3) family history of colon cancer, (4) family history of inflammatory bowel disease, and (5) abdominal mass palpable on exam. Those recommendations were made for chronic constipation; however, they provide a guide for patients who require more urgent follow-up when such testing is not required for evaluation and treatment in the ED. Patients with alarm symptoms can be expected to have a higher rate of colon cancer, and therefore require more urgent follow-up. For patients who are stable and discharge home is planned, the presence of alarm symptoms should prompt follow-up within 1 to 2 weeks so further testing can be initiated.

EMERGENCY DEPARTMENT CARE AND DISPOSITION

The most important management decision on behalf of patients presenting with a complaint of constipation is not what agent to use to relieve the symptoms, but the decision to further investigate with diagnostic testing as outlined above. The second task is manual disimpaction as needed. After this has been accomplished or the rectum has been found to be empty of hard stool, a logical treatment plan can be initiated.

TREATMENT OF FECAL IMPACTION

Patients with fecal impaction require manual removal.[5,10] Topical anesthetic lubricant, such as viscous lidocaine should be used to provide local anesthesia. Consideration should be given to sedation as well. The anus should be dilated using two fingers, and the stool broken up using a scissoring motion. As much stool as possible should be removed manually. These efforts can be followed by an enema; however, enemas are only helpful if the patient can retain it, making this treatment less useful in debilitated patients. Tap water or oil retention enemas should be used. Soapsuds enema can be a local irritant to the rectal mucosa, and therefore is discouraged by some authors,[5] despite the fact that it has been used in EDs for decades. An enema of water soluble contrast material (meglumine diatrizoate, or Gastrografin) may be of some benefit for diagnosis and as an osmotic cathartic, but generally requires movement to a radiology suite.[5] If stool is higher than what can be reached with enemas, polyethylene glycol balanced solution is recommended as the best studied agent in the setting of fecal impaction.[26,27] Administration typically requires an inpatient setting for patients with disability (the dose is listed in Table 8-4). Oral treatment, with or without the balanced electrolytes, is recommended in children for the treatment of fecal impaction.[28]

GENERAL TREATMENT MEASURES

The American College of Gastroenterology Chronic Constipation Task Force evaluated treatments for chronic constipation, which provides a guide for outpatient treatment of constipation after the ED visit. The upper portion of Table 8-4 is based on that report; recommended treatments are "grade B" or better.[23] Many other agents are used frequently, but have not been demonstrated to be effective in well designed clinical trials, or evidence is conflicting in trials. Increasing dietary fiber would seem to be a sensible recommendation to patients with simple constipation,[29] yet dietary fiber is not as effective as the first three agents listed in Table 8-4. It appears that all dietary fiber is equally effective in the treatment of mild constipation.[30] Introduction of fiber to a patient's diet typically results in bloating that resolves over 3 to 4 weeks, and when introduced slowly is better tolerated. Dietary fiber, as well as psyllium, undergoes bacterial degradation in the intestine, which contributes to bloating and flatus. Methycellulose and polycarbophil are semisynthetic fiber, that are relatively resistant to bacterial degradation (and less prone to bloating) but have not been shown to be as effective as psyllium.[23] For simple transient constipation, dietary fiber will help the patient without significant pathology, and continues to be recommended in the literature, even if limitations of its effectiveness are acknowledged.[4,31,32] Since the publication of the American College of Gastroenterology Chronic Constipation Task Force document, a double-blind, randomized, placebo-controlled trial assessing bisacodyl has been published.[33] Patients in the treatment group had twice the number of stools as the placebo group. Incidence of adverse events was similar between groups.

Polyethylene glycol without electrolytes (such as Miralax) is an effective treatment, lacks the advantage of the balanced electrolytes, but is an acceptable alternative for short periods in patients unlikely to have preexisting electrolyte abnormalities or comorbidities, for both children and adults.[34,35] Stool softeners such as docusate sodium have been shown to no more effective than placebo.[23] Mineral oil has been reported to be helpful by softening and lubricating stool, but is contraindicated in patients with swallowing disorders and may prevent the absorption of soluble vitamins. Glycerin suppositories may be effective in mild cases, but also may cause local irritation and cramping. Sodium phosphate enemas are used frequently, but can lead to significant local trauma, cramping, and hyperphosphatemia, especially in patients with renal insufficiency. Magnesium citrate, or milk of magnesia, is widely used; magnesium toxicity is a potential adverse effect along with cramping and flatulence. Stimulant laxatives such as senna or cascara sagrada are converted to their active form by colonic bacteria and stimulate motility of the large bowel. These drugs have been thought to cause cathartic bowel, but pathologic confirmation of these changes are lacking.[36] They cause a condition known as melanosis coli, which darkens the colonic mucosa, and resolves after discontinuation of the laxatives.[37] There is no known association of cancer with melanosis coli.[38]

SPECIFIC TREATMENTS FOR ASSOCIATED DISORDERS

Anal lesions may need local care. Hemorrhoids that are thrombosed will need excision and drainage. A meta-analysis has shown fiber to be an effective adjunct to the treatment of hemorrhoids, reducing bleeding and discomfort.[39] Anal fissures will benefit from stool softeners (as contrasted to chronic constipation, where they have little benefit). If discovered, electrolyte disorders will need treatment, as well as other metabolic or hormonal disorders (i.e., hypothyroidism).

Rectal abscesses will need drainage. Perianal abscesses typically can be drained in the ED, while for deeper perirectal, or ischiorectal abscesses, consultation with surgery is typically recommended. Metabolic disorders will need correction, but this process will require time, and possibly admission to the hospital as the clinical situation demands.

The majority of life-threatening disorders discussed will require surgical or gastroenterology consultation.

DISPOSITION

While no patient with simple constipation should be admitted to the hospital, no patient with unresolved or undiagnosed abdominal pain and distension should be discharged home. The need to admit a patient complaining of constipation depends almost entirely on the underlying cause and the certainty of the diagnosis. A patient with a fecal impaction who is successfully treated with disimpaction and subsequently has a large stool output with or without enema, may be considered for discharge provided the patient is sufficiently mobile and abdominal pain has resolved completely. However, the patient may still require close follow-up. In general, the greater the patient's disability, the more likely that the patient will require admission for treatment for fecal impaction or continued diagnostic testing. Functional, independent patients with simple constipation will be well served with a treatment plan and recommendations for follow-up, with the presence or absence of alarm symptoms to guide the urgency of follow-up. Patients over the age of 50, even those without alarm symptoms, should eventually have colonoscopy.[40]

PITFALLS

- Assuming the patient's chief complaint is the diagnosis rather than looking for a potential serious cause of constipation.

- Failing to recommend follow-up for all patients who present with constipation, as colon cancer is always a possible cause.

- Recommending a treatment with no efficacy (i.e., stool softeners) because of a belief that recommending a laxative will promote abuse.

REFERENCES

1. Higgins PD, Johanson JF. Epidemiology of Constipation in North America: A systematic review. *Am J Gastoenterol.* 2004;99:750.
2. Lembo A, Camilleri M. Chronic constipation. *N Engl J Med.* 2003;349:1360.
3. Campbell, AJ, Busby WJ, Horwath CC. Factors associated with constipation in a community based sample aged 70 years and older. *J Epidemiol Community Health.* 1993;47:23.
4. Towers AL, Burgio KL Locher IS, et al. Constipation in the elderly: influence of dietary, psychological, and physiological factors. *J Am Geriatr Soc.* 1994;42:701.
5. Pather CM, Ortiz-Camocho CP. Evaluation and treatment of constipation and fecal impaction in adults. *Mayo Clin Proc.* 1998;73:881.
6. Muller-Lissner SA, Kamm MA, Scarpignato C, Wald A. Myths and misconceptions about chronic constipation. *Am J Gastoenterol.* 2005;100:232.
7. Roberts MC, Millikan RC, Galanko JA, et al. Constipation, laxative use, and colon cancer in a North Carolina population. *Am J Gastoenterol.* 2003;98:857.
8. Aalten CM, Samson MM, Jansen PAF. Diagnostic errors; the need to have autopsies. *Netherlands J Med.* 2006; 64:186.
9. Voderholzer WA, Schatke W, Muhdorfer, et al. Clinical response to dietary fiber treatment of chronic constipation. *Am J Gastoenterol.* 1997;92:95.
10. Wrenn K: Fecal impaction. *N Engl J Med.* 1989;321:658.
11. Bobba RK, Arsura EL, Amire KA, et al. Rectosigmoid stricture probably from ischemia presenting as constipation in an elderly patient. *J Am Geriatr Soc.* 2005; 53:1634.
12. Mallo RD, Salem L, Lalani T, Flum DR. Computed tomography diagnosis of ischemia and complete obstruction in small bowel obstruction: A systematic review. *J Gastrointest Surg.* 2005;9:690.
13. Pepin C, Ladabaum U. The yield of lower endoscopy in patients with constipation: Survey of a university hospital, a public county hospital, and a Veterans Administration medical center. *Gastrointest Endosc.* 2002;56:325.
14. Waseem M, Hipp A. Megacolon: Constipation or volvulus? *Ped Emerg Care.* 2006;22:346.
15. Jalan K, Sircus W, Card WI, et al. An experience of ulcerative colitis. I. Toxic dilatation in 55 cases. *Gastroenterology.* 1969;57:68.
16. Gan SI, Beck PL. A new look at toxic megacolon; An update and review of incidence, etiology, pathogenesis, and management. *Am J Gastoenterol.* 2003;98:2363.
17. Imbriaco M, Balthazar EJ. Toxic megacolon: Role of CT in the evaluation and detection of complications. *Clin Imaging.* 2001;25:349.
18. Camilleri M, Choi MG. Irritable bowel syndrome. *Aliment Pharmacol Ther.* 1997;11:3.
19. Drossman DA, Whitehead WE, Camilleri M. Irritable bowel syndrome: a technical review of practice guideline development. *Gastroenterology.* 1997;112:2120.
20. Horwitz BJ, Fisher RS. The irritable bowel syndrome. *N Engl J Med.* 2001;344:1846.
21. Evans BW, Clark WK, Moore DJ, Whorwell PJ. Tegaserod for the treatment of irritable bowel syndrome. *Cochrane Database Syst Rev.* 2004;1:1.
22. Kamm MA, Muller-Lissner S, Talley NJ, et al. Tegaserod for the treatment of chronic constipation: A randomized, double blind, placebo-controlled multinational study. *Am J Gastoenterol.* 2005;100:362.
23. Brandt LJ, Prather CM, Quigley EMM, et al. Systematic review on the management of chronic constipation in North America. *Am J Gastoenterol.* 2005;100:S1.
24. Rao SSC Ozturk R, Laine L. Clinical utility of diagnostic tests for constipation in adults: A systematic review. *Am J Gastoenterol.* 2005;100:1605.
25. Reuchlin-Vroklage LM, Bierma-Zeinstra S, Benninga MA, Berger MY. Diagnostic value of abdominal radiography in constipated children: A systematic review. *Arch Pediatr Adolesc Med.* 2005;159:671.
26. Chen CC, Su MY, Tung SY, et al. Evaluation of polyethylene glycol plus electrolytes in the treatment of severe constipation and fecal impaction in adults. *Curr Med Res Opin.* 2005;21:1595.
27. Culbert P, Gillett H, Ferguson A. Highly effective new oral therapy for faecal impaction. *Brit J Gen Pract.* 1998; 48:1599.

28. Rasquin A, Di Lorenzo C, Forbes D, et al. Childhood functional gastrointestinal disorders: Child/adolescent. *Gastroenterology.* 2006;130:1527.

29. Badiali D, Corazziari E, Habib FI, et al. Effect of wheat bran in the treatment of chronic nonorganic constipation: a double blind controlled trial. *Dig Dis Sci.* 1995;40:349.

30. James SL, Muir JG, Curtis SL, Gibson PR. Dietary fibre: a roughage guide. *Intern Med J.* 2003;33:291.

31. Hsieh C. Treatment of constipation in older adults. *Am Fam Physician.* 2005;72:2277.

32. Tramonte SM, Brand MB, Mulrow CD, et al. The treatment of chronic constipation in adults: A systematic review. *J Gen Intern Med.* 1997;12:15.

33. Keinzle-Horn S, Vix JM, Schuijt C, et al. Efficiency and safety of bisacodyl in the acute treatment of constipation: a double-blind, randomized, placebo-controlled study. *Aliment Pharmacol Ther.* 2006;23:1479.

34. Youssef NN, Peters JM, Henderson W, et al. Dose response of PEG 3350 for the treatment of childhood fecal impaction. *J Pediatr.* 2002;141:410.

35. Cleveland MvB, Flavin DP, Ruben RA, et al. New polyethylene glycol laxative for treatment of constipation in adults: A randomized, double blind, placebo-controlled study. *Southern Med J.* 2001;94:478.

36. Tzavella K, Reipl RL, Klauser AG, et al. Decreased substance P levels in rectal biopsies from patients with slow transit constipation. *Eur J Gastroenterol Hepatol.* 1996;8:207.

37. Badiali D, Marcheggiano A, Pallone F, et al. Melanosis of the rectum in patients with chronic constipation. *Dis Colon Rectum.* 1985;28:241.

38. van Gorkom BA, de Vries EG, Karrenbeld A, et al. Anthranoid laxatives and their potential carcinogenic effects. *Aliment Pharmacol Ther.* 1999;13:443.

39. Alonso-Coello P, Mills E, Heels-Ansdell D, et al. Fiber for the treatment of hemorrhoids complications: A systematic review and meta-analysis. *Am J Gastroenterol.* 2006; 101:181.

40. Lieberman DA, Weiss DG. One-time screening for colorectal cancer with combined fecal occult-blood testing and examination of the distal colon. *N Engl J Med.* 2001;345:555.

9

Acute Appendicitis

Mitchell C. Sokolosky

HIGH YIELD FACTS

- The clinical presentation of acute appendicitis is highly variable.
- No single test is highly sensitive or specific for the diagnosis of acute appendicitis.
- History and physical exam remain cornerstones for diagnosis.
- Factors associated with a missed diagnosis of appendicitis on computed tomography (CT) include a misleading clinical history, paucity of intraabdominal fat, and presence of small bowel ileus.
- Adequate analgesia with narcotics is underutilized.

EPIDEMIOLOGY

Acute appendicitis is among the most frequent causes of surgical abdominal disease worldwide with an annual incidence of 1.1:1000 population, with a lifetime risk of 8.6% for males and 6.7% for females.[1] In the United States in 1997, there were an estimated 252,682 appendicitis-related hospitalizations.[2]

PATHOPHYSIOLOGY

The appendix is a blind-ended, tubular structure attached to the base of the cecum near the ileocecal valve. The usual appendiceal length is several centimeters long but may vary up to 30 cm. This variability in length displaces the appendix to various positions in the abdomen and pelvis, which may explain some atypical presentations. The appendix functions as an immunologic organ that actively secretes immunoglobulin (IG), particularly IgA. However, its function is not essential, and appendectomy is not associated with any predisposition of immune compromise. Obstruction of the lumen is the dominant cause of acute appendicitis with fecaliths being the usual cause of obstruction in older patients.

Lymphoid follicular hyperplasia is usually the cause in children, and parasites can also cause obstruction in endemic areas in all age groups. Other causes of obstruction include tumors, foreign bodies, and calculi. Obstruction of the lumen leads to increased intraluminal pressures because of ongoing mucosal secretions. The patient, at this point, usually develops a dull, poorly localized pain due to stimulation of the visceral afferent pathways. Ischemia eventually develops leading to invasion of bacteria and inflammatory cells. As the appendix becomes more inflamed and swollen, the patient will start to develop localized abdominal pain as the appendix irritates adjacent structures. Progression of swelling and ischemia may result in necrosis and perforation. Time to perforation is highly variable.

CLINICAL FEATURES

The clinical presentation of acute appendicitis is highly variable. Pain is commonly the first symptom of appendicitis. The classic presentation of initial generalized abdominal pain that localizes to the right lower quadrant is not universal but, if present, is highly suggestive of acute appendicitis. Patients may complain of anorexia, nausea, vomiting (frequently after the onset of pain), and fever but often these symptoms are absent. Physical exam is often unrevealing early on but patients usually develop localized abdominal tenderness as the disease progresses. Classic teaching emphasized tenderness at McBurney point (an area 2 cm from the anterosuperior iliac spine) as being the rule; however, a recent study reveals that the positions of the lower pole of the cecum and base of the appendix may be lower and more medial than previously described.[3] Therefore, it is not uncommon for pain to be localized elsewhere in the abdomen other than the McBurney point. Other signs of peritoneal inflammation include the presence of guarding, rebound tenderness (often a late finding), Rovsing sign (palpation of left lower quadrant causes pain in right lower quadrant indicative of right-sided local peritoneal irritation), psoas sign (extension of hip causes increased pain when psoas muscle is stretched associated with a retrocecal appendix) (Figure 9-1), and obturator sign (pain with hip flexion and internal rotation) (Figure 9-2). Routine rectal exam does not appear to increase diagnostic sensitivity but may aid in ruling in or out other conditions; however repeated exams, especially on children are discouraged.[4,5] Pain on rectal examination has no discriminatory or predictive power for diagnosing acute appendicitis.[6]

Psoas Sign

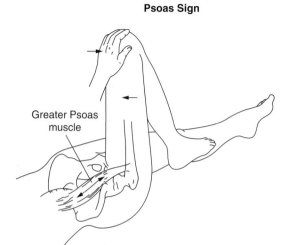

Greater Psoas muscle

Fig. 9-1. A Psoas sign. Used with permission from Wagner et al.[7]

Certain clinical examination findings do identify the patient at increased likelihood for appendicitis (Table 9-1) and includes: right lower quadrant pain (positive likelihood ratio, [LR+] = 8.0), rigidity (LR+ = 4.0), and migration of initial periumbilical pain to the right lower quadrant (LR+ = 3.1).[7] The absence of certain clinical examination findings decrease the likelihood of

Obturator Sign

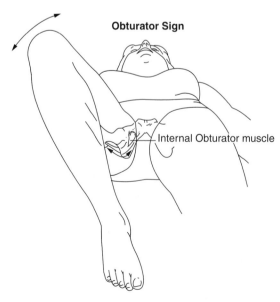

Internal Obturator muscle

Fig. 9-2. Obturator sign.

acute appendicitis and includes: absence of right lower quadrant pain (negative likelihood ratio, [LR–] = 0.2), the presence of similar previous pain (LR– = 0.3), and the absence of the classic migration of pain (LR– = 0.5). The presence of vomiting before pain was highly efficient in ruling out appendicitis. The absence of anorexia, nausea, or vomiting has little impact on the likelihood of appendicitis.

Clinical diagnostic scoring systems have been developed for the diagnosis of appendicitis (Table 9-2) but have not been shown prospectively to improve diagnostic accuracy in the emergency department (ED).[8]

DIAGNOSIS AND DIFFERENTIAL

The diagnosis of acute appendicitis is primarily a clinical diagnosis based on history and physical exam findings. Surgery consultation is all that is required in the patient who presents with the classic symptoms and exam. However, because of frequent atypical presentations, ancillary testing, particularly CT, have become an integral part of the evaluation.

No single ancillary test is highly sensitive or specific for acute appendicitis. Elevated total white blood cell (WBC) count >10,000 cells/mm, while statistically associated with the presence of appendicitis, has very poor sensitivity (76%, 95% confidence interval [CI] = 65% to 84%) and specificity (52%, 95% CI = 45% to 60%) and has almost no clinical utility when used alone.[9] The proportion of gangrenous and perforated appendixes in patients with a normal WBC count is the same as in patients with an elevated WBC count.[10] A temperature >99.0°F has a sensitivity of 47% (95% CI = 36% to 57%) and a specificity of 64% (95% CI = 57% to 71%)[9]. Therefore, clinicians should not rely on the presence or absence of either an elevated total WBC count or temperature to diagnose or exclude the presence of appendicitis. C-reactive protein (CRP) is a nonspecific inflammatory marker that may be used in the evaluation of patients with suspected appendicitis. C-reactive protein has a reported sensitivity of 62% to 76% and specificity of 56% to 84% for diagnosing acute appendicitis.[11,12] A urinalysis is frequently obtained to rule out a urinary tract infection. However, microscopic hematuria and pyuria can be found in up to one third of patients with acute appendicitis due to close proximity of the inflamed appendix to the bladder and ureter.[13] According to a recent metaanalysis,[6] appendicitis was likely when two or more inflammatory variables (WBC count, granulocyte count, proportion of polymorphonuclear blood cells, and CRPin) were increased

Table 9-1. History and Examination Operating Characteristics for Appendicitis

Characteristic	Sensitivity	Specificity	LR+ (95% CI)	LR– (95% CI)
Right Lower quadrant pain	0.81	0.53	7.31–8.46†	0.28†
Rigidity	0.27	0.83	3.76 (2.96–4.78)	0.82 (0.79–0.85)
Migration	0.64	0.82	3.18 (2.41–4.21)	0.50 (0.42–0.59)
Pain before vomiting‡	1.00	0.64	2.76 (1.94–3.94)	NA
Psoas sign	0.16	0.95	2.38 (1.21–4.67)	0.90 (0.83–0.98)
Fever	0.67	0.79	1.94 (1.63–2.32)	0.58 (0.51–0.67)
Rebound tenderness test	0.63	0.69	1.10–6.30†	0–0.86†
Guarding	0.74	0.57	1.65–1.78†	0–0.54†
No similar pain previously	0.81	0.41	1.50 (1.36–1.66)	0.323 (0.246–0.424)
Rectal tenderness	0.41	0.77	0.83–5.34†	0.36–1.15†
Anorexia	0.68	0.36	1.27 (1.16–1.38)	0.64 (0.54–0.750
Nausea	0.58	0.37	0.69–1.2†	0.70-0.84†
Vomiting	0.51	0.45	0.92 (0.82–1.04)	1.12 (0.95–1.33)

All studies used to create two by two tables and then tested for homogeneity of the odds ratio using the Breslow-Day statistic. If studies were not rejected as heterogeneous by this statistic, P=0.05, confidence intervals (CI) were manually reviewed to exclude type II errors. Studies satisfying both criteria were combined and likelihood ratios (LRs) were calculated using the Mantel-Haenszel method. Only one study evaluated pain before vomiting. LR+ indicates the positive likelihood ratio with its 95% CI, and LR–, the negative likelihood ratio with its 95% CI.

† In heterogeneous studies, the LRs are reported as ranges.

‡ Only one study on this metaanalysis.

(LR+ = >10) and unlikely when all were normal (LR– = <0.10). An elevated WBC and granulocyte count, and CRP are relatively strong predictors of perforated appendicitis (LR+ = 7.20). Whereas, perforated appendicitis is unlikely with a low WBC and granulocyte count, and a CRP concentration of less than 10 g/L (LR– = 0.11 – 0.20).

Table 9-2. MANTRELS Clinical Scoring System

Characteristic	Score
M = migration of pain to RLQ	1
A = anorexia	1
N = nausea and vomiting	1
T = tenderness in RLQ	2
R = rebound tenderness	1
E = elevated temperature	1
L = leukocytosis	2
S = shift of WBC to left	1
Total	10

Score of 5-6 is compatible with the diagnosis of acute appendicitis, score of 7-8 indicates a probable appendicitis, and a score of 9-10 indicates a very probable appendicitis.

In summary, although all clinical and laboratory variables are weak discriminators individually, their predictive values increase when combined.

Plain film radiography is rarely useful in the diagnosis of acute appendicitis and may not be necessary for all patients. Positive findings may include the presence of an appendicolith, focal ileus, loss of the psoas shadow, deformity of cecal outline, or a soft tissue density representing a phlegmon.

Ultrasound has been used successfully in the diagnosis of acute appendicitis, especially in children, with sensitivity 76% to 86% and a specificity of 89% to 98%.[14-16] Ultrasound findings of acute appendicitis include diameter of 6 mm or larger, intraluminal fluid, lack of compressibility, and periappendical inflammatory changes (Figures 9-3 and 9-4). Ultrasound may also be preferred over CT for use in the pregnant patient to avoid radiation exposure. Ultrasound is very user dependent and may be difficult in persons of large body habitus and those with overlying bowel gas.

Figures 9-3 and 9-4, ultrasound findings of acute appendicitis. (Compliments of Manoj Pariyadath, MD)

Computed tomography has been shown to be helpful in the diagnosis of appendicitis, especially in atypical presentations. Computed tomography can also provide an alternative diagnosis in some cases and has been

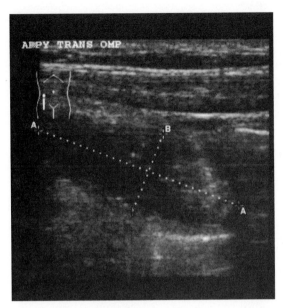

Fig. 9-3. Ultrasound image, long axis view of noncompressible, fluid filled, distended appendix.

shown to decrease the negative appendectomy rate in women.[17,18] A recent systematic review reported the aggregated diagnostic performance characteristics of all modes of CT scanning were excellent with a range of

sensitivity (83%–97%), specificity (93%–98%), positive predictive value (86%–98%), negative predictive value (94%–99%), and accuracy (92%–97%).[6] Computed tomography findings suggestive of the diagnosis include increased appendiceal size (6 mm or more), thickened wall (>2 mm), target structure (concentric thickening of inflamed appendix, Figure 9-5), absence of intraluminal gas, presence of an appendicolith, and periappendiceal and cecal inflammatory changes (stranding in fat) (Figure 9-6). Abscesses and phlegmons can also be identified. Controversy exists over which type of contrast should be used. The downside to oral and rectal contrast is that it can obscure appendicoliths and oral contrast requires time for digestion.[19] Intravenous (IV) contrast, on the other hand, can improve the diagnostic accuracy by enhancing the presence of periappendiceal or pericecal inflammation.[20,21] Thin CT sections (2.5–5.0 mm) allow for better delineation of anatomy and separate bowel loops. However, CT can miss acute appendicitis that is later confirmed by pathology. Factors associated with a missed diagnosis of appendicitis on CT include a misleading clinical history, paucity of intraabdominal fat (common in children), incomplete contrast opacification of the cecum and distal small bowel (if used), presence of small bowel ileus, and lack of the typical CT signs of appendicitis.[22] Other CT pitfalls include failure to recognize an unusual location of an inflamed appendix, or images may appear normal if only a small portion of the distal appendix is involved (tip appendicitis).[23] The presence of intraluminal air or contrast is usually a reassuring sign. However, intraluminal air can be seen in

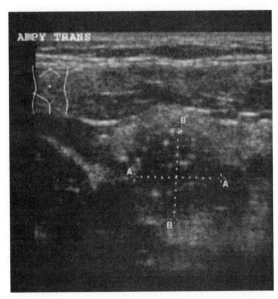

Fig. 9-4. Ultrasound image, short axis view of noncompressible, fluid filled, distended appendix.

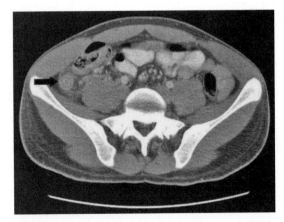

Fig. 9-5. Computed tomography findings of acute appendicitis illustrating a concentrically inflamed appendix referred to as the "target sign," see arrow.

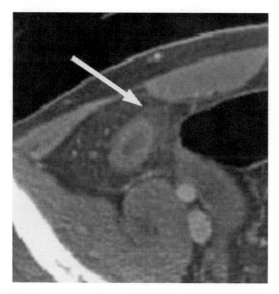

Fig. 9-6. Computed tomography of abdomen illustrating a thick appendiceal wall and periappendiceal interstitial inflammation (arrow) consistent with acute appendicitis.

cases of appendicial perforation. Appendicitis is encountered in about 30% of patients with equivocal findings on CT.[24] The diagnosis should be considered in most of these patients if they are appropriately symptomatic. In the absence of a distinctly visualized appendix and secondary inflammatory changes, the incidence of appendicitis is low.[25] In summary, beyond IV contrast and thin sections, there are pros and cons to all approaches and familiarization with your hospital's protocol is recommended.

Magnetic resonance imaging (MRI) has shown some promise in the evaluation of pregnant patients with possible appendicitis.[26] More scientific data are needed before a firm recommendation on the use of MRI for diagnosing acute appendicitis is made.

Nuclear medicine imaging utilizing a radiolabeled monoclonal antibody directed against polymorphonuclear neutrophils has been used previously to localize infection but a recent metaanalysis provided no clear role for its use.[27]

The differential diagnosis for anyone with undifferentiated abdominal pain should include the possibility of acute appendicitis because of the variability in its clinical presentations. Although very rare, this includes even those patients who have had a prior appendectomy because of the possibility of "stump

appendicitis" which can occur after either laparoscopic or open appendectomy. Twenty-nine cases of stump appendicitis have been reported in the world literature, and it is felt to be an underreported entity.[28] Differential diagnosis of acute appendicitis includes ureterolithiasis, diverticulitis (cecal or Meckel), regional enteritis, mesenteric adenitis, inflammatory bowel disease, incarcerated hernia, psoas abscess, symptomatic aortic aneurysm, abdominal wall hematoma, and bowel obstruction. In females, one must also consider ectopic pregnancy, ovarian torsion or cyst rupture, pelvic inflammatory disease, and endometriosis. A common misdiagnosis is gastroenteritis.[29] Physicians should be wary of this diagnosis in any patient complaining of significant pain or abdominal tenderness and who lacks the typical diagnostic criteria (diarrhea and the typical prodrome).

The diagnosis of acute appendicitis in the very young (preschool age) and elderly (>50–60 years) is very difficult and associated with significant morbidity and mortality including a high perforation rate.[30–34] Clinical presentations are often very atypical in these age groups and a high index of suspicion is warranted. Factors associated with a misdiagnosis in children include: vomiting before pain onset, constipation, diarrhea, dysuria, signs and symptoms of upper respiratory infection, absence of right lower quadrant tenderness, and pain duration of more than two days.[35] The absence of intraperitoneal fat in some children may also make the diagnosis by CT more technically difficult.[36] Interestingly, the liberal use of CT scans in diagnosing appendicitis in children has not resulted in a decreased negative appendectomy rate.[37]

The pregnant patient also provides a diagnostic challenge. The clinical presentation varies and often the diagnosis is delayed. The clinical features vary with the stage of pregnancy. The location of pain and tenderness will vary as the location of the appendix migrates upward due to the enlarging uterus. Right-sided abdominal pain is the principal basis for diagnosis, while an elevated WBC count and low level fever, as in the nonpregnant state, are unreliable for diagnosis.[38]

EMERGENCY DEPARTMENT CARE AND DISPOSITION

Airway, breathing, and circulation should be assessed initially on all ED patients. Those patients suspected of having acute appendicitis should be placed on the proper monitors and have an IV started. Patients should be kept NPO (nothing by mouth) except for radiographic contrast if used. The patient's pain should be treated with adequate doses of narcotic analgesia. The practice of withholding narcotic analgesia is archaic and lacks support in the literature. Many studies have concluded that adequate narcotic analgesia does not adversely affect the clinical exam, diagnostic accuracy, or outcome of acute appendicitis.[39–41] However, physicians should be prudent not to oversedate the patient so they may follow their clinical exam. Antiemetics (e.g., promethazine, etc.) should be used with caution since they may potentate the sedative effects of narcotics if given concurrently. Broad spectrum, gram negative, and anaerobic antibiotics (e.g., Cefoxitin, etc.) should be initiated once the decision is made to go to the operating room or if the patient appears septic from a perforation.

Acute appendicitis is a surgical problem. Surgery consultation should be obtained as early as possible in any patient suspected of having acute appendicitis. Appendectomy can be performed by either an open incision or by laparoscopy. The surgical technique used depends upon physician preference, certainty of diagnosis, history of prior surgery, patient's age, gender, and body habitus. Some patients with equivocal findings may require admission to the hospital for further observation. For those patients in whom the diagnosis is unlikely but still possible, they may be discharged home with mandatory follow-up in 12 hours, provided they have a benign clinical exam. Patients should be instructed to return to the ED if they worsen. All patients discharged home should receive clear verbal and written instructions that early appendicitis is a possibility and the importance of the follow-up exam.

PITFALLS

- Failure to consider the diagnosis of acute appendicitis in any patient with undifferentiated abdominal pain.

- Excluding appendicitis based on the absence of fever or leukocytosis.

- Misdiagnosing acute appendicitis as gastroenteritis even when patients lack the typical diagnostic criteria.

- Computed tomography scans are not 100% sensitive for appendicitis and can miss cases later confirmed by pathology.

- Failure to provide appropriate verbal and written instructions to the patient discharged home with possible early appendicitis or abdominal pain of unknown etiology.

REFERENCES

1. Addiss D, Shaffer N, Fowler BS, et al. The epidemiology of appendicitis and appendectomy in the United States. *Am J Epidemiol* 1990;132:910.
2. Davies GM, Dasbach EJ, Teutsch S. The burden of appendicitis-related hospitalizations in the United States in 1997. *Surg Infect.* 2004;5:160.
3. Karim OM, Boothroyd AE, Wyllie JH. McBurney's point . . . fact or fiction? *Ann R Coll Engl.* 1991;73:65.
4. Manimaran N, Galland RB. Significance of routine digital rectal examination in adults presenting with abdominal pain. *Ann R Coll Surg Engl.* 2004;86:292.
5. Dunning PG, Goldman MD. The incidence and value of rectal examination in children with suspected appendicitis. *Ann R Coll Surg Engl.* 1991;73:399.
6. Andersson RE. Meta-analysis of the clinical and laboratory diagnosis of appendicitis. *Br J Surg.* 2004;91:28.
7. Wagner JM, Mckinney PW, Carpenter JL. Does this patient have appendicitis? The rational clinical exam. *JAMA.* 1996;276:1589.
8. Alvarado A. A practical score for the early diagnosis of acute appendicitis. *Ann Emerg Med.* 1986;15:557.
9. Cardell T, Glasser J, Guss DA. Clinical value of the total white blood cell count and temperature in the elevation of patients with suspected appendicitis. *Acad Emerg Med.* 2004;11:1021.
10. Coleman C, Thompson JE Jr. Bennion RS, et al. White blood cell count is a poor predictor of severity of disease in the diagnosis of appendicitis. *Am Surg.* 1998;64:983.
11. Khan MN, Davie E, Irshad K. The role of white cell count and C-reactive protein in the diagnosis of acute appendicitis. *J Ayub Med Coll Abbottabad.* 2004;16:17.
12. Pruekprasert P, Maipang T, Geater A, et al. Accuracy in diagnosis of acute appendicitis by comparing serum C-reactive protein measurements, Alvarado score and clinical impressions of surgeons. *J Med Assoc Thai.* 2004; 87:296.
13. Bell RH, Rikkers LF, Mulholland MW. Digestive Tract Surgery: A Text and Atlas, 1st ed. Lippincott-Raven Publishers, Philadelphia. 1996:1316.
14. Balthazar EJ, Birnbaum BA, Yee J, et al. Acute Appendicitis: CT and US correlation in 100 patients. *Radiology.* 1994;190:31.
15. Schwerk WB, Wichtrup B, Rothmund M. Ultrasonography in the diagnosis of acute appendicitis: a prospective study. *Gastroenterology.* 1989;97:630.
16. Soda K, Nemoto K, Yoshizawa S. Detection of pinpoint tenderness on the appendix under ultrasonography is useful to confirm acute appendicitis. *Arch Surg.* 2001;136:1136.
17. Antevil J, Rivera L, Langenberg B, Brown CV. The influence of age and gender on the utility of computed tomography to diagnose acute appendicitis. *Am Surg.* 2004;70:850.
18. Bendeck SE, Nino-Murcia M, Berry GJ, et al. Imaging for suspected appendicitis: Negative appendectomy and perforation rates. *Radiology.* 2002;225:131.

19. Anderson BA, Salem L, Flum DR. A systematic review of whether oral contrast is necessary for the computed tomography diagnosis of appendicitis in adults. *Am J Surg.* 2005;190:474.

20. Jacobs JE, Birnbaum BA, Macari M, et al. Acute appendicitis: Comparison of helical CT diagnosis-focused technique with oral contrast material versus nonfocused technique with oral and intravenous contrast material. *Radiology.* 2001;220:683.

21. Balthazar, Megibow AJ, Hulnick D, et al. CT of appendicitis. *AJR Am J Roentgenol.* 1986;147:705.

22. Levine CD, Aizenstein O, Lehavi O, et al. Why we miss the diagnosis of appendicitis on abdominal CT: evaluation of imaging features of appendicitis incorrectly diagnosed on CT. *AJR Am J Roentgenol.* 2005;184:855.

23. Levine CD, Aizenstein O, Wachsberg RH. Pitfalls in the CT diagnosis of appendicitis. *Br J Radiol.* 2004;77:792.

24. Daly DP, Cohan RH, Francis IR, et al. Incidence of acute appendicitis in patients with equivocal CT findings. *AJR Am J Roentgenol.* 2005;184:1813.

25. Nikolaidis P, Hwang CM, Miller FH, et al. The nonvisualized appendix: incidence of acute appendicitis when secondary inflammatory changes are absent. *AJR Am J Roentgenol.* 2004;183:889.

26. Oto A, Ernst RD, Shah R, et al. Right lower quadrant pain and suspected appendicitis in pregnant women: evaluation with MR imaging—initial experience. *Radiology.* 2004;234:445.

27. Annovazzi A, Bagni B, Burroni L, et al. Nuclear medicine imaging of inflammatory/infective disorders of the abdomen. *Nucl Med Commun.* 2005;26:657.

28. Watkins BP, Kothari SN, Landercasper J. Stump appendicitis: case report and review. *Surg Laparosc Endosc Percutan Tech.* 2004;14:167.

29. Rusnak RA, Borer JM, Fastow JS. Misdiagnosis of acute appendicitis: common features discovered in cases after litigation. *Am J Emerg Med.* 1994;12:397.

30. Sakellaris G, Tilemis S, Charissis G. Acute appendicitis in preschool-age children. *Eur J Pediatr.* 2005;164:80.

31. Gurleyik G, Gurleyik E. Age-related clinical features in older patients with acute appendicitis. *Eur J Emerg Med.* 2003;10:200.

32. Lunca S, Bouras G, Romedea NS. Acute appendicitis in the elderly patient: diagnostic problems, prognostic factors and outcomes. *Rom J Gastroenterol.* 2004;13:299.

33. Burns RP, Cochran JL, Russell WL, et al. Appendicitis in mature adults. *Ann Surg.* 1985;201:695.

34. Daehlin L. Acute appendicitis during the first three years of life. *Acta Chir Scand.* 1982;148:291.

35. Rothrock SG, Skeoch G, Rush JJ, et al. Clinical features of misdiagnoses appendicitis in children. *Ann Emerg Med.* 1991;20:45.

36. Grayson DE, Wettlaufer JR, Dalrmple NC, et al. Appendiceal CT in pediatric patients: relationship of visualization to amount of peritoneal fat. *AJR Am J Roentgenol.* 2001;176:497.

37. Martin AE, Vollman D, Adler B, Caniano DA. CT scans may not reduce the negative appendectomy rate in children. *J Pediatr Surg.* 2004;39:886.

38. Duqoum W. Appendicitis in pregnancy. *East Mediterr Health J.* 2001;7:642.

39. Wolfe JM, Smithline HA, Phipen S, et al. Does morphine change the physical examination in patients with acute appendicitis? *Am J Emerg Med.* 2004;22:280.

40. Aydelotte JD, Collen JF, Martin RR. Analgesic administration prior to surgical evaluation for acute appendicitis. *Curr Surg.* 2004;61:373.

41. Kokki H, Lintula H, Vanamo K, et al. Oxycodone vs placebo in children with undifferentiated abdominal pain: A randomized, double-blind clinical trial of the effect of analgesia on diagnostic accuracy. *Arch Pediatr Adolesc* Med. 2005; 159:320.

10

Peptic Ulcer Disease

Catherine A. Marco
Randall W. King

HIGH YIELD FACTS

- Peptic ulcer disease is more common among patients with *Helicobacter pylori* infection, patients who use of nonsteroidal anti-inflammatory drugs (NSAIDs), aspirin, steroids, alcohol, coffee, tea, and patients with family history, advanced age, smoking, obesity, trauma, or surgery.

- *Helicobacter pylori* infection should be considered in all patients with suspected peptic ulcer disease.

- Medical management of peptic ulcer disease may include proton pump inhibitors, H2 receptor antagonists, and antacids.

- *Helicobacter pylori* infection should be treated with triple therapy, including a proton pump inhibitor and two antibiotics, such as clarithromycin, amoxicillin, and/or metronidazole.

EPIDEMIOLOGY

Gastrointestinal (GI) complaints comprise approximately 13% of emergency department (ED) visits, with abdominal pain comprising 6.5% of ED visits.[1] Peptic ulcer disease is the most common etiology of upper GI hemorrhage. Upper gastrointestinal (UGI) hemorrhage is a common disease state, with an incidence of approximately 50 to 150 per 100,000 adults per year. Mortality has been estimated between 10 and 40% of patients with UGI hemorrhage and significantly lower for stable patients.[2] Risk factors for peptic ulcer disease include *H. pylori* infection, use of nonsteroidal anti-inflammatory drugs (NSAIDs), aspirin, steroids, alcohol, coffee, tea, family history, advanced age, smoking, obesity, trauma, or surgery.[3–5] Nonulcer dyspepsia is more common than peptic ulcer disease, especially in patients under 40 years of age.

PATHOPHYSIOLOGY

Peptic ulcer disease is the pathologic formation of an ulcer in the lining of the stomach or duodenum. The ulcer results from the action of the gastric juice (hydrochloric acid, proteases) on the mucous membrane when the membrane is rendered susceptible or when there is excessive production of gastric acid effectively overwhelming the epithelium's resistance to the damaging effects of gastric acid.

The normal digestive process involves the secretion of hydrochloric acid by parietal cells combined with protease (primarily pepsinogen) secretion by the chief cells. These acids and proteases combine to form a digestive gastric juice with a pH as low as 0.8. The primary structure supporting acid secretion is the "proton pump" (H^+/K^+ ATPase) located in the parietal cells. The epithelial lining of the stomach and duodenum is protected from this corrosive juice by mucous formation and bicarbonate ion secretion from the mucous cells.

The most common cause of peptic ulcer disease is bacterial infection of the GI tract by *H. pylori*.[6,7] *H. pylori* is thought to be responsible for or associated with the majority of duodenal and gastric ulcers. The bacteria are motile coccoid or spiral-shaped organisms that reside between the mucous layer and the superficial layer of the gastric epithelium. *H. pylori* produce enzymes including urease, which facilitate the metabolism of urea. The exact mechanism of the *H. pylori* associated ulcer formation is still unclear but is thought to be related to inflammation and injury due to production of urease and other toxins resulting in a breakdown of the protective mucosal layer, thereby allowing corrosive gastric juice access to the epithelial lining. Regardless of mechanism, eradication of *H. pylori* in patients with peptic ulcer disease effectively reduces the rate of ulcer recurrence from a range of 60 to 80% down to a range of to 10 to 15%.[8,9]

The second most common cause of gastric ulcers, and possibly duodenal ulcers, is chronic use of acetylsalicylic acid (ASA) or other (NSAIDS). Nonsteroidal anti-inflammatory drugs act to inhibit prostaglandin synthesis leading to decreases in mucous secretion and bicarbonate production and also cause a decrease in mucosal blood flow to the gastric epithelium and direct topical injury.

The third leading cause of ulcer disease is Zollinger-Ellison syndrome (gastrinoma) which, due to hyperelevated gastrin secretion, essentially floods the stomach and duodenum with an overproduction of hydrochloric acid effectively overwhelming the mucous protective barrier.

Other contributing factors include cigarette smoking, emotional stress, and shock states leading to decreased mesenteric blood flow.[10]

CLINICAL FEATURES

Patients with peptic ulcer disease may present with a variety of symptoms, including abdominal pain, chest discomfort, heartburn, dysphagia, belching, abdominal distension, and early satiety. Patients with a gastric ulcer may experience pain with eating, while patients with a duodenal ulcer may experience postprandial pain. Many patients (up to 40 to 50%) with peptic ulcer disease are completely asymptomatic.

DIAGNOSIS AND DIFFERENTIAL

The diagnosis of new-onset peptic ulcer disease can be difficult in the emergency medicine setting. The disease is usually suspected based on the patient's clinical presentation of dyspepsia without other demonstrated or obvious cause for the presenting symptoms. Although not tested in the ED setting, certain symptom clusters make peptic ulcer disease less likely. In patients younger than 40 years of age presenting with dyspepsia, if food or milk aggravates pain, the patient has no night pain, no vomiting, and no weight loss, the patient is likely to have nonulcer dyspepsia with specificity of 94%.[11] Testing can be performed to rule out complications of peptic ulcer disease or to determine the presence of "alarm symptoms," and to narrow the differential list. These studies include electrocardiogram (ECG) and cardiac enzymes for possible acute coronary syndrome, complete blood count (CBC) to investigate anemia from chronic blood loss, amylase and/or lipase for possible pancreatitis, and liver function tests for hepatitis.

Noninvasive laboratory testing includes serology for *H. pylori* antibodies, stool evaluation for *H. pylori* antibodies, and breath testing for urease activity using special carbon isotopes. Positive tests predict the need for "triple therapy" (see below).

Serologic tests for *H. pylori* detect the presence or absence of IgG antibodies to *H. pylori*. The test is positive 21 days after infection and remains positive after treatment. It cannot differentiate between active disease and past disease, which limits its usefulness. Sensitivity is 85.0% and specificity is 79.0 %. Turnaround time for the test is usually hours to one day. Cost is approximately $95.00. Due to its poor performance compared to breath tests and stool antigen in populations with low and intermediate prevalence, some authors believe serology should no longer be done in the United States. [12,13]

Urea breath test indicates the presence of active disease by demonstrating the presence of urease. The patient ingests labeled carbon isotope (either radioactive 14 or nonradioactive 13) which is hydrolyzed by the bacteria urease and then detected in the breath. Sensitivity is 94.7% and specificity is 95.7%. The test takes several hours to complete. The cost is approximately $104.00.

Stool antigen testing is an ELISA (enzyme immunoassay) test, which identifies a polyclonal anti-*H. pylori* antibody. It is positive for active disease. The test takes approximately 10 minutes and has a sensitivity of 93.1% and specificity of 92.8%. The test requires a stool sample and takes minutes to complete. The cost is approximately $50.00 to $126.00.

Plain radiography abdominal series with chest radiography can potentially indicate peptic ulcer disease complications, such as presence of free air indicating ulcer, evidence of obstruction, or it may demonstrate the presence of other disease, such as lower lobe pneumonia. However, only patients with more severe symptoms will require x-rays.

Ultrasonography can be used to demonstrate presence of gallbladder disease, pancreatic disease, aortic aneurysm, or pericardial effusion. Direct confirmation and diagnosis of peptic ulcer can occur through either barium UGI radiography or through endoscopy. Neither of these are routinely done in the ED setting unless complications of ulcer such as significant hemorrhage or other "alarm symptoms" are present.

Upper gastrointestinal diagnosis is accomplished by demonstrating barium within an ulcer with typical radiographic characteristics. Sensitivity of UGI for peptic ulcer disease is variable. Simple, single-contrast UGI studies may miss up to 50% of duodenal ulcers. Special techniques such as double contrast and compression can improve the sensitivity to 80 to 90% while also increasing the ability to differentiate benign from malignant ulcers.[14]

Endoscopy is sensitive and specific for the direct diagnosis of peptic ulcer disease. The procedure involves direct visualization, inspection, multiple biopsies, and testing for the presence of urease followed by possible direct culture for *H. pylori*. Sensitivity is approximately 95%.[15,16]

The differential list is long and includes gastroesophageal reflux disease (GERD), gastritis, hiatal hernia, gallbladder disease, partial bowel obstruction, pancreatitis, gastroenteritis, hepatitis, pneumonia, acute coronary syndrome, pericarditis, aortic dissection, aortic aneurysm, and renal colic.

Table 10-1. Medical Therapy of Peptic Ulcer Disease

Agent (Trade Names)	Dose Range	Mechanism of Action
Omeprazole (Prilosec)	20–40 mg daily	PPI
Lanzoprazole (Prevacid)	15–30 mg daily	PPI
Pantoprazole (Protonix)	40 mg daily	PPI
Esomeprazole (Nexium)	40 mg daily	PPI
Rabeprazole (Aciphex)	20 mg daily	PPI
Ranitidine (Zantac)	300 mg daily	H2-receptor antagonist
Famotidine (Pepcid)	20–40 mg daily	H2-receptor antagonist
Nizatidine (Axid)	300 mg nightly	H2-receptor antagonist
Cimetidine (Tagamet)	300 mg nightly	H2-receptor antagonist
Bismuth subsalicylate (Pepto-Bismol)	2 tabs bid	Part of quadruple therapy regiment
Octreotide (Sandostatin)	50–100 mcg bolus IV, then 25–50 mcg/h	Hemostatic agent
Vasopressin (Pitressin)	0.2–0.4 units/min IV initial dose	Vasoconstrictor
Clarithromycin (Biaxin)	500 mg bid	Antibiotics
Metronidazole (Flagyl)	Part of Helidac	Antibiotic
Amoxicillin (Amoxil)	1000 mg bid	Antibiotic
Sucralfate (Carafate)	1 gm qid	Ulcer coating complex
Misoprostol (Cytotec)	200 mg.qid	Prostaglandin analog
Antacids (Mylanta, Maalox, etc)	After meals and nightly	Antacids

Abbreviations: PPI, proton pump inhibitors; bid, two times per day; qid, four times per day.

EMERGENCY DEPARTMENT CARE AND DISPOSITION

Initial management of the patient with peptic ulcer disease consists of stabilization, including airway intervention, intravenous access, fluid resuscitation, and administration of packed red blood cells, if indicated.

Following stabilization, a determination of severity of illness is indicated. For patients with unstable vital signs or active UGI hemorrhage, urgent endoscopy may be indicated. A variety of endoscopic interventions may be utilized to limit hemorrhage and inflammation, including injection of epinephrine, sclerosants, alcohol, thrombin, or fibrin glue; thermal interventions, including heater probe, electrocoagulation, Nd-Yag (neodymium-doped yttrium aluminum garnet) laser, or argon plasma coagulation (APC); and mechanical interventions, including hemoclips, banding, staples, and sutures.[17] On rare occasions, surgical intervention may be necessary.

For stable patients, medical management may include acid-reducing agents, octreotide, and antibiotics effective against *H. pylori*. Agents that reduce the pH of gastric contents include proton pump inhibitors and H2-receptor antagonists.[18–20] Proton pump inhibitors include omeprazole, lanzoprazole, pantoprazole, esomeprazole, and rabeprazole. Mechanisms of action and efficacy are similar among this class of drugs[21] (Table 10-1).

Treatment for the eradication of *H. pylori* infection typically includes either triple or quadruple therapy. Triple therapy includes a proton pump inhibitor (*H. pylori* eradication doses are at the upper dosing range, [Table 10-1]), and dual antibiotic therapy, including two agents such as clarithromycin, amoxicillin, and metronidazole. Quadruple therapy consists of the above with the addition of bismuth subsalicylate. Therapy should be instituted for 7 to 14 days.[22–24]

PITFALLS

- Failure to consider risk factors for peptic ulcer disease and address them in discharge instructions.
- Failure to diagnose peptic ulcer disease in UGI hemorrhage.
- Failure to initiate prompt therapy to eradicate *H. pylori* infection in suspected peptic ulcer disease.

REFERENCES

1. McCaig LF, Burt CW. National Hospital Ambulatory Medical Care Survey: 2002 Emergency Department Summary. *Advance Data from Vital and Health Statistics* 2004;340:15.
2. Rockall TA, Logan RFA, Devlin HB, et al. Incidence of and mortality from acute upper gastrointestinal haemorrhage. *BMJ* 1995;311:222.
3. Greenwald DA. Aging, the gastrointestinal tract, and risk of acid-related disease. *Am J Med* 2004;117(Suppl 5A):8S.
4. Lu CL, Chang SS, Wang SS, et al. Silent peptic ulcer disease: frequency, factors leading to "silence," and implications regarding the pathogenesis of visceral symptoms. *Gastrointest Endosc*. 2004;60:34.
5. Svoboda P, Kantorova I, Scheer P, et al. Helicobacter pylori is not a risk factor for stress ulcer bleeding in polytraumatized patients. *Hepatogastroenterology*. 2004;51:476.
6. Sung, JJ, Chung, SC, Ling SK, et al. Antibacterial treatment of gastric ulcers associated with Helicobacter pylori. *N Engl J Med*. 1995;332:139.
7. Seppala K, Pikkarainen P, Sipponen P, et al. Cure of peptic gastric ulcer associated with eradication of Helicobacter pylori. Finnish Gastric Ulcer Study Group. *Gut*. 1995; 36:834.
8. Pohle T, Domschke WK. Results of short- and long-term medical treatment of gastroesophageal reflux disease (GERD). Langenbecks *Arch Surg*. 2000;385:317.
9. Hopkins RJ, Girardi LS, Turney EA. Relationship between Helicobacter pylori eradication and reduced duodenal and gastric ulcer recurrence: a review. *Gastroenterology*. 1996; 110:1244.
10. Parasher G, Eastwood GL. Smoking and peptic ulcer in the Helicobacter pylori era. *Eur J Gastroenterol Hepatol*. 2000;12:843.
11. Muris JWM, Starmans R, Pop P, et al. Discriminate value of symptoms in patients with dyspepsia. *J Fam Prac*. 1994; 38:139.
12. Vakil N, Fendrick AM. How to test for Helicobacter pylori in 2005. *Cleve Clin J Med*. 2005;72(Suppl 2):S8.
13. Loy CT, Irwig LM, Katelaris PH, et al. Do commercial serological kits for Helicobacter pylori infection differ in accuracy? A meta-analysis. *Am J Gastroenterol*. 1996; 91:1138.
14. Levine MS. Role of the double-contrast upper gastrointestinal series in the 1990s. *Gastroenterol Clin North Am*. 1995;24:289.
15. Ford AC, Qume M, Moayyedi P, et al. Helicobacter pylori "test and treat" or endoscopy for managing dyspepsia: an individual patient data meta-analysis. *Gastroenterology*. 2005;128:838.
16. Mones J, Gisbert JP, Borda F, et al. Indications, diagnostic tests and Helicobacter pylori eradication therapy. Recommendations by the 2nd Spanish Consensus Conference. *Rev Esp Enferm Dig*. 2005;97:348.
17. Arasaradnam RP, Donnelly MT. Acute endoscopic intervention in non-variceal upper gastrointestinal bleeding. *Postgrad Med J*. 2005;81:92.
18. Leontiadis GI, Sharma VK, Howden W. Systematic review and meta-analysis of proton pump inhibitor therapy in peptic ulcer bleeding. *BMJ*. 2005;330:568.
19. Robinson M. Review article: the pharmacodynamics and pharmacokinetics of proton pump inhibitors—overview and clinical implications. *Aliment Pharmacol Ther*. 2004;20 (Suppl 6):1.
20. Leontiadis GI, McIntyre L, Sharma VK, et al. Proton pump inhibitor treatment for acute peptic ulcer bleeding. *Cochrane Database Syst Rev*. 2004;CD002094.
21. Hellstrom PM, Vitols S. The choice of proton pump inhibitor: does it matter? *Basic Clin Pharmacol Toxicol*. 2004;94:106.
22. Drugs for peptic ulcers. *Treat Guidel Med Lett*. 2004;2:9.
23. Conway BR. Drug delivery strategies for the treatment of Helicobacter pylori infections. *Curr Pharmaceut Design*. 2005;11:775.
24. Gisbert JP, Pajares JM. Systematic review and meta-analysis: is 1-week proton pump inhibitor-based triple therapy sufficient to heal peptic ulcer? *Aliment Pharmacol Ther*. 2005;21:795.

11

Gastroesophageal Reflux Disease and Gastritis

David M. Barrett

GASTROESOPHAGEAL REFLUX DISEASE

High Yield Facts

- The classic symptoms of GERD are heartburn and acid regurgitation. Both have a high specificity for GERD, although they lack sensitivity.
- In patients with a predominant symptom of heartburn, the specificity for GERD is 89%. The specificity of heartburn for GERD is lower when it is not the predominant complaint.
- In patients with suspected GERD but without symptoms suggesting complications, a therapeutic trial of acid suppressive therapy is recommended.
- Patients with symptoms of GERD who respond to empiric therapy do not need routine follow-up testing.

Epidemiology

Gastroesophageal reflux disease (GERD) is one of the most prevalent illnesses in the United States and is frequently encountered in both the emergency department (ED) and primary care setting. According to a 1999 survey, the prevalence of GERD in the United States was estimated at 18.6 million.[1] In a population-based survey of patients in Olmstead County, Minnesota, the overall prevalence of heartburn and acid regurgitation within the prior 12 months was 42.4% and 45% of respondents, respectively.[2] Heartburn that occurred weekly was reported by 17.8% and daily by 7%.[3] Prevalence rates of 5% to 13% have been reported in European populations[4] and 1.6% to 5.7% in Asian populations.[5] Gastroesophageal reflux disease occurs at a similar rate across age groups and gender.[2] Environmental factors such as smoking, consumption of certain foods, alcohol, and obesity have been associated with GERD,[6] and it occurs with an increased frequency in pregnancy, scleroderma, and Zollinger-Ellison syndrome.

Pathophysiology

Gastroesophageal reflux disease is caused by reflux of gastric contents into the lower esophagus. Although reflux episodes occur in otherwise normal healthy individuals, they are considered pathologic when they produce frequent or severe symptoms or mucosal damage.[7] Changes in lower esophageal sphincter function and structural changes in the gastroesophageal junction are both involved in producing GERD,[8,9] and particularly severe symptoms may be seen in patients with hiatal hernia.[10] Persistent reflux of acidic gastric contents may produce inflammatory changes of the lower esophagus (i.e., esophagitis) or symptoms of GERD. Increased sensitivity of the lower esophagus to acid is the predominant mechanism of GERD in patients without demonstrable esophagitis.[11]

Clinical Features

Heartburn is the cardinal symptom of GERD. Patients may describe a burning feeling, rising from the stomach or lower chest, and radiating to the neck.[12] Heartburn is generally exacerbated by meals, particularly large meals, spicy foods, high-fat foods, alcohol, and the recumbent position. It is generally relieved by antacids. Acid regurgitation, the effortless return of gastric contents into the pharynx without nausea or vomiting, is also highly suggestive of GERD. Belching, bending, or coughing may provoke acid regurgitation. When heartburn is the predominant symptom, it has been shown to have a specificity of 89% and a positive predictive vale of 81% for GERD as determined by abnormal esophageal pH monitoring.[13] Acid regurgitation as the predominant symptom had a specificity of 95% and a positive predictive value of 57% for GERD when it is the predominant symptom.[13] The sensitivity and negative predictive values of both symptoms are poor. Dysphagia for solids has been reported in 13% to 39% of patients with GERD.[14] Odynophagia is a less common presentation of GERD (10%) but when present is suggestive of esophagitis. Gastroesophageal reflux disease may present with nonspecific symptoms such as epigastric pain, nausea, and belching,[13] sometimes referred to as dyspepsia.[15] Gastroesophageal reflux disease also has been reported to cause a wide variety of extraesophageal manifestations including hoarseness, globus sensation, cough laryngitis, and asthma,[16,17] and it may also present as retrosternal chest pain and at times may be clinically indistinguishable from unstable angina.[18]

Abnormal signs on physical examination of patients with GERD are typically absent. The presence of abnormal vital signs, significant abdominal tenderness, pallor, or an abdominal mass may indicate a complication of GERD or the presence of an alternative diagnosis.

The complications of GERD include hemorrhage, esophageal perforation, esophageal stricture, Barrett esophagus, and esophageal adenocarcinoma. Esophageal strictures in GERD result from prolonged inflammation and fibrosis.[19] Barrett esophagus is replacement of the normal squamous columnar epithelium of the esophagus with metaplastic intestinal epithelium and is a precursor for esophageal adenocarcinoma.[20]

Diagnosis and Differential

Gastroesophageal reflux disease has been defined as symptoms or mucosal damage produced by the abnormal reflux of gastric contents in to the esophagus.[21] Given the wide spectrum of severity and clinical manifestations of GERD, there is no single criterion for the diagnosis of GERD. In the ED, GERD may be diagnosed clinically on the basis of the typical symptoms of heartburn and acid regurgitation, both of which have high specificity for reflux.[7]

Laboratory tests including a white blood count, hemoglobin level, and hematocrit, may be useful for detecting complications of GERD or for identifying an alternative diagnosis.

Plain radiographs may identify patients with a hiatal hernia but are not useful in identifying patients with GERD. Barium esophagrams may identify patients with dysphagia and have an overall sensitivity of 60% to 80% and a specificity of 90% for detecting esophagitis as compared to endoscopy.[22] The sensitivity of barium esophagrams decreases in milder cases of esophagitis and is poor for detecting pathologic reflux as measured by 24-hour pH monitoring.[23]

Endoscopy is the preferred method for detection of esophagitis, Barrett esophagus, and complications of GERD,[24] although it is not routinely available in the emergency setting. When esophagitis is present on endoscopic examination, the procedure is considered diagnostic. The absence of esophagitis on endoscopy, however, does not exclude the diagnosis of GERD as up to 61% of patients with GERD have a normal esophagus at endoscopy.[25] Patients with symptoms suggestive of severe or complicated disease, including dysphagia or odynophagia; weight loss; evidence of gastrointestinal bleeding or iron deficiency anemia; over the age of 55; and with symptoms of long duration or persistent symptoms despite therapy should be referred to a gastroenterologist for urgent endoscopy.[26]

Twenty-four hour ambulatory pH monitoring is widely available on an outpatient basis for the diagnosis of GERD although it is neither practical nor feasible in the ED. It may be indicated following initial ED evaluation for patients with poor response to therapy or unclear symptoms, patients who are symptomatic but with a negative endoscopy, or patients prior to antireflux surgery.[27]

A therapeutic trial of acid suppression is the initial diagnostic method favored for patients with symptoms of GERD who do not have symptoms suggestive of complications.[21] Response to a 1-week trial of omeprazole 20 mg twice a day showed 75% sensitivity and 55% specificity for identifying reflux in patients with heartburn using ambulatory pH monitoring as the reference standard.[28] Tests with other doses of omeprazole in patients with noncardiac chest pain, dyspepsia, or other symptoms of GERD have yielded sensitivities from 70% to 90% and specificities of 55% to 85% depending on the dosage used and study population.[22] The methodological problems of using a therapeutic trial as a diagnostic test may be weighed against the ease of use and decreased costs associated with this approach.[29]

The differential diagnosis of GERD includes other causes of esophagitis such as infectious and pill esophagitis, peptic ulcer disease, cholelithiasis, achalasia, functional dyspepsia, and angina pectoris.

Emergency Department Care and Disposition

Gastroesophageal reflux disease itself is rarely life-threatening.[30] Treatment of patients with GERD primarily involves identification of patients with possible complications and alleviation of symptoms. The cornerstone of treatment of GERD is acid suppressive therapy.[21] In a systematic review of proton pump inhibitors (PPIs) versus histamine 2 receptor antagonists (H2RAs), PPIs were more effective in reducing symptoms of heartburn in endoscopically negative reflux disease.[31] A recent metaanalysis showed that PPIs resulted in a rate of healing nearly twice as fast as H2RAs in patients with esophagitis.[32]

Antacids are effective in reducing heartburn symptoms but do not promote healing of esophagitis.[33] H2RAs reduce symptoms of heartburn and promote healing of esophagitis.[34] While not as effective as PPIs, they may be useful as patient-directed or intermittent therapy in cases of mild GERD.[35]

Lifestyle modifications, including elevation of the head of the bed, decreased fat intake, cessation of smoking, weight loss, and avoidance of the recumbent position after meals have been recommended to help control symptoms of GERD. Although such modifications alone are not likely to control symptoms of GERD and have limited evidence to support them, they may still be of benefit to patients.[21]

Pitfalls

- Alarm symptoms of GERD are suggestive of complicated disease and include dysphagia, vomiting, unintentional weight loss, gastrointestinal bleeding, or iron deficiency anemia. Patients with alarm symptoms, patients over the age of 55, and patients with a history of prolonged symptoms should receive a referral to a gastroenterologist for urgent endoscopy.

- Although many patients with GERD have classic symptoms, GERD has been linked to a wide variety of extraesophageal manifestations, including chest pain. In patients presenting with unexplained chest pain, especially those with risk factors for coronary artery disease, GERD is a diagnosis of exclusion. Evaluation and treatment for life-threatening causes of chest pain including acute coronary syndrome (ACS) should occur prior to treatment of GERD.

GASTRITIS

High Yield Facts

- Gastritis refers to inflammation of the gastric mucosa. It is not a disease but rather a condition that may result from a variety of disease processes. Gastric mucosal damage without inflammation may occur in response to a variety of chemical agents or other insults and is sometimes termed acute erosive gastritis but is more accurately referred to as gastropathy.

- Clinicians often use the term gastritis to refer to vague symptoms of epigastric discomfort or fullness. Such symptoms are more appropriately termed dyspepsia as the presence of gastritis cannot be reliably determined on the basis of the history and physical examination.

Epidemiology

Both gastritis and gastropathy are extremely common conditions. *Helicobacter pylori* is the most common cause of gastritis in adults worldwide.[36] In developed countries, prevalence rates of 20% to 50% have been reported[37-39] and are inversely correlated with socioeconomic status.[37] Autoimmune gastritis is an autosomal dominant disorder seen most commonly in northern Europeans and is a risk factor for development of pernicious anemia. Less common forms of gastritis include postantrectomy gastritis, eosinophilic gastritis, cytomegalovirus gastritis in patients with acquired immunodeficiency syndrome (AIDS) or other immunodeficiencies, lymphocytic gastritis in association with celiac disease, and bacterial gastritis due to *Helicobacter heilmannii*. Granulomatous gastritis may be seen in patients with tuberculosis, sarcoidosis, and Crohn disease. Phlegmonous gastritis is a rare but often severe bacterial infection of the stomach seen more often in elderly debilitated patients, alcoholics, and patients with immunocompromise.[40] Emphysematous gastritis is an even more rare and lethal form of phlegmonous gastritis caused by gas-forming organisms.[41] Anisakiasis is a helminthic infection of the stomach occurring in patients who have ingested raw or undercooked fish.

Acute erosive gastropathy may result from a variety of conditions that produce gastric mucosal ischemia including sepsis, shock, trauma, and burns. Nonsteroidal antiinflammatory medications (NSAIDs) are the most common cause of acute erosive gastropathy overall. Other common causes of gastropathy include trauma, sepsis, and burns, often referred to as stress gastritis.[42] Alcohol, iron, potassium, chemotherapy agents, and cocaine are substances known to cause acute gastric mucosal injury.[43]

Pathophysiology

The pathophysiology of gastritis varies according to the underlying etiology. Any process that disrupts normal gastric mucosal defense mechanisms leads to increased vulnerability of the gastric mucosa to damage from acid, bile salts, and digestive enzymes.

Clinical Features

Gastritis and gastropathy do not have characteristic clinical symptoms. Acute infection with *H. pylori* produces acute gastritis in some patients with epigastric pain, nausea, and vomiting—symptoms that are entirely nonspecific.[44] Most patients with acute or chronic infection with *H. pylori* are asymptomatic.[38] In the setting of *H. pylori* infection, abdominal pain is suggestive of a complication such as ulceration. Acute phlegmonous gastritis causes epigastric abdominal pain and vomiting, often with fever. Patients are acutely ill and overall mortality rates of 40% have been reported even with aggressive treatment.[45]

A careful history may elicit features which are suggestive of a causative agent for dyspepsia.[46] Patients may complain of abdominal discomfort in the setting of acute or chronic ingestion of substances known to cause gastric mucosal injury, such as alcohol or NSAIDs. Mild epigastric abdominal tenderness may be present. The presence of significant vomiting or abdominal tenderness should prompt a search for an alternative diagnosis.

Diagnosis and Differential

Gastritis is a histological diagnosis.[43] Endoscopy with gastric mucosal biopsy is essential for identification and classification of gastritis;[47] however, endoscopy would not be performed during an ED visit. Laboratory tests may be useful for detecting complications such as anemia or in identifying another etiology but have no utility for the diagnosis of gastritis with the possible exception of serologic tests for *H. pylori*.[39] Radiologic tests are not accurate for the routine detection of gastritis. Plain radiographs and abdominal computed tomography (CT) scanning may be used to exclude causes such as perforation from a suspected ulcer. In cases of suspected phlegmonous gastritis, abdominal CT scanning may identify a thickened, edematous stomach wall.[45] The differential diagnosis of gastritis includes other causes of epigastric pain, gastric or duodenal ulcer, pancreatitis, chololithiasis and cholecystitis, GERD, and nonulcer dyspepsia.

Emergency Department Care and Disposition

Treatment of gastritis depends on the underlying etiology. The ED evaluation should focus on excluding other causes of abdominal pain and identifying complications such as anemia. In patients taking NSAIDs with symptoms of dyspepsia, treatment with misoprostol, a histamine receptor antagonist, or a PPI, may be helpful in relieving some symptoms.[48] Discontinuation of medications known to cause dyspepsia or moderation of alcohol intake also may relieve symptoms in some patients.

The ED evaluation may not identify the cause of dyspeptic symptoms in many patients. Patients with uncomplicated dyspepsia should be referred to a primary care provider. As with patients with GERD, patients with symptoms suggesting complicated disease, such as weight loss or anemia, should be referred to a gastroenterologist for prompt endoscopy.[15]

Pitfalls

- While certain forms of gastritis may be suspected based on a clinical history, it remains a diagnosis of exclusion. The symptoms if any are nonspecific; therefore the ED evaluation of dyspepsia should exclude serious causes of abdominal pain.

REFERENCES

1. Frank L, Kleinman L, Ganoczy D, et al. Upper gastrointestinal symptoms in North America: prevalence and relationship to healthcare utilization and quality of life. *Dig Dis Sci.* 2000;45:809.
2. Locke GR, 3rd, Talley NJ, Fett SL, et al. Prevalence and clinical spectrum of gastroesophageal reflux: a population-based study in Olmsted County, Minnesota. *Gastroenterology.* 1997;112:1448.
3. Nebel OT, Fornes MF, Castell DO. Symptomatic gastroesophageal reflux: incidence and precipitating factors. *Am J Dig Dis.* 1976;21:953.
4. Stanghellini V. Three-month prevalence rates of gastrointestinal symptoms and the influence of demographic factors: results from the Domestic/International Gastroenterology Surveillance Study (DIGEST). *Scand J Gastroenterol Suppl.* 1999;231:20.
5. Ho KY, Kang JY, Seow A. Prevalence of gastrointestinal symptoms in a multiracial Asian population, with particular reference to reflux-type symptoms. *Am J Gastroenterol.* 1998;93:1816.
6. Dent J, El-Serag HB, Wallander MA, et al. Epidemiology of gastro-oesophageal reflux disease: a systematic review. *Gut.* 2005;54:710.
7. An evidence-based appraisal of reflux disease management—the Genval Workshop Report. *Gut.* 1999;44 (Suppl 2):S1.
8. Dent J, Holloway RH, Toouli J, et al. Mechanisms of lower oesophageal sphincter incompetence in patients with symptomatic gastrooesophageal reflux. *Gut.* 1988;29:1020.
9. Pandolfino JE, Shi G, Curry J, et al. Esophagogastric junction distensibility: a factor contributing to sphincter incompetence. *Am J Physiol Gastrointest Liver Physiol.* 2002;282:G1052.
10. Van Herwaarden MA, Samsom M, Smout AJ. Excess gastroesophageal reflux in patients with hiatus hernia is caused by mechanisms other than transient LES relaxations. *Gastroenterology.* 2000;119:1439.
11. Trimble KC, Pryde A, Heading RC. Lowered oesophageal sensory thresholds in patients with symptomatic but not excess gastro-oesophageal reflux: evidence for a spectrum of visceral sensitivity in GORD. *Gut.* 1995;37:7.
12. Smith L. Updated ACG Guidelines for Diagnosis and Treatment of GERD. *Am Fam Physician.* 2005;71:2376.

13. Klauser AG, Schindlbeck NE, Muller-Lissner SA. Symptoms in gastro-oesophageal reflux disease. *Lancet.* 1990; 335:205.

14. Jacob P, Kahrilas PJ, Vanagunas A. Peristaltic dysfunction associated with nonobstructive dysphagia in reflux disease. *Dig Dis Sci.* 1990;35:939.

15. Talley NJ, Vakil N. Guidelines for the management of dyspepsia. *Am J Gastroenterol.* 2005;100:2324.

16. Richter JE. Extraesophageal presentations of gastroesophageal reflux disease: an overview. *Am J Gastroenterol.* 2000;95:S1.

17. Harding SM, Guzzo MR, Richter JE. The prevalence of gastroesophageal reflux in asthma patients without reflux symptoms. *Am J Respir Crit Care Med.* 2000;162:34.

18. Richter JE. Chest pain and gastroesophageal reflux disease. *J Clin Gastroenterol.* 2000;30:S39.

19. Richter JE. Peptic strictures of the esophagus. *Gastroenterol Clin North Am.* 1999;28:875.

20. Solaymani-Dodaran M, Logan RF, West J, et al. Risk of oesophageal cancer in Barrett's oesophagus and gastro-oesophageal reflux. *Gut.* 2004;53:1070.

21. DeVault KR, Castell DO. Updated guidelines for the diagnosis and treatment of gastroesophageal reflux disease. *Am J Gastroenterol.* 2005;100:190.

22. Van Herwaarden MA, Smout AJ. Diagnosis of reflux disease. *Baillieres Best Pract Res Clin Gastroenterol.* 2000;14:759.

23. Chen MY, Ott DJ, Sinclair JW, et al. Gastroesophageal reflux disease: correlation of esophageal pH testing and radiographic findings. *Radiology.* 1992;185:483.

24. The role of endoscopy in the management of GERD: guidelines for clinical application. From the ASGE. American Society for Gastrointestinal Endoscopy. *Gastrointest Endosc.* 1999;49:834.

25. Masclee AA, de Best AC, de Graaf R, et al. Ambulatory 24-hour pH-metry in the diagnosis of gastroesophageal reflux disease: determination of criteria and relation to endoscopy. *Scand J Gastroenterol.* 1990;25:225.

26. Kapoor N, Bassi A, Sturgess R, et al. Predictive value of alarm features in a rapid access upper gastrointestinal cancer service. *Gut.* 2005;54:40.

27. American Gastroenterological Association medical position statement: guidelines on the use of esophageal pH recording. *Gastroenterology.* 1996;110:1981.

28. Johnsson F, Weywadt L, Solhaug JH, et al. One-week omeprazole treatment in the diagnosis of gastro-oesophageal reflux disease. *Scand J Gastroenterol.* 1998;33:15.

29. Numans ME, Lau J, de Wit NJ, et al. Short-term treatment with proton-pump inhibitors as a test for gastroesophageal reflux disease: a meta-analysis of diagnostic test characteristics. *Ann Intern Med.* 2004;140:518.

30. *The burden of gastrointestinal diseases.* American Gastroenterological Association, Bethesda, MD 2001.

31. Van Pinxteren B, Numans ME, Bonis PA, et al. Short-term treatment with proton pump inhibitors, H2-receptor antagonists and prokinetics for gastro-oesophageal reflux disease-like symptoms and endoscopy negative reflux disease. *Cochrane Database Syst Rev.* 2004;CD002095.

32. Chiba N, De Gara CJ, Wilkinson JM, et al. Speed of healing and symptom relief in grade II to IV gastroesophageal reflux disease: a meta-analysis. *Gastroenterology.* 1997;112:1798.

33. Farup PG, Weberg R, Berstad A, et al. Low-dose antacids versus 400 mg cimetidine twice daily for reflux oesophagitis. A comparative, placebo-controlled, multicentre study. *Scand J Gastroenterol.* 1990;25:315.

34. Earnest D, Robinson M, Rodriguez-Stanley S, et al. Managing heartburn at the 'base' of the GERD 'iceberg': effervescent ranitidine 150 mg b.d. provides faster and better heartburn relief than antacids. *Aliment Pharmacol Ther.* 2000;14:911.

35. Xue S, Katz PO, Banerjee P, et al. Bedtime H2 blockers improve nocturnal gastric acid control in GERD patients on proton pump inhibitors. *Aliment Pharmacol Ther.* 2001; 15:1351.

36. Graham DY, Go MF. Helicobacter pylori: current status. *Gastroenterology.* 1993;105:279.

37. Graham DY, Malaty HM, Evans DG, et al. Epidemiology of Helicobacter pylori in an asymptomatic population in the United States: Effect of age, race, and socioeconomic status. *Gastroenterology.* 1991;100:1495.

38. Dooley CP, Cohen H, Fitzgibbons PL, et al. Prevalence of Helicobacter pylori infection and histologic gastritis in asymptomatic persons. *N Engl J Med* 1989;321:1562.

39. Suerbaum S, Michetti P. Helicobacter pylori infection. *N Engl J Med* 2002;347:1175.

40. Schultz MJ, van der Hulst RW, Tytgat GN. Acute phlegmonous gastritis. *Gastrointest Endosc.* 1996;44:80.

41. Allan K, Barriga J, Afshani M, et al. Emphysematous gastritis. *Am J Med Sci.* 2005;329:205.

42. Sugawa C, Lucas CE, Rosenberg BF, et al. Differential topography of acute erosive gastritis due to trauma or sepsis, ethanol and aspirin. *Gastrointest Endosc.* 1973;19:127.

43. Rubesin SE, Furth EE, Levine MS. Gastritis from NSAIDS to Helicobacter pylori. *Abdom Imaging.* 2005;30:142.

44. Marshall BJ, Armstrong JA, McGechie DB, et al. Attempt to fulfil Koch's postulates for pyloric Campylobacter. *Med J Aust.* 1985;142:436.

45. Kim GY, Ward J, Henessey B, et al. Phlegmonous gastritis: case report and review. *Gastrointest Endosc.* 2005;61:168.

46. Richter JE. Dyspepsia: organic causes and differential characteristics from functional dyspepsia. *Scand J Gastroenterol Suppl.* 1991;182:11.

47. Dixon MF, Genta RM, Yardley JH, et al. Classification and grading of gastritis: The updated Sydney System. International Workshop on the Histopathology of Gastritis, Houston 1994. *Am J Surg Pathol.* 1996;20:1161.

48. Cappell MS, Schein JR. Diagnosis and treatment of nonsteroidal anti-inflammatory drug-associated upper gastrointestinal toxicity. *Gastroenterol Clin North Am.* 2000; 29:97.

12

Gastrointestinal Bleeding

Angela M. Mills

HIGH YIELD FACTS

- As gastrointestinal (GI) bleeding carries a 10% overall mortality rate, patients require prompt diagnosis, aggressive resuscitation, risk stratification, and timely consultation.
- Advanced age, serious comorbid conditions, hemodynamic instability, esophageal varices, significant hematemesis or melena, and marked anemia are important risk factors leading to increased morbidity and mortality in patients with GI bleeding.

EPIDEMIOLOGY

Gastrointestinal bleeding (GIB) is a common complaint in the emergency department with an overall mortality rate of up to 10%, which has not changed greatly over the past several decades.[1–3] Gastrointestinal bleeding may be divided into upper and lower gastrointestinal bleeding (UGIB and LGIB, respectively) as defined by hemorrhage originating proximal or distal to the ligament of Treitz. Upper gastrointestinal bleeding is much more common and accounts for a greater proportion of admissions in adults. The annual incidence for UGIB is estimated at 50 to 150 per 100,000 population,[2,4] while that of LGIB is much lower at approximately 20 to 27 per 100,000 population.[3,5] Most cases of bleeding are self-limited, with the majority of patients having only one episode of bleeding.[3] Both UGIB and LGIB are more common in males and the elderly.[2,4,5]

In addition to age greater than 60, other independent markers of increased morbidity and mortality include presence of comorbid conditions, requirement of more than 5 units of packed red blood cells, hemodynamic instability, recurrent bleeding, endoscopic stigmata of recent hemorrhage, melena or hematochezia, esophageal varices, and bloody nasogastric aspirate.[1,6,7]

PATHOPHYSIOLOGY

The most common cause of UGIB is peptic ulcer disease comprising approximately 60% of cases. While the overall mortality of UGIB may be about 10%, there are significant differences in mortality according to the etiology of bleeding. Those patients with portal hypertension-related bleeding, which includes esophageal and gastric varices and portal hypertensive gastropathy, have mortality rates of greater than 50% as compared to a 4% rate with peptic ulcer bleeding.[2] Bleeding is rarely the cause of death in cases of nonvariceal bleeding in contrast to those with portal hypertension. Variceal bleeding is also the most common cause of persistent and severe UGIB and more often presents with bright red or red hematemesis.[3] A list of UGIB causes may be found in Table 12-1.

The most common causes of LGIB include colonic diverticulosis and angiodysplasia, and patients tend to be older than those with UGIB. It is estimated that 75% to 85% of patients with lower hemorrhage resolve spontaneously.[3,8] Diagnosis may be difficult as lower bleeding may be intermittent or may originate from the small intestine or an upper tract source of brisk bleeding. Lower tract sources of hemorrhage have a rebleeding rate of 10% to 20%, require surgery in 10% to 15% of cases, and have a 4% mortality rate.[2,3,5] A list of LGIB causes may be found in Table 12-2.

CLINICAL FEATURES

While many patients may present with hematemesis or blood in the stool, clinical suspicion for GIB must remain high in patients with signs or symptoms of hypovolemia or more subtle presentations, including hypotension, tachycardia, dizziness, angina, confusion, or syncope. Important historical features to obtain include time of onset, amount of bleeding, and associated symptoms. Patients should be asked about symptoms of volume depletion, including lightheadedness or dizziness, and symptoms of anemia, including fatigue, dyspnea, and chest pain.

History of coagulopathy, past GIB, liver disease, or hemorrhoids may be helpful. Medication history should be obtained including aspirin, nonsteroidal anti-inflammatory medications (NSAID), glucocorticoids, and anticoagulants. Aspirin and NSAID use have been shown to contribute to both upper and lower GIB and are dose and duration of use dependent.[9–11] A history of alcohol abuse may also lead to various causes of GIB such as peptic ulcer disease or varices. Patients with prior aortic graft surgery may present with an aortoenteric fistula.

Hematemesis is a complaint that usually signifies UGIB and may be bright red or darker such as "coffee-ground" emesis. Approximately 50% of patients with UGIB present with hematemesis.[3] Patients may also complain of hematochezia, which may be bright red or

Table 12-1. Causes of Upper Gastrointestinal Bleeding*

Peptic ulcer disease
Gastroduodenal erosions
Esophagitis
Varices
Mallory-Weiss tear
Vascular malformation
Neoplasm/Tumor

*Other less common etiologies exist.

maroon-colored blood in the stool, which may signify a lower tract source of hemorrhage, but is caused by a brisk upper source with rapid transit in approximately 14% of cases.[12] Hematochezia due to UGIB has been shown to be associated with a higher transfusion requirement, need for surgery, and mortality rate.[3,12] Melena, or black tarry stool, may also be seen with upper and lower sources of bleeding, but has a lower mortality rate when compared to hematochezia.[3] Approximately 70% of patients with UGIB present with melena in contrast to only 20% to 30% of patients with LGIB.[3,11]

Table 12-2. Causes of Lower Gastrointestinal Bleeding*

Diverticular disease
Arteriovenous malformations
Colitis
    Inflammatory bowel disease
    Ischemia
    Radiation
Neoplasm/Tumor
Postpolypectomy bleeding
Anorectal causes
    Hemorrhoids
    Rectal varices
    Fissures
Colonic ulcers
Small bowel etiologies
    Angiodysplasia,
    Jejunoileal diverticula
    Meckel diverticulum
    Enteritis
    Aortoduodenal fistula

*Other less common etiologies exist.

While vital sign abnormalities such as hypotension and tachycardia may indicate significant blood loss, normal vital signs do not rule out significant GIB. Physical examination should include assessment of general appearance, mental status, examination of the conjunctiva (with pale color suggesting anemia), and skin characteristics including color, temperature, presence of petechiae, and stigmata of liver disease. Examination of the nasopharynx and oropharynx may reveal a source of blood that is being swallowed. A thorough abdominal exam is important to check for tenderness, masses, and peritoneal signs. Rectal examination should include assessment for anal fissures, hemorrhoids, and rectal masses. Stool should be examined for color and tested for occult blood. Extremities should be evaluated for character of pulses and adequacy of capillary refill.

DIAGNOSIS AND DIFFERENTIAL

Important laboratory studies to obtain in the patient with GIB include a type and crossmatch, hemoglobin and hematocrit, blood urea nitrogen (BUN), and creatinine. The initial hemoglobin obtained in an ED setting may not adequately reflect the true amount of blood loss. A hemoglobin <10 g/dL has been correlated with increased rebleeding and mortality rates.[6] As UGIB is associated with an elevation of the BUN concentration, the BUN to creatinine ratio has been used to discriminate UGIB from LGIB. A ratio greater than 36, in patients without renal failure, has a sensitivity of 90% to 95% in predicting UGIB.[13,14] Patients on anticoagulation therapy or with liver disease may also benefit from coagulation studies and platelet count.

An electrocardiogram and cardiac markers should be obtained in those patients at risk for acute coronary syndrome, as GIB may lead to decreased oxygen delivery and resultant myocardial ischemia.[15,16] Routine abdominal radiographs in patients with GIB have been shown to be of limited value.[17] In the absence of pulmonary exam findings or known pulmonary disease, routine chest radiographs do not alter clinical outcomes or management decisions.[18]

In patients with hematemesis and a clear upper source of GIB, nasogastric aspiration with lavage may be used to detect and quantify active bleeding. In those patients without hematemesis and an unclear source of bleeding, a positive nasogastric aspirate often indicates an upper source of bleeding. A bloody aspirate has been shown to be associated with the presence of a high-risk lesion at endoscopy.[19] In contrast, a negative nasogastric aspirate is not as helpful as it may miss various sources of UGIB and has been shown to miss up to 50% of patients with recent duodenal bleeding.[20,21]

Some patients who complain of vomiting blood or passing blood in the stool may not have GIB. Red-colored food products may cause vomitus to appear as hematemesis. The appearance of melena may be due to the presence of iron or bismuth ingestion, while that of hematochezia may be due to beets. In these cases, stool will be heme negative on testing. Suspected UGIB may actually be due to a source of bleeding from the nasopharynx or oropharynx that is being swallowed.

EMERGENCY DEPARTMENT CARE AND DISPOSITION

Emergency department care encompasses timely diagnosis, immediate resuscitation, assessment of risk factors, and prompt consultation when required. Patients may need definitive airway management to prevent aspiration, and aggressive resuscitation may be initiated with crystalloid fluids via large-bore intravenous catheters. As hemorrhage can lead to decreased oxygen delivery, supplemental oxygen and cardiac monitoring are recommended. Transfusion of blood products is recommended in those patients who continue with hemodynamic instability despite crystalloid resuscitation and in those with continuous bleeding. Patients requiring more than 5 units of packed red cells have a much higher mortality rate and often require surgery.[1]

Various medical therapies have been shown to improve outcome in GIB. Somatostatin and octreotide, its longer-acting derivative, have been shown to reduce the risk for continued bleeding and rebleeding in patients with UGIB.[22,23] A large systematic review of the use of somatostatin analogues for acute bleeding due to esophageal varices showed no significant reduction in mortality but did show a reduction in bleeding and transfusion requirement.[24] The standard dose for octreotide is a 50 μg bolus intravenously followed by a continuous infusion of 25 to 50 μg/hour.

Proton pump inhibitors have been shown to reduce bleeding and the need for surgery, with conflicting evidence for mortality reduction, in patients with non-variceal UGIB.[25–27] Vasopressin has been used in GIB, most often for variceal bleeding, but is associated with a significant rebleeding rate and high rate of complication including hypertension, dysrhythmias, myocardial and peripheral ischemia, and decreased cardiac output.[28] The use of H2-receptor antagonists in UGIB has not been shown to be of significant value, with no benefit in bleeding duodenal ulcers and possibly weak benefit in bleeding gastric ulcers.[29,30]

After hemodynamic stabilization, upper endoscopy is the most accurate intervention in cases of UGIB allowing for diagnosis of the site of bleeding and achievement of hemostasis in greater than 90% of cases.[31] Endoscopic therapies such as sclerotherapy and band ligation are useful in acute variceal bleeding. Early endoscopy, performed within 12 to 24 hours of bleeding, reduces the risk of rebleeding and hospital length of stay in patients with UGIB.[32] Endoscopic findings are also important for risk stratification and allow for decisions on patient disposition.[33,34]

The goal in treating active LGIB is localization of the site of bleeding for therapy to ultimately avoid a subtotal colectomy. Requiring both rapid bowel preparation and availability of the endoscopist, urgent colonoscopy may be both diagnostic and therapeutic in cases of LGIB.[5,35] Colonoscopy is often performed in stabilized patients with self-limited bleeding or in those with a higher likelihood of a localized lesion. Patients with clinical signs of severe hemorrhage may be more likely to undergo radiographic interventions rather than urgent colonoscopy.[36]

Technetium-labeled red cell scanning is a noninvasive technique that may be used in localizing an obscure source of LGIB. The technetium scan requires active hemorrhage at a rate of at least 0.1 mL/min.[3,37,38] This method is then used to direct therapy either by angiography or surgery.

Angiography may also be used to localize obscure lower bleeding but requires a brisker rate of hemorrhage of at least 0.5 to 1 mL/min. It has the advantage of allowing for therapeutic intervention but the disadvantage of complications including acute renal failure, contrast reactions, and arterial thrombosis or dissection. Angiography is often reserved for severe continuous LGIB.[3,39]

There is controversy in the management of LGIB as to which diagnostic test should be implemented first, and management may be influenced by institutional availability and expertise, and the consulting clinician's preference.

Balloon tamponade with a Sengstaken-Blakemore tube is rarely used due to its high rate of complications, but it may be used for active variceal bleeding in the exsanguinating patient when endoscopy is not available. Patients with UGIB or LGIB who fail to respond to the therapies described may require surgery for continued hemorrhage. Early consultation with a surgeon is advisable.

Hospital admission is required for patients with significant GIB. Various studies have demonstrated a subset of low-risk patients who may be safely discharged home with UGIB, although short observation and endoscopy was performed in all of these study patients prior to discharge. These low-risk patients were age <60 years of age and had no significant comorbidities, no signs of shock, no history of varices or liver disease, no severe anemia, no frequent hematemesis or melena, and had follow-up care.[33,34,40] Risk stratification for patients with LGIB has not been well studied and therefore most patients with significant lower sources of bleeding are admitted for further management.

PITFALLS

- Normal vital signs do not rule out a life-threatening episode of GIB.
- Failure to adequately and aggressively resuscitate and obtain prompt consultation in patients with GIB may lead to increased morbidity and mortality.

REFERENCES

1. Hussain H, Lapin S and Cappell MS. Clinical scoring systems for determining the prognosis of gastrointestinal bleeding. *Gastroenterol Clin North Am.* 2000;29:445.
2. Wilcox CM, Clark WS. Causes and outcome of upper and lower gastrointestinal bleeding: the Grady Hospital experience. *South Med J.* 1999;92:44.
3. Peter DJ, Dougherty JM. Evaluation of the patient with gastrointestinal bleeding: an evidence based approach. *Emerg Med Clin North Am.* 1999;17:239.
4. Longstreth GF. Epidemiology of hospitalization for acute upper gastrointestinal hemorrhage: a population-based study. *Am J Gastroenterol.* 1995;90:206.
5. Longstreth GF. Epidemiology and outcome of patients hospitalized with acute lower gastrointestinal hemorrhage: a population-based study. *Am J Gastroenterol.* 1997;92:419.
6. Rockall TA, Logan RF, Devlin HB, et al. Risk assessment after acute upper gastrointestinal haemorrhage. *Gut.* 1996; 38:316.
7. Kollef MH, O'Brien JD, Zuckerman GR, et al. BLEED: a classification tool to predict outcomes in patients with acute upper and lower gastrointestinal hemorrhage. *Crit Care Med.* 1997;25:1125.
8. Jensen DM, Machicado GA. Colonoscopy for diagnosis and treatment of severe lower gastrointestinal bleeding. Routine outcomes and cost analysis. *Gastrointest Endosc Clin N Am.* 1997;7:477.
9. Hernandez-Diaz S, Rodriguez LA. Association between nonsteroidal anti-inflammatory drugs and upper gastrointestinal tract bleeding/perforation: an overview of epidemiologic studies published in the 1990s. *Arch Intern Med.* 2000;160:2093.
10. Foutch PG. Diverticular bleeding: are nonsteroidal anti-inflammatory drugs risk factors for hemorrhage and can colonoscopy predict outcome for patients? *Am J Gastroenterol.* 1995;90:1779.
11. Peura DA, Lanza FL, Gostout CJ, et al. The American College of Gastroenterology Bleeding Registry: preliminary findings. *Am J Gastroenterol.* 1997;92:924.
12. Wilcox CM, Alexander LN, Cotsonis G. A prospective characterization of upper gastrointestinal hemorrhage presenting with hematochezia. *Am J Gastroenterol.* 1997; 92:231.
13. Ernst AA, Haynes ML, Nick TG, et al. Usefulness of the blood urea nitrogen/creatinine ratio in gastrointestinal bleeding. *Am J Emerg Med.* 1999;17:70.
14. Chalasani N, Clark WS, Wilcox CM: blood urea nitrogen to creatinine concentration in gastrointestinal bleeding: a reappraisal. *Am J Gastroenterol.* 1997;92:1796.
15. Bellotto F, Fagiuoli S, Pavei A, et al. Anemia and ischemia: myocardial injury in patients with gastrointestinal bleeding. *Am J Med.* 2005;118:548.
16. Prendergast HM, Sloan EP, Cumpston K, et al. Myocardial infarction and cardiac complications in emergency department patients admitted to the intensive care unit with gastrointestinal hemorrhage. *J Emerg Med.* 2005;28:19.
17. Andrews AH, Lake JM, Shorr AF. Ineffectiveness of routine abdominal radiography in patients with gastrointestinal hemorrhage admitted to an intensive care unit. *J Clin Gastroenterol.* 2005;39:228.
18. Tobin K, Klein J, Barbieri C, et al. Utility of routine admission chest radiographs in patients with acute gastrointestinal hemorrhage admitted to an intensive care unit. *Am J Med.* 1996;101:349.
19. Aljebreen AM, Fallone CA, Barkun AN. Nasogastric aspirate predicts high-risk endoscopic lesions in patients with acute upper-GI bleeding. *Gastrointestinal Endoscopy.* 2004;59:172.
20. Witting MD, Magder L, Heins AE, et al. Usefulness and validity of diagnostic nasogastric aspiration in patients without hematemesis. *Ann Emerg Med.* 2004;43:525.
21. Leung FW. The venerable nasogastric tube. *Gastrointest Endosc.* 2004;59:255.
22. Imperiale TF, Birgisson S. Somatostatin or octreotide compared with H2 antagonists and placebo in the management of acute nonvariceal upper gastrointestinal hemorrhage: a meta-analysis. *Ann Intern Med.* 1997;127:1062.
23. Jenkins SA, Shields R, Davies M, et al. A multicentre randomised trial comparing octreotide and injection sclerotherapy in the management and outcome of acute variceal haemorrhage. *Gut.* 1997;41:526.
24. Gotzsche PC. Somatostatin or octreotide for acute bleeding oesophageal varices.[update in Cochrane Database Syst Rev. 2002;(1):CD000193; PMID: 11869569]. *Cochrane Database Syst Rev.* 2000;CD000193.
25. Khuroo MS, Khuroo MS, Farahat KL, et al. Treatment with proton pump inhibitors in acute non-variceal upper gastrointestinal bleeding: a meta-analysis. *J Gastroenterol Hepatol.* 2005;20:11.
26. Bardou M, Toubouti Y, Benhaberou-Brun D, et al. Meta-analysis: proton-pump inhibition in high-risk patients with acute peptic ulcer bleeding. *Aliment Pharmacol Ther.* 2005; 21:677.

27. Leontiadis GI, McIntyre L, Sharma VK, et al. Proton pump inhibitor treatment for acute peptic ulcer bleeding. *Cochrane Database Syst Rev.* 2004;CD002094.

28. Grace ND, Bhattacharya K. Pharmacologic therapy of portal hypertension and variceal hemorrhage. *Clin Liver Dis.* 1997;1:59.

29. Levine JE, Leontiadis GI, Sharma VK, et al. Meta-analysis: the efficacy of intravenous H2-receptor antagonists in bleeding peptic ulcer. *Aliment Pharmacol Ther.* 2002;16:1137.

30. Walt RP, Cottrell J, Mann SG, et al. Continuous intravenous famotidine for haemorrhage from peptic ulcer. *Lancet.* 1992;340:1058.

31. Van Dam J, Brugge WR. Endoscopy of the upper gastrointestinal tract. *N Engl J Med.* 1999;341:1738.

32. Cooper GS, Chak A, Way LE, et al. Early endoscopy in upper gastrointestinal hemorrhage: associations with recurrent bleeding, surgery, and length of hospital stay. *Gastrointest Endosc.* 1999;49:145.

33. Rockall TA, Logan RF, Devlin HB, et al. Selection of patients for early discharge or outpatient care after acute upper gastrointestinal haemorrhage. National Audit of Acute Upper Gastrointestinal Haemorrhage. *Lancet.* 1996; 347:1138.

34. Longstreth GF, Feitelberg SP. Outpatient care of selected patients with acute non-variceal upper gastrointestinal haemorrhage. *Lancet.* 1995;345:108.

35. Jensen DM, Machicado GA, Jutabha R, et al. Urgent colonoscopy for the diagnosis and treatment of severe diverticular hemorrhage. *N Engl J Med.* 2000;342:78.

36. Strate LL, Orav EJ, Syngal S. Early predictors of severity in acute lower intestinal tract bleeding. *Arch Intern Med.* 2003; 163:838.

37. Levy R, Barto W, Gani J. Retrospective study of the utility of nuclear scintigraphic-labelled red cell scanning for lower gastrointestinal bleeding. *ANZ J Surg.* 2003;73:205.

38. Suzman MS, Talmor M, Jennis R, et al. Accurate localization and surgical management of active lower gastrointestinal hemorrhage with technetium-labeled erythrocyte scintigraphy. *Ann Surg.* 1996;224:29.

39. Fallah MA, Prakash C, Edmundowicz S. Acute gastrointestinal bleeding. *Med Clin North Am.* 2000;84:1183.

40. Courtney AE, Mitchell RM, Rocke L, et al. Proposed risk stratification in upper gastrointestinal haemorrhage: is hospitalisation essential? *Emerg Med J.* 2004;21:39.

13

Bowel Obstruction and Volvulus

David M. Cline

Roy L. Alson

HIGH YIELD FACTS

- The sensitivity of plain abdominal radiographs for bowel obstruction is 77%, while the sensitivity for computed tomography (CT) scan is 93%.
- The sensitivity of CT scan for the diagnosis of ischemia associated with bowel obstruction is 83%, with a specificity of 92%, a positive predictive value of 79%, and a negative predictive value of 93%.
- Plain films of the abdomen miss sigmoid volvulus in 44% of cases.

The presentation of small bowel obstruction (SBO) is similar to that of large bowel obstruction (LBO); however, the epidemiology of each is significantly different and, therefore, the patients represented by each diagnostic entity are different. This chapter will contrast small and large bowel obstruction and each of its major classifications, including volvulus. Mechanical obstruction is defined by the presence of a physical barrier to passage of the intraluminal contents of the bowel. Simple obstruction refers to the partial or complete blockage to flow, but without vascular compromise. Closed loop obstruction is defined by complete obstruction at two sequential points, typically by a twisted loop of bowel. Strangulated bowel implies complete obstruction with compromise of the vascular supply and proceeds to perforation without intervention.

EPIDEMIOLOGY

The etiology of bowel obstruction differs in developed countries compared to third-world countries were most hernias remain untreated and strangulated hernia is more common, and outcomes are worse. In developed countries, small bowel obstruction (SBO) accounts for approximately 1% of all hospital admissions and 28.8% of major laparotomies.[1] The ratio of SBO to LBO is 3:1 to 4:1.[2,3] Overall mortality for SBO is 5% for those treated surgically, and 8% for those treated nonsurgically.[4] In contrast, for those patients sustaining strangulation and perforation, the mortality rate approaches 30%.[1] Readmission rate after the index admission for SBO is 15% for those treated surgically and 19% for those treated nonsurgically.[4] Mortality for LBO varies, but may be as high as 19%.[5] Table 13-1 lists the causes of SBO, and Table 13-2 lists the causes of LBO; etiologies are listed in decreasing order of frequency, referenced to developed countries.[1–6] Although fecal impaction is listed last as a cause of LBO, it is a common cause of partial bowel obstruction. By definition, pseudo-obstruction (Ogilvie syndrome), is not a cause of colonic obstruction, but may present with identical symptoms.

PATHOPHYSIOLOGY

Obstruction can be caused by intrinsic lesions (involving the bowel wall), extrinsic lesions (outside the bowel), or intraluminal lesions, such as foreign bodies. Physical obstruction initially causes the accumulation of intraluminal contents with associated distension of the proximal portion of the intestines. Secondary increased peristalsis occurs both above and below the site of obstruction, which explains the loose stools that may be seen early in the course of the disease. Increased secretory activity follows, further distending the bowel proximal to the obstruction, which impairs the ability of the bowel wall to absorb the extra fluid. These factors increase vascular and lymphatic pressures, prompting edema of the bowel wall, further exacerbating distension and vascular compromise. Microvascular changes may allow entry of gut flora into the circulation, resulting in bacteremia. If the situation does not resolve, or is left untreated, perforation follows. The associated vomiting, intraperitoneal fluid sequestration, and eventual sepsis further lead to hypovolemia and ultimately shock. The patient's course and symptoms are affected by the comorbid conditions and the site of obstruction. Older patients are more likely to sustain obstruction and to be subject to complications. In general, the more distal the obstruction, the longer the period is between the onset of obstruction and presentation. Closed loop obstruction prevents retrograde flow and has a more rapid course for both symptoms and serious complications.

Table 13-1. Causes of Small Bowel Obstruction

Adhesions
Strangulated hernia
Crohn disease
Neoplasia
Radiation
Intussusception
Volvulus
Gallstones
Bezoar
Foreign body

Table 13-3. Clinical Findings in Bowel Obstruction[2]

Clinical Finding	Percent of Patients with Finding
Symptom	
Absence of passage of flatus	90%
Absence of passage of feces	81%
Vomiting	77%
Abdominal discomfort	66%
Nausea	59%
Sign	
Abdominal distention	66%
Guarding	37%
Rebound tenderness	5%

CLINICAL FEATURES

The symptoms of bowel obstruction in decreasing order are: absence of passage of flatus, and/or feces, vomiting, abdominal discomfort, and nausea, see Table 13-3.[2] Colicky pain, seen in 74% of those with pain, is more common in SBO, while constant pain is seen in 14.6% of patients.[2] Small bowel obstruction more commonly results in periumbilical pain versus hypogastric pain, which is more common with LBO.[7] The most common sign is abdominal distension; guarding is seen in 37%, while rebound tenderness is seen in only 5%.[2] Peritoneal signs suggest perforation. Early in the disease course, bowel sounds have high-pitched rushes, but this finding diminishes with time. The patient may have surgical scars, hernias, or intraabdominal masses associated with the obstruction. Clinical signs of dehydration and/or shock may be present (tachycardia, hypotension, and delayed capillary refill). Rectal exam may reveal impaction, occult blood, or carcinoma. Passage of stool does not rule out obstruction as 19% of those with obstruction will report continued passage of feces. Women may have palpable gynecologic neoplasms on pelvic exam. Large bowel obstruction is more common in the elderly and the institutionalized patient.

Table 13-2. Causes of Large Bowel Obstruction

Colon cancer
Adhesions
Hernias
Extrinsic cancer
Diverticulitis
Volvulus
Fecal impaction

Historical variables can be used to predict bowel obstruction. Böhner and colleagues studied 704 patients with abdominal pain. Clinical findings with the highest sensitivity for bowel obstruction included a distended abdomen, increased bowel sounds, a history of constipation, previous abdominal surgery, age over 50, and a history of vomiting. If only patients with 2 of these symptoms were sent for films, 42% of radiographs could be avoided, and no patient would be missed.[8] Eskelinin and colleagues found the strongest predictor of SBO was a history of previous abdominal surgery with a relative risk (RR) of 12.1. Other predictors include colicky versus steady pain, (RR = 2.4), abdominal distension, (RR = 13.1), and abnormal bowel sounds (RR = 9.0).[9] An earlier study looked for predictors of strangulation and found a positive correlation with age (greater than 70 years), feculent vomiting, peristaltic sounds, and a white blood cell count higher than 18,000/mm.[3,10] Strangulation shows no correlation with onset, localization or type of pain, duration of symptoms, temperature, tachycardia, or plain x-ray findings.[10]

DIAGNOSIS AND DIFFERENTIAL

Bowel obstruction is suspected clinically and diagnosed primarily by radiographs (Figures 13-1–13-4). Laboratory analysis plays little role in the diagnosis, but may aid in determining the severity in associated complications, dehydration, or shock. Suspicion of bowel obstruction remains one of the few clear indications for plain abdominal radiography or the acute obstruction series, a supine film, an upright abdominal film, and a posterior-anterior chest radiograph. The sensitivity of plain films

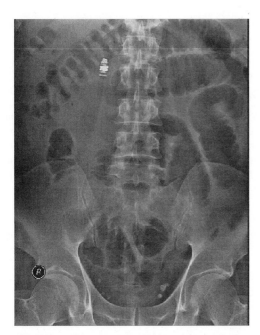

Fig. 13-1. Supine abdomen of bowel obstruction. Supine abdomen showing multiple dilated loops of small bowel. Additionally, a metallic foreign body is seen.

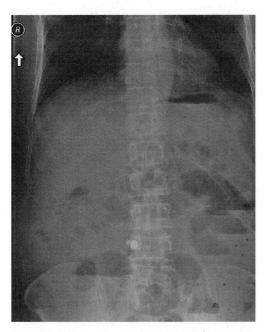

Fig. 13-2. Upright abdomen of bowel obstruction. Upright view of abdomen showing dilated loops of small bowel with multiple air fluid levels. Additionally, a metallic foreign body is seen.

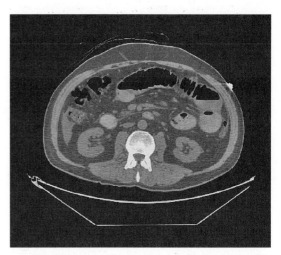

Fig. 13-3. CT Image of small bowel obstruction. CT image of a patient with small bowel obstruction showing dilated loops of small bowel with air fluid levels.

for bowel obstruction is 77%, while the sensitivity for CT scan is 93%.[11] In a study of pretest diagnostic accuracy, the pre-CT suspicion of bowel obstruction was accurate in only 39% of cases; conversely, 50% of those found to have bowel obstruction by CT exam were suspected of other disorders prior to scan.[12] Based on 743 patients in a 2005 metaanalysis, the sensitivity of CT for the diagnosis of bowel obstruction with ischemia was 83%, the

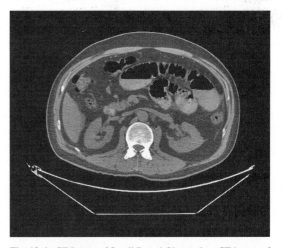

Fig. 13-4. CT Image of Small Bowel Obstruction. CT image of the abdomen showing dilated loops of small bowel and the beginning of the transition point in the right abdomen (left hand portion of the image). Beyond this point, the bowel collapsed indicating the transition point.

specificity was 92%, the positive predictive value was 79%, and the negative predictive value was 93%.[13] Enteroclysis (oral contrast given with the assistance of a tube passed beyond the pylorus) with CT has been recommended in this setting, but may be beyond the capability of many emergency departments.[14]

Volvulus

Chronic constipation is a risk factor for sigmoid volvulus as a large redundant colon is produced and is more likely to twist.[15,16] Other risk factors for sigmoid volvulus include advancing age, institutionalization, and prolonged bed rest. Volvulus occurs when a loop of large bowel twists on a fixed point at the base. Most commonly this occurs at the sigmoid, but also at the cecum and rarely in the transverse colon. Sigmoid volvulus presents identically to other forms of LBO. Volvulus is frequently missed or misinterpreted on plain films. A 2006 retrospective study found that plain films of the abdomen missed 44% of 29 cases of sigmoid volvulus.[16] In that review, it was found that only 58% of patients with sigmoid volvulus complained of pain, while 79% complained of abdominal distension and 55% complained of obstipation. In a Veterans Affairs study, 22% of patients with sigmoid volvulus presented with a clinical picture of constipation with nausea, vomiting, and abdominal pain; 67% had abdominal distension.[15] Sigmoid volvulus is treated first with endoscopic detorsion, and is successful in approximately 81% of cases,[15] unless the patient has signs of gangrene or peritonitis, in which case surgery is indicated. There is a high recurrence rate, as much as 43%.[16] Constipation is not a clear risk factor for cecal volvulus; however, it is frequently misdiagnosed and should be considered in patients thought clinically to have bowel obstruction.[16,17]

Pseudoobstruction (Ogilvie Syndrome)

Colonic pseudoobstruction or Ogilvie syndrome may present with symptoms identical to colonic obstruction: vomiting, abdominal distension, and cramping pain. However, it typically has a more prolonged onset, occurring over several weeks or even months. On investigation with CT scanning or at surgery, no mechanical obstruction is found. It can lead to chronic dilation of the colon and can be fatal. Initial treatment consists of cessation of any drugs that may be causing the disorder (i.e., narcotics, anticholinergics) bowel rest and intravenous fluids and enemas as needed. Consultation for colonoscopic decompression may be needed. Exclusion of true obstruction may require Gastrografin or barium enema.

EMERGENCY DEPARTMENT CARE AND DISPOSITION

With mechanical bowel obstruction, prompt surgical consultation is required, although, approximately three fourths of patients with SBO can be treated nonsurgically while being observed in-hospital.[4] If surgery is being considered, it should be accomplished within 24 hours, as further delays lead to significant complications.[18] A nasogastric tube is used to decompress the bowel. Use of long intestinal tubes in the emergency department is not indicated. Fluid resuscitation should be started using crystalloid. Monitor vital signs and urine output to measure response to fluids. Appropriate antibiotic therapy (such as piperacillin-tazobactam 3.375 g, or ampicillin-sulbactam 3.0 g IV) should be started if perforation is suspected or surgery is anticipated (use should be discussed with surgical consultant). For adynamic ileus, conservative treatment including nasogastric decompression, fluid replacement, and observation are usually effective.

PITFALLS

- Using the passage of stool to rule out obstruction (19% of those with obstruction will report continued passage of feces).
- Ruling out strangulation on clinical grounds alone. (Strangulation shows no correlation with onset, localization or type of pain, duration of symptoms, temperature, tachycardia, or plain x-ray findings.)

REFERENCES

1. Ellis H. The clinical significance of adhesions: focus on intestinal obstruction. *Eur J Surg Supp.* 1997;577:5.
2. Markogiannakis H, Messaris E, Dardamanis D, et al. Acute mechanical bowel obstruction: clinical presentation, etiology, management and outcome. *World J Gastroenterol.* 2007;13:432.
3. Mohamed AY, al-Ghaithi A, Langevin JM, et al. Causes and management of intestinal obstruction in a Saudi Arabian hospital. *J R Coll Surg Edinb.* 1997;42:21.
4. Foster NM, McGory JL, Zingmond DS, et al. Small bowel obstruction: a population-based appraisal. *J Am Coll Surg.* 2006;203:170.

5. Biondo S, Pares D, Frago R, et al. Large bowel obstruction: predictive factors for postoperative mortality. *Dis Colon Rectum.* 2004;47:1889.

6. Miller G, Boman J, Shrier I, et al. Etiology of small bowel obstruction. *Am J Surg.* 2000;180:33.

7. Becker WF. Intestinal obstruction: an analysis of 1007 cases. *South Med J.* 1955;48:41.

8. Bohner H, Yang Q, Franke C, et al. Simple data from history and physical examination help to exclude bowel obstruction and to avoid radiographic studies in patients with acute abdominal pain. *Eur J Surg.* 1998;164:777.

9. Eskelinen M, Ikonen J, Lipponen P. Contributions of history-taking, physical examination, and computer assistance to diagnosis of acute small-bowel obstruction: a prospective study of 1333 patients with acute abdominal pain. *Scand J Gastroenterol.* 1994;29:715.

10. Bizer LS, Liebling RW, Delany HM. Small bowel obstruction: the role of nonoperative treatment in simple intestinal obstruction and predictive criteria for strangulation obstruction. *Surgery.* 1981;89:407.

11. Suri S, Gupta S, Sudhakar PJ, et al. Comparative evaluation of plain films, ultrasound and CT in the diagnosis of intestinal obstruction. *Acta Radiol.* 1999;40:422.

12. Rosen MP, Siewert B, Sands DZ, et al. Value of abdominal CT in the emergency department for patients with abdominal pain. *Eur Radiol.* 2003;13:418.

13. Mallo RD, Salem L, Lalani T, Flum DR. Computed tomography diagnosis of ischemia and complete obstruction in small bowel obstruction: A systematic review. *J Gastrointest Surg.* 2005;9:690.

14. Gollub MJ. Multidetector computed tomography enteroclysis of patients with small bowel obstruction: A volume-rendered "surgical perspective." *J Comput Assist Tomogr.* 2005;29:401.

15. Grossman EM, Longo WE, Stratton MP, et al. Sigmoid volvulus in Department of Veterans Affairs Medical Centers. *Dis Colon Rectum.* 2000;43:414.

16. Lau KC, Miller BJ, Schache DJ, Cohen JR. A study of large-bowel volvulus in urban Australia *Can J Surg.* 2006; 49:203.

17. Anderson JR, Mills JO. Caecal volvulus: a frequently missed diagnosis? *Clin Radiol.* 1984;35:65.

18. Bickell NA, Federman AD, Aufses AH. Influence of time on risk of bowel resection in complete small bowel obstruction. *J Am Coll Surg.* 2005;201:847.

14

Hernia in Adults and Children

Joseph C. Schmidt

HIGH YIELD FACTS

- In the United States hernia repair is the most common major general surgical procedure with approximately 1.2 million performed annually.
- No imaging modality possesses the sensitivity and specificity to reliably eliminate hernia as a potential diagnosis.

EPIDEMIOLOGY

The term hernia describes the protrusion of all or part of an organ through a defect in its surrounding support structure. This discussion is limited to the herniation of abdominal contents through defects in the abdominal wall, diaphragm, or other internal structures.

In the United States approximately1.2-million abdominal wall hernia repairs are performed each year, making this the most common major operation performed by general surgeons.[1] Groin hernias account for 75% with the vast majority being inguinal (direct or indirect) and a much smaller proportion being femoral. Umbilical hernias are also common with 175,000 annual repairs. It should be noted that the majority of umbilical hernias do not require surgical repair and therefore the actual incidence is much greater. Incisional hernias account for approximately 10% of all repairs.[1]

Inguinal hernias have a male to female ratio of 9:1 while femoral hernias are more common in women with a 1:3 ratio.[2,3] Risk of herniation increases with age and the lifetime risk in men approaches 25%.[4] Anterior abdominal wall hernias including incisional occur equally in men and women with increased frequency over the age of 40 years. Children may present with life-threatening diaphragmatic hernias at birth but more commonly they have congenital inguinal or umbilical hernias.

PATHOPHYSIOLOGY

The process of herniation begins with all or part of an abdominal organ passing into a defect in a surrounding structure. If the affected organ can freely return to its original position, then minimal symptoms are usually present, with the possible exception of a bulge or mass. If the hernia becomes entrapped in the defect, swelling and pain occur and the hernia is considered to be incarcerated. Persistent swelling or twisting of the neck of the hernia can compromise the vascular supply and lead to ischemia and eventual death of the organ. This condition is referred to as strangulation.

The etiology of hernia development is more complex (Table 14-1) but falls into three major categories: congenital predisposition, increased intraabdominal pressure, and trauma. Family history, connective tissue diseases, and low birth weight have been associated with increased incidence of hernias.[4,5] Increased intraabdominal pressure as a predisposing factor is well accepted but not well studied. Iatrogenic trauma, in the form of incisional hernias, account for nearly 10% of all hernia repairs.[1] A direct blow can cause a hernia without the presence of an open wound as described in cases of "handlebar" hernias.[6]

The anatomic location of the hernia can be a key feature in the presentation. Groin hernias are most common and fall into three major categories. Indirect inguinal hernias pass through a patent internal (deep) inguinal ring and into the inguinal canal. Direct inguinal hernias pass directly though the fascial and muscular structures of the abdominal wall medial to the inferior epigastric vessels. A pantaloon hernia is a combination of both direct and indirect features. Femoral hernias protrude through a defect in the transversalis fascia inferior to the inguinal ligament.

A hernia though the ventral abdominal wall can occur in the superior midline (epigastric), around the umbilicus (umbilical) , along the lateral edge of the rectus muscle (Spigelian) ,or anywhere a surgical incision has been made (incisional). Although uncommon, hernias can occur in the pelvic floor (pelvic), the superior or inferior lumbar triangles (lumbar), the obturator foramen (obturator), or through various structures completely contained within the abdomen (internal).

CLINICAL FEATURES

Patients may present with a constellation of symptoms ranging from none to mesenteric ischemia induced septic shock. Typical historical features include pain at the site

Table 14-1. Causative Factors Associated with Abdominal Wall Hernias*

Coughing	Obesity
COPD	Pregnancy
Family history of hernia	Low birth weight
Straining (constipation/ prostatism)	Valsalva maneuvers
	Ascites
Heavy lifting	Connective tissue disorders
Peritoneal dialysis	Trauma
Previous surgery	

*Other less common etiologies exist.
Abbreviation: COPD, chronic obstructive pulmonary disease.

of the hernia with an associated mass. The symptoms are often intermittent and get progressively worse later in the day. Maneuvers that increase intraabdominal pressure often exacerbate symptoms. Resting in the supine position will often improve the pain. Inguinal hernias will frequently have referred pain to the testicle. Hernias in the pelvic floor, lumbar triangle, and obturator foramen will present atypically and are often missed until complications arise.

The physical exam in a patient suspected of having a hernia consists of a careful inspection of the area in question, and the examiner should attempt to define the borders of the defect. Significant tenderness, discoloration, or generalized abdominal signs may indicate ischemia or obstruction. Examination of the inguinal canal should be accomplished with the patient both supine and standing. The examiner places the tip of the index finger at the most dependant part of the scrotum and directs it to the external inguinal ring. The patient is asked to strain but the practice of having the patient cough is discouraged as it leads to the overdiagnosis of hernia.[7] The overall accuracy of physical exam has been estimated to have a sensitivity of 74.5% and a specificity of 96.3%.[8] The ability to accurately diagnose indirect and direct hernias is lower and estimated to be 80% and 60%, respectively.[9,10] This may be important because direct hernias are presumed to have a lower complication rate and surgical referral may be delayed.

The complications of hernia include chronic pain, bowel obstruction, and ischemia of abdominal contents. The complication rate is highest when the defect is small.[11] Ischemia may be present in the absence of obstruction when only part of the bowel wall (Richter

hernia) or other abdominal structures, such as the omentum, are involved.

DIAGNOSIS AND DIFFERENTIAL

The gold standard for the diagnosis of hernias is surgery. Suggestive features in the history and physical may be sufficient to warrant surgical evaluation and repair. When the diagnosis is in doubt, additional investigations may be helpful.

Laboratory analysis will be normal unless the hernia is complicated by obstruction or bowel ischemia, and these complications are often associated with a leukocytosis. Early bowel obstruction will present with laboratory findings consistent with vomiting and volume depletion. Progression to bowel ischemia may produce metabolic acidosis, further leukocytosis with left shift, azotemia, or elevated phosphate levels but none of these tests is sensitive or specific.[12,13]

Plain radiography is helpful only in the diagnosis of complications and alternate diagnoses. Upright abdominal films may reveal free air and preempt any further evaluation. Small bowel obstruction may be evidenced by dilated loops of small bowel, air fluid levels, and a paucity of distal air (Figure 14-1). Ultrasound may add considerable information in questionable cases. Diagnostic accuracy in children was improved from 84% to 97.9% when ultrasound was added to clinical assessment.[14] Other investigations have determined ultrasound to have a sensitivity of 92.7% and specificity of 81.5% in diagnosing inguinal hernias based on size of the inguinal ring.[8] Ultrasound has also proved useful in determining incarceration,[15] uncommon hernias,[16] alternate diagnoses,[17] and in assisting in manual reduction thereby decreasing emergency surgery rates.[18]

Computed tomography (CT) has demonstrated particular usefulness in diagnosing unusual hernia locations (i.e., internal),[19] complicated presentations like acute appendicitis in a femoral hernia,[20] or in patients who are difficult to assess because of obesity.[21] Hernia complications were also aided with the addition of CT scanning (Figure 14-2). Several investigations have found the sensitivity and specificity of CT in diagnosing small bowel obstruction to range from 87% to 94% and 86% to 96%, respectively.[22,23] Additional sensitivity for hernia detection can be gained with the increased use of multidetector helical scanners allowing dynamic scanning during a Valsalva maneuver,[24] yielding a sensitivity for hernia detection of approximately 83%.[24,25]

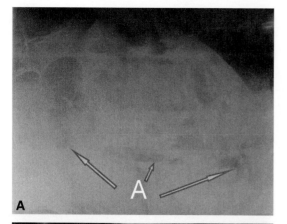

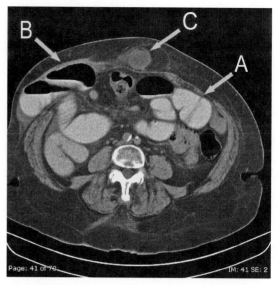

Fig. 14-2. CT findings of incarcerated hernia complicated by small bowel obstruction. The CT of the same patient demonstrates dilated, contrast filled loops of small bowel (A) with associated air fluid levels passing through an unobstructed ventral hernia (B) with no contrast beyond a presumed incarcerated portion of bowel in a second ventral hernia (C).

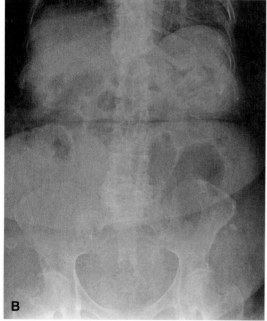

Fig. 14-1. A and B. Abdominal series (left lateral decubitus and supine views) findings of incarcerated hernia complicated by small bowel obstruction. The abdominal series; the left lateral decubitus view demonstrates air fluid levels in loops of small bowel (A) indicative of small bowel obstruction, and the supine view demonstrates a paucity of distal air (B).

Other imaging modalities have been employed with success. Dynamic magnetic resonance imaging (MRI) has been reported to detect hernias with a sensitivity of 94.5% and specificity of 96.3%.[8] Herniography has also been suggested when the diagnosis remains unclear, but may be limited by its invasive nature.[26]

The differential diagnosis of hernias is extensive (Table 14-2). Primary scrotal pathology can be difficult to distinguish from hernia and consideration of testicular torsion is particularly important because of its time sensitive nature. Lymphadenopathy is also commonly a confounding diagnosis. A generous femoral fat pad (femoral pseudohernia) can be misdiagnosed as a hernia.[27]

EMERGENCY DEPARTMENT CARE AND DISPOSITION

The primary goal in the emergency treatment of hernias is to identify those patients who have strangulation physiology. These patients require aggressive

Table 14-2. Differential Diagnosis of Hernias

Lymph node	Spermatocele
Varicocele	Epididymitis
Testicular torsion	Testicular tumor
Hydrocele	Ectopic testicle
Undescended testicle	Sebaceous cyst
Hematoma	Ascites
Abscess	Femoral artery aneurysm
Lipoma	Lymphogranuloma venereum
Hydradenitis suppurativa	Epidermal inclusion
Femoral fat pad (pseudohernia) cyst	

fluid resuscitation, electrolyte replacement, nasogastric decompression, broad spectrum antibiotics, and emergent surgical consultation. Surgical consultation should occur prior to attempting manual reduction if the duration and severity of symptoms suggest the presence of ischemic or necrotic tissue in the hernia.

Patients presenting with incarcerated hernias require urgent reduction to avoid further complications. An initial trial of passive reduction can be attempted. Gravity alone may reduce the hernia if the patient is comfortable and placed in proper position. Trendelenburg position should be employed for groin hernias, while ventral wall hernias may be left supine. Adequate sedation and analgesia is key. A cool compress over the hernia may reduce swelling. If passive reduction is unsuccessful, manual reduction may be attempted.

Manual reduction requires a comfortable and cooperative patient. Following adequate sedation the examiner should locate the defect and position one hand at the edge opposite the reducing hand. This will help to prevent the hernia contents from expanding around the defect and will facilitate reduction.[28] Gentle, constant pressure can then be applied to the hernia. Multiple or vigorous attempts at manual reduction are not recommended. If manual reduction is successful, a period of observation is warranted but if symptoms persist or progress, a diagnosis of partial reduction or the reduction of strangulated contents must be considered. Successful reduction of hernias with the highest rate of recurrence, namely pediatric inguinal and all femoral hernias, requires urgent surgical referral to reduce the risk of intervening complications.[11,29,30] Telephone consultation with a surgeon is recommended in these situations if follow-up cannot be otherwise arranged in 1 week. If manual reduction fails, a surgeon should be consulted in the emergency department.

Patients who present with spontaneously reduced or asymptomatic hernias require little emergent care. If there is no evidence of complications, the patient can be discharged home with primary care or surgical referral and precautions.

PITFALLS

- Failure to recognize and adequately resuscitate patients with strangulated hernias.

- Failure to provide adequate sedation and analgesia when attempting manual hernia reduction.

- Failure to refer for urgent surgical repair successful manual reductions that have the highest rate of recurrent complications, namely pediatric inguinal and all femoral hernias.

REFERENCES

1. Rutkow IM. Demographic and socioeconomic aspects of hernia repair in the United States in 2003. *Surg Clin North Am.* 2003;83:1045.
2. Rutkow IM. Epidemiologic, economic, and sociologic aspects of hernia surgery in the United States in the 1990's. *Surg Clin North Am.* 1998;78:941.
3. Rutkow IM. Demographic, classificatory, and socioeconomic aspects of hernia repair in the United States. *Surg Clin North Am.* 1993;73:413.
4. Abramson JH, Gofin J, Hopp C, et al. The epidemiology of inguinal hernia. A survey in western Jerusalem. *J Epidemiol Community Health.* 1978;32:59.
5. Kitchen WH, Doyle LW, Ford GW. Inguinal hernia in very low birthweight children: a continuing risk to 8 years. *J Paediatr Child Health.* 1991;27:300.
6. Perez VM, McDonald D, Ghani A, et al. Handlebar hernia: A rare traumatic abdominal wall hernia. *J Trauma.* 1998;44:568.
7. Fitsgibbons RJ, Filipi CJ, Quinn TH. Inguinal hernias. In *Schwartz's Principles of Surgery.* 8th ed. New York:-McGraw-Hill, 2004:1365.
8. van den Berg JC, de Valois JC, Go PM, et al. Detection of groin hernia with physical examination, ultrasound, and MRI compared with laparoscopic findings. *Invest Radiol.* 1999; 34:739.
9. Kark AE, Kurzer M, Waters KJ. Accuracy of clinical diagnosis of direct and indirect inguinal hernia. *Br J Surg.* 1994;81:1082.
10. Ralphs DNL, Brain AJL, Grundy DJ, et al. How accurately can direct and indirect inguinal hernias be distinguished? *BMJ.* 1980;12:1039.
11. Gallegos NC, Dawson J, Jarvis M, et al. Risk of strangulation in groin hernias. *Br J Surg.* 1991;78:1171.
12. Kumar S, Sarr MG, Kamath PS. Mesenteric venous thrombosis. *N Engl J Med.* 2001;345:1683.
13. Sreenarasimhaiah J. Diagnosis and management of intestinal ischaemic disorders. *BMJ.* 2003;326:1372.
14. Chen KC, Chu CC, Chou TY, et al. Ultrasonography for inguinal hernias in boys. *J Pediatr Surg.* 1998;33:1784.
15. Rettenbacher T, Hollerweger A, Macheiner P, et al. Abdominal wall hernias: cross-sectional imaging signs of incarceration determined with sonography. *AJR Am J Roentgenol.* 2001; 177:1061.
16. Mufid MM, Abu-yousef MM, Kakish ME, et al. Spigelian hernia: diagnosis by high-resolution real-time sonography. *J Ultrasound Med.* 1997;16:183.
17. Klingler PJ, Wetscher G, Glaser K, et al. The use of ultrasound to differentiate rectus sheath hematoma from other acute disorders. *Surg Endosc.* 1999;13:1129.
18. Chen SC, Lee CC, Liu YP, et al. Ultrasound may decrease the emergency surgery rate of incarcerated inguinal hernia. *Scand J Gastroenterol.* 2005;40:721.
19. Blachar A, Federle MP, Brancatelli G, et al. Radiologist performance in the diagnosis of internal hernia by using specific CT findings with emphasis on transmesenteric hernia. *Radiology.* 2001;221:422.

20. Zissen R, Brautbar O, Shapiro-Feinberg M. CT diagnosis of acute appendicitis in a femoral hernia. *Br JRadiol.* 2000; 73:1013.

21. Rose M, Eliakim R, Bar-Ziv Y, et al. Abdominal wall hernias: The value of computed tomography diagnosis in the obese patient. *J Clin Gastroenterol.* 1994;19:94.

22. Megibow AJ, Balthazar EJ, Cho KC, et al. Bowel obstruction: Evaluation with CT. *Radiology.* 1991;180:313.

23. Jabra AA, Eng J, Zalenski CG, et al. CT of small-bowel obstruction in children: sensitivity and specificity. *AJR Am J Roentogenol.* 2001;177:431.

24. Jaffe TA, O'Connell MJ, Harris JP, et al. MDCT of abdominal wall hernias: is there a role for Valsalva's maneuver? *AJR Am J Roentogenol.* 2005;184:847.

25. Hojer AM, Rygaard H, Jess P. CT in the diagnosis of abdominal wall hernias: a preliminary study. *Eur Radiol.* 1997;7:1416.

26. Hamlin JA, Kahn AM. Herniography: A review of 333 herniograms. *Am Surg.* 1998;64:965.

27. Bendavid R. Femoral pseudi-hernias. *Hernia.* 2002;6:141.

28. Manthey DE. Abdominal hernia reduction. In Robert JR, Hedges JR (eds.): *Clinical Procedures in Emergency Medicine.* 4th ed. Philadelphia: Saunders, 2004:860.

29. Naude GP, Ocon S, Bongard F. Femoral hernia: the dire consequences of a missed diagnosis. *Am J Emerg Med.* 1997; 15:680.

30. Gahukamble DB, Khamage AS. Early versus delayed repair of reduced incarcerated inguinal hernias in the pediatric population. *J Pediatr Surg.* 1996;31:1218.

15

Inflammatory Bowel Disease

Joshua Broder
Christopher Reynolds

HIGH YIELD FACTS

- Computed tomography (CT) scan of the abdomen has a 90% sensitivity for delineating the complications of both Crohn's disease and ulcerative colitis (abscess or obstruction) but only a 70% sensitivity for detecting the associated inflammation.

- Systemic steroids are a mainstay of therapy in Crohn disease and ulcerative colitis (UC) patients requiring hospitalization.

- Although certain ethnic, gender, and age groups are at increased risk, patients of any age, gender, or ethnicity may be affected.

- Laboratory tests are of limited value in predicting severity of illness.

- Physical exam findings are neither sensitive nor specific in determining severity of illness.

Inflammatory bowel diseases (IBDs), including UC and Crohn disease, are characterized by recurring noninfectious inflammatory reactions of the intestine. Ulcerative colitis involves solely the mucosal layer of the large bowel, extending proximally from the rectum in a continuous fashion. Crohn disease may involve any portion of the alimentary tract from mouth to anus, may be transmural, and is noncontiguous.[1]

EPIDEMIOLOGY

Inflammatory bowel diseases are common in North America. For example, in 2001 CDC data indicate 301,000 U.S. admissions for noninfectious enteritis and colitis, compared with 283,000 for appendicitis.[2]

Crohn Disease

Crohn disease affects approximately 400,000 to 600,000 patients, with an incidence of approximately 3.1 to 14.6 cases per 100,000 person-years and a prevalence as high as 144 to 198.5 cases per 100,000 persons. New diagnoses of Crohn disease are made in an estimated 9000 to 44,000 patients per year in North America. Incidence of these diseases has been linked to Caucasian ethnicity, with Caucasians suffering an incidence 10 times higher than Hispanics. Ashkenazi Jews are also at significantly increased risk for both Crohn and UC.[1]

Environmental links have also been implicated, with higher prevalence rates noted in northern latitudes.[3] Cigarette smoking is a well-described risk factor for Crohn disease but may actually reduce the risk of UC.[4] Nonsteroidal anti-inflammatory drugs (NSAIDs) may also be a risk factor and have been linked to disease flares.[4] A slight female predominance has been noted, though estimates range from 48% to 66%. A contributory genetic basis is likely as well, with first degree relatives of patients with IBD having a risk of disease 4 to 20 times higher than the general population. Genetic background does not fully determine the presence of disease, however, as only 45% of identical twin pairs are concordant for Crohn disease.[4]

Mean age at first diagnosis of Crohn is between 33 and 39 years in most studies. However, patients of any age may be affected. Crohn disease may have a bimodal onset, with peaks in incidence in the second or third decade and again, to a lesser degree, in the sixth and seventh decades. The natural history of Crohn disease is one of remission and frequent exacerbation, with up to 10% of patients annually having active disease requiring corticosteroid or other immune modifier therapy, and 30% requiring 5-aminosalicylate therapy. Surgery is commonly required, with between 41% and 57% of patients requiring at least one bowel resection.[3]

Ulcerative Colitis

Ulcerative colitis affects 250,000 to 500,000 individuals in the United States, with an incidence of 2 to 7 per 100,000 per year. It results in 250,000 physician visits annually, with 20,000 hospitalizations.[5] Geographic variations have been noted: in Baltimore, rates of 1 to 3 cases per 100,000 person-years,[6] compared to Sweden with a rate of 7 to 12 cases per 100,000 person-years [7] and Minnesota with a rate of 7.6 cases per 100,000 person-years. Incidence increased from the 1940s to the 1970s and has remained stable since that time. Men and urban dwellers are at increased risk.[8]

PATHOPHYSIOLOGY

Crohn disease and UC are chronic disorders caused by inappropriate activation of the intestinal immune system in the presence of normal bowel flora. There is strong evidence for a genetic component to IBD. Family history is the strongest risk factor for the development of IBD, especially for Crohn disease.[4] Multiple gene mutations have been shown to alter gut immunity and increase the risk of IBD.[9] Genetic heterogeneity may account for the heterogeneous pattern of clinical disease. One widely accepted hypothesis holds that mucosal resistance to bacterial invasion is compromised in susceptible individuals. Environmental factors, such as smoking and exposure to NSAIDs, may also play a role in allowing gut bacteria to penetrate the mucosal layer and stimulate an immune response.[4,10] Although the details are not well understood, there is evidence that different subsets of T-lymphocytes are involved in Crohn disease and UC.[9] Activation of Th-1 lymphocytes in Crohn disease leads to stimulation of macrophages and release of tumor necrosis factor (TNF)-α. This immune response may be responsible for the typical Crohn pattern of discontinuous transmural inflammation and granuloma formation affecting any portion of the gastrointestinal tract. In contrast, UC may be associated with a Th-2 lymphocyte response leading to superficial mucosal and submucosal inflammation limited to the colon and rectum.

CLINICAL FEATURES

Crohn Disease

The classic presentation of Crohn disease is chronic diarrhea and crampy abdominal pain. Diarrhea is reported by over 90% of patients. The incidence of abdominal pain at initial diagnosis ranges from 60% to 95%.[11–13] Although these symptoms are nonspecific, suspicion for Crohn disease should be raised when fever, fatigue, and weight loss are present. Additional features of the disease have been correlated with the anatomic site of involvement.[12] Ileocolic inflammation is present in 41% of patients at presentation and is associated with increased incidence of perianal, internal, and cutaneous fistula formation (34%–38%). Ileocolic and small bowel disease (present in 28.6%) are associated with intestinal obstruction in 35% to 44% of patients. Crohn colitis (present in 27%) is associated with perianal fistulae (36%), arthritis (16%),

and toxic megacolon (11%). Clinical features are presented in Table 15-1.

Patients with mild disease may appear well while others appear fatigued, anemic, or malnourished from anorexia and malabsorption. Abdominal examination is generally nonspecific but may reveal tenderness or a palpable mass. Upper abdominal pain suggests gastric inflammation or duodenitis. Ileocolitis can cause right lower quadrant pain that mimics appendicitis. Fistulizing disease may present with skin findings if enterocutaneous, as recurrent urinary tract infections if enterovesicular, or with abscess formation. Symptoms of obstruction, such as nausea, vomiting, and abdominal distension may be present. Stool will frequently contain occult blood, but gross rectal bleeding is uncommon except in cases of Crohn colitis (46%).[12]

Extraintestinal manifestations of Crohn disease and UC are divided into colitis-associated and small bowel-associated disorders.[14] The colitis-associated disorders tend to worsen with IBD exacerbation and improve with treatment of the underlying disease. These disorders include migratory arthritis, typically of the larger peripheral joints (23%), erythema nodosum or the pustular lesions of pyoderma gangrenosum (15%), and oral (4%) or eye lesions, such as uveitis and episcleritis (4%). A small number of patients experience axial arthritis in the form of sacroileitis or ankylosing spondylitis. The small-bowel associated disorders do not respond to therapy and include malabsorption (10%), gallstones (11%), and renal stones (9%). Patients with IBD are also at increased risk of early osteoporosis, liver disease, pericholangitis, primary sclerosing cholangitis, peptic ulcer disease, amyloidosis, and venous thromboembolism.[14,15]

With current therapy, the life expectancy of patients with Crohn disease approaches that of the general

Table 15-1. Clinical Features of Inflammatory Bowel Diseases

Clinical Features	Ulcerative Colitis	Crohn Disease
Fever	Fairly common	Common
Abdominal pain	Varies	Common
Diarrhea	Very common	Fairly common
Rectal bleeding	Very common	Fairly common
Weight loss	Fairly common	Common
Malnutrition	Fairly common	Common
Perianal disease	Absent	Fairly common
Abdominal mass	Absent	Common
Growth failure (children)	Occasional	Common

population.[16] Most patients have a chronic relapsing and remitting course with long disease-free periods. Crohn disease is not curable, and most patients will require surgical intervention for hemorrhage, perforation, abscess, obstruction, or severe medically refractory disease.

Ulcerative Colitis

The clinical hallmark of UC is rectal bleeding. Abdominal pain in UC is less common and less severe than in Crohn disease. Pain in the abdomen or rectum is reported by 53% of patients at the time of diagnosis.[11] Many patients will also note a change in bowel patterns or tenesmus, weight loss (43%), and fever (27%). Patients with severe exacerbations report six or more diarrheal stools per day with evidence of gross blood, and have fever, tachycardia, anemia, and elevated serum inflammatory markers.[17] Seventy percent of patients present with moderate to severe disease.[11] Ulcerative colitis may present as isolated colonic disease (41%), isolated rectal disease (41%), or pancolitis (16%). Clinical features of UC are presented in Table 15-1.

The physical examination is unremarkable or nonspecific in many patients. Pallor, fatigue, and tachycardia may be present if rectal bleeding has been brisk or prolonged. Abnormal findings on abdominal and rectal examination correspond to the location and severity of disease. Abdominal tenderness and distension are present in fulminant disease and may be present in milder forms unless disease is limited to the rectum.[5] Rectal examination will reveal gross blood in moderate and severe attacks. Rectal fullness or tenderness is present except in some cases of isolated colonic disease. An important complication of fulminant UC is toxic megacolon, defined as tachycardia, fever, leukocytosis, hypoalbuminemia, and colonic dilatation greater than 5 cm in diameter with loss of haustral markings on plain x-ray.[13] Ulcerative colitis and Crohn disease share many extraintestinal complications as discussed above.

Many patients have an indolent form of UC, characterized by chronic recurrent exacerbations, and are able to lead long, productive lives.[5,18] Young age at presentation and severe initial attack are correlated with increased morbidity and mortality.[13,19] Patients with UC are at increased risk for colon cancer.

DIAGNOSIS AND DIFFERENTIAL

The diagnosis of suspected IBD or complications of known disease may require clinical features from history and physical exam, laboratory tests, diagnostic imaging exams, and endoscopy, though not all may be necessary in the emergency department (ED). Ulcerative colitis and Crohn disease are diagnosed based on clinical history and findings on endoscopy or biopsy, as well as negative stool studies for infectious causes of inflammation.[5,16] In the ED, a typical scenario will be the presentation of a patient with previously confirmed disease, or a new presentation with history, exam, and ED work-up suspicious for IBD.

History and Exam

A complete history of present illness is indicated as for any patient with abdominal pain. In UC, younger age may be a risk factor for failure to respond to medical therapy. The duration of the patient's disease and the duration of the current attack do not predict failure of medical therapy. Number of stools per day, fever (>99°F or 37.2°C), and tachycardia greater than 90 beats per minute do not predict outcome.[20] Patients with continued frequent stools, hematochezia, and elevated C-reactive protein (CRP) after admission have an increased risk of requiring colectomy.[21]

Clinical Activity Scores

Multiple clinical activity scores have been described, though none are well validated. The Truelove-Witt class and Clinical Activity Index have been advocated to identify UC patients likely to fail medical therapy.[20] However, clinical activity scores have high variability, and may be poor predictors of an individual patient's clinical course.[22]

Laboratory Evaluation

Serologic markers may assist in the specific diagnosis of Crohn disease and UC, but these tests have little role in the ED. Serologic tests include perinuclear-staining antineutrophil cytoplasmic antibodies, present in 70% of UC, and anti-*Saccharomyces cerevisiae* antibody, found in 50% of Crohn cases.[4]

In the ED, laboratory values including complete blood count, standard chemistry studies, coagulation studies, and markers of inflammatory response such as CRP and sedimentation rate may play a role in assessment. However, total leukocyte count, platelet count, sedimentation rate, potassium, albumin, and fibrin degradation products have not been shown to predict failure of medical therapy for patients with UC. C-reactive protein, hemoglobin, prothrombin time (PT), and fibrinogen levels do appear predictive of response to medical therapy (Table 15-2).[20] Stool studies for ova and parasites, bacteria including *Clostridium difficile*, and viruses are recommended, as superimposed infection may be the cause of flares of both UC and Crohn disease.[21,23]

Table 15-2. Independent Predictors of Treatment Failure in Ulcerative Colitis

Characteristic	Sensitivity	Specificity	P Value
Pedal edema	NR	NR	0.02
Transverse colon diameter >5 cm	NR	NR	<0.0001
Hemoglobin <9 g/dL	80%	73%	0.01
C reactive protein >1.86 mg/dL	89%	59%	0.04
Prothrombin time >14 sec (control 12 sec)	60%	75%	0.002
Fibrinogen <220 mg/dL	75%	90%	0.006

Abbreviation: NR, not reported.

Imaging

Standard x-ray has a limited role in the evaluation of patients, although it may be useful in identifying frank pneumoperitoneum, small bowel obstruction, or toxic megacolon. Studies suggest that the presence of three or more distended loops of small bowel on plain film predict failure of medical management in UC.[24,25] Ultrasound has been described in the evaluation of Crohn disease, having high sensitivity (90%) for the detection of abscesses.[26] Graded compression ultrasonography with color Doppler may also allow detection of stenotic bowel, fistulous tracts, and inflammatory changes marked by increased blood flow.[27] Traditionally, air contrast barium enema or small bowel series were performed and might demonstrate cobblestones, pseudopolyps, separation of bowel loops, or a narrow terminal ileum "string sign."[28,29]

In the ED, cross-sectional imaging methods (CT and magnetic resonance imaging [MRI]) have largely supplanted the above techniques, because of the ability of these tests to diagnose luminal and extraluminal complications, as well as unrelated abdominal emergencies. Computed tomography can detect free air, moderate to high grade stenosis or obstruction, thickened bowel segments representing active disease, abscesses, and fistulas. MRI shares these advantages and does not expose the patient to radiation, making it the diagnostic test of choice for pregnant patients. Early or mild disease may be better diagnosed by traditional methods than by CT or MRI, as these latter methods show poor detail of mucosal abnormalities, which may be the only findings in early disease. Computed tomography may also allow needle or catheter drainage of abscesses. A number of studies have compared the sensitivity and specificity of CT and MR to conventional imaging techniques. Although CT and MR have only an approximately 70% sensitivity for detection of inflammation, when compared with endoscopy, both have excellent sensitivity, in the 90% range, for obstruction and abscess.[27,28] Radiographs of UC and Crohn disease are shown in Figures 15-1 to 15-3.

Enteroclysis, a long-standing technique for evaluation of bowel abnormalities, involves the insertion of a nasojejunal tube and rapid infusion of contrast material to distend the small bowel. Computed tomography and MR enteroclysis show great promise for delineating mucosal abnormalities, although they face the same issues of patient discomfort as traditional enteroclysis.[28,29]

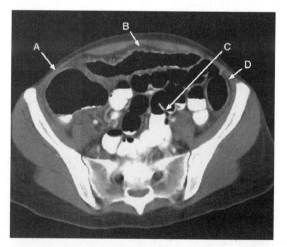

Fig. 15-1. CT scan of the abdomen in a patient with ulcerative colitis. This CT demonstrates diffuse thickening of the ascending, transverse, and descending colon, consistent with pancolitis. This patient developed hemodynamic instability and required emergent colectomy. (A) Ascending colon, (B) Transverse colon, (C) Prominent small bowel loops, consistent with ileus (D) descending colon.

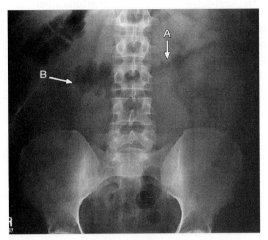

Fig. 15-2. Abdominal radiograph demonstrating colitis. The patient underwent endoscopy which confirmed Crohn disease. (A) Narrowing of the distal transverse colon with thumbprinting (mucosal edema) and featureless descending colon. (B) Proximal transverse colon shows normal haustral markings.

Endoscopy

Though not usually an ED diagnostic procedure, endoscopy may confirm the diagnosis of UC or Crohn disease and may determine clinical severity. Ulcerative colitis is described as demonstrating superficial ulcerations, a friable mucosal surface, altered vascularity of the mucosa, and exudates. Mucosal bleeding is common. Continuous involvement from the rectum is usual in UC but may be altered by medical therapy. Endoscopic findings in Crohn disease include ulcerations, skip areas, cobblestones, pseudopolyps, and rectal sparing.[30]

DIFFERENTIAL DIAGNOSIS

The differential diagnosis of IBD in the ED varies depending on whether the patient being evaluated has a known history of IBD. In patients with abdominal pain but no prior history of IBD, the diagnosis should be considered, particularly in those with a history of indolent or recurring symptoms. Abdominal pain associated with weight loss, diarrhea, bloody stools, and fever should heighten suspicion of IBD. The clinical features of Crohn disease and UC are similar though not identical (Table 15-1).

In patients with a history of IBD, particular attention should be given to known intestinal complications of these diseases, although the broader differential for all abdominal pain must be considered. Intestinal

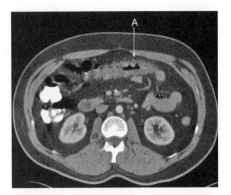

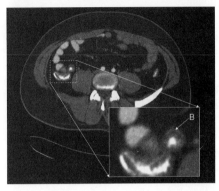

Fig. 15-3. A and B Abdominal CT from patient in figure 15-2. Same patient as shown in Figure 15-2. CT confirms colitis and demonstrates terminal ileitis. The patient underwent endoscopy which confirmed Crohn disease. (A) Thickened transverse colon, corresponding to A in Figure 15-2. (B) Thickened terminal ileum consistent with terminal ileitis of Crohn disease.

complications of Crohn disease and UC are shown in Table 15-3. Extraintestinal complications may also occur, including primary sclerosing cholangitis in a smaller number of Crohn patients. Medication-related and immunosuppression-related derangements should

Table 15-3. Surgical Complications of Inflammatory Bowel Diseases

Intestinal Complications	Ulcerative Colitis	Crohn Disease
Stricture	Unknown	Common
Fistula	Absent	Fairly common
Toxic megacolon	Unknown	Absent
Perforation	Unknown	Uncommon
Cancer	Common	Fairly common

Table 15-4. Pharmacologic Therapy of Inflammatory Bowel Disease

Drug	Dose/Route	Mechanism(s)	Disease/Indication
5-aminosalicylates • Mesalamine • "Rowasa" (rectal suspension enema) • Asacol (delayed release oral form) • Pentasa • Sulfasalzine • Olsalazine • Balsalazide	• Dose varies with agent, from 2.4 g–4.8 g per day divided tid PO/PR (enema) • Specific medication and route chosen to target disease location	• Blocks prostaglandin and leukotriene production, inhibits neutrophil chemotaxis and secretion, scavenges reactive oxygen species	• Mild to moderate UC, distal/left side • Mild to moderate CD
Steroid enemas/foams • Cortifoam	• PR	• Multiple	• Mild to moderate UC, distal/left side • Alternative to 5-ASA for distal disease
Proton pump inhibitors	• PO	• Alteration in gut pH	• Gastroduodenal CD
Oral steroids • Prednisone • Budesonide	• 40 mg PO qd • 9 mg PO qd	• Multiple • Topically active steroid; deactivated by first-pass hepatic metabolism	• UC unresponsive to 5-ASA • Moderate to severe CD • Mild to moderate CD
Purine analogues • 6-mercaptopurine • Azathioprine	• 1.5 mg/kg PO qd • Up to 2.5 mg/kg PO qd	• Inhibit T lymphocyte proliferation	• Moderate to severe CD and UC • Failed response to steroids • Onset takes weeks • Not helpful in acute exacerbation
Methotrexate	• 15 mg/week IM • 25 mg/week SC	• Folate metabolism inhibitor • Inhibits leukocyte proliferation • Multiple	• Moderate to severe CD • Steroid-resistant or dependent • Severe UC and CD • Refractory to oral therapy
IV steroids* • Hydrocortisone* • Methylprednisolone*	• 100 mg IV q8h • 40 mg IV qd		
Antibiotics • Ciprofloxacin • Metronidazole	• 400 mg IV q8 • 750 mg IV q8h	• Treat concurrent infection • Limit bacterial invasion of damaged mucosa	• Empirical use to prevent peritonitis or treat superimposed infection • Likely helpful in CD • Not likely helpful in UC • Limited demonstrated benefit in controlled randomized trials.

*Rule out infection or abscess first; advanced imaging such as CT recommended.
Abbreviations: UC, ulcerative colitis; CD, Crohn disease.

also be suspected. Patients with both UC and Crohn are at increased risk of colon cancer. Infectious mimics of UC include colitis due to *Escherichia coli* O157:H7, and *C. difficile*. Crohn disease may resemble terminal ileitis due to *Yersinia enterocolitica* or *Mycobacterium tuberculosis*. Intestinal lymphomas, celiac sprue, radiation enteropathy, and NSAID-induced enteropathy may have similar presentations. Appendicitis can present with an identical clinical picture to Crohn-related terminal ileitis.[1]

EMERGENCY DEPARTMENT CARE AND DISPOSITION

Emergency department care of UC and Crohn disease focuses on hemodynamic support, antibiotic therapy of acute infectious complications, surgical therapy of structural abnormalities, and immune modulation to induce remission of disease. Intensity of therapy should be modified to fit the clinical severity of the individual patient.

Hemodynamic Support

Intravenous fluid therapy should be guided by clinical judgment and titrated to parameters such as heart rate, blood pressure, and urine output. Transfusion may be necessary in patients with chronic anemia or acute blood loss.

Pharmacologic Therapy

Treatment guidelines for Crohn disease and UC are published by the American College of Gastroenterology.[5,31] Pharmacologic therapy for UC and Crohn disease includes high-dose steroids, other immune modifiers, and antibiotics. A tiered approach to therapy is indicated in Table 15-4. For other treatment options such as cyclosporine and infliximab, consultation with gastroenterology is recommended.[31,32] Antibiotic therapy is recommended for severe exacerbations of IBD with signs of infection. In UC, ciprofloxacin has been used in randomized controlled trials but has not been shown to improve outcome when compared with steroid therapy alone.[33] In Crohn disease, therapy with ciprofloxacin and metronidazole has not been shown to be helpful when added to steroids for ileal disease, but may improve outcome in colonic disease.[34]

Surgical therapy for acute flares of IBD is often required. One-third of patients with acute exacerbation of UC undergo colectomy despite medical therapy, and 1 % to 3% die. No validated objective predictors of the need for surgery exist, although there are generally agreed upon indications for surgery, including perforation, obstruction, abscess, toxic megacolon, massive hemorrhage, fistula,

and failed medical therapy. In a recent multivariate analysis, factors associated with poor response to medical therapy within 48 hours of admission included pedal edema, transverse colonic diameter greater than 5 cm on abdominal radiograph, low hemoglobin, high CRP, low serum fibrinogen, and prolonged PT.[20]

Disposition

Indications for admission include surgical complications, dehydration, refractory pain, vomiting, and failure of oral therapies aimed at inducing disease remission. Patients with mild symptoms may be managed as outpatients with close follow-up.

PITFALLS

- Failure to recognize surgical complications of UC or Crohn disease.
- Overreliance on plain film to exclude pathology.
- Use of normal laboratory values to exclude pathology.
- Failure to administer steroids for severe exacerbations.
- Failure to exclude concurrent infection.

REFERENCES

1. Lasher BA. Inflammatory Bowel Disease. The Cleveland Clinic Disease Management Project. Available at thttp://www.clevelandclinicmeded.com/diseasemanagement/gastro/inflammatory_bowel/inflammatory_bowel1. htm. Accessed August 21, 2007.
2. Kozak LJ, Owings MF, Hall MJ. National Hospital Discharge Survey: 2001 annual summary with detailed diagnosis and procedure data. National Center for Health Statistics. *Vital Health Stat.* 2004;13.
3. Loftus EV, Schoenfled P, Sandborn WJ. The epidemiology and natural history of Crohn's disease in population-based patient cohorts from North America: a systematic review. *Aliment Pharmacol Ther.* 2002;16:51.
4. Podolsky DK. Inflammatory bowel disease. *N Engl J Med.* 2002;347:417.
5. Kornbluth A, Sachar DB. Practice Parameters Committee of the American College of Gastroenterology. Ulcerative colitis practice guidelines in adults (update): American College of Gastroenterology, Practice Parameters Committee. *Am J Gastroenterol.* 2004;99:1371.
6. Calkins BM, Lilienfeld AM, Garland CF, Mendeloff AI. Trends in incidence rates of ulcerative colitis and Crohn's disease. *Dig Dis Sci.* 1984;10:913.
7. Ekbom A, Helmick C, Zack M, Adami HO. The epidemiology of inflammatory bowel disease: a large, population-based study in Sweden. *Gastroenterology.* 1991;100:350.

8. Loftus EV Jr, Silverstein MD, Sandborn WJ, et al. Ulcerative colitis in Olmsted County, Minnesota, 1940–1993: incidence, prevalence, and survival. *Gut.* 2000;46:336.

9. Melmed GY, Abreu MT. New insights into the pathogenesis of inflammatory bowel disease. *Curr Gastroenterol Rep.* 2004;6:474.

10. Garcia Rodriguez LA, Gonzalez-Perez A, Johansson S, et al. Risk factors for inflammatory bowel disease in the general population. *Aliment Pharmacol Ther.* 2005;22:309.

11. Both H, Torp-Pedersen K, Kreiner S, et al. Clinical appearance at diagnosis of ulcerative colitis and Crohn's disease in a regional patient group. *Scand J Gastroenterol.* 1983;18:987.

12. Farmer RG, Hawk WA, Turnbull RB. Clinical patterns in Crohn's disease: a statistical study of 615 cases. *Gastroenterology.* 1975;68:627.

13. Farmer RG. Clinical features and natural history of inflammatory bowel disease. *Med Clin North Am.* 1980;64:1103.

14. Greenstein AJ, Janowitz HD, Sachar DB. The extraintestinal complications of Crohn's disease and ulcerative colitis: a study of 700 patients. *Medicine (Baltimore).* 1976;55:401.

15. Talbot RW, Heppell J, Dozois RR, et al. Vascular complications of inflammatory bowel disease. *Mayo Clin Proc.* 1986;61:140.

16. Hanauer SB, Sandborn W. Practice Parameters Committee of the American College of Gastroenterology. Management of Crohn's disease in adults. *Am J Gastroenterol.* 2001; 96:635.

17. Truelove SC, Witts LJ. Cortisone in ulcerative colitis: final report on a therapeutic trial. *BMJ.* 1955;2:1041.

18. Hendriksen C, Kreiners S, Binder V. Long-term prognosis in ulcerative colitis: based on results from a regional patient group from the county of Copenhagen. *Gut.* 1985;26:158.

19. Edwards FC, Truelove SC. The course and prognosis of ulcerative colitis. *Gut.* 1963;4:299.

20. Kumar S, Ghoshal UC, Aggarwal R, et al. Severe ulcerative colitis: prospective study of parameters determining outcome. *J Gastroenterol Hepatol.* 2004;19:1247.

21. Travis SP, Farrant JM, Ricketts C, et al. Predicting outcome in severe ulcerative colitis. *Gut.* 1996;38:905.

22. Sostegni R, Daperno M, Scaglione N, Lavagna A, Rocca R, Pera A. Review article: Crohn's disease: monitoring disease activity. *Aliment Pharmacol Ther.* 2003;17(Suppl 2):11.

23. Linskens RK, van Bodegraven AA, Schoorl M, Baak JP, et al. Predictive value of inflammatory and coagulation parameters in the course of severe ulcerative colitis. *Dig Dis Sci.* 2001;46:644.

24. Latella G, Vernia P, Viscido A, et al. GI distension in severe ulcerative colitis. *Am J Gastroenterol.* 2002;97:1169.

25. Chew CN, Nolan DJ, Jewell DP. Small bowel gas in severe ulcerative colitis. *Gut.* 1991;32:1535.

26. Maconi G, Sampietro GM, Parente F, et al. Contrast radiology, computed tomography and ultrasonography in detecting internal fistulas and intra-abdominal abscesses in Crohn's disease: A prospective comparative study. *Am J Gastroenterol.* 2003;98.

27. Tarjan Z, Toth G, Gyorke T, et al. Ultrasound in Crohn's disease of the small bowel. *Eur J Radiol.* 2000;35:176.

28. Schreyer AG, Seitz J, Feuerbach S, Rogler G, Herfarth H. Modern imaging using computed tomography and magnetic resonance imaging for inflammatory bowel disease (IBD). *Inflamm Bowel Dis.* 2004;10.

29. Furukawa A, Saotome T, Yamasaki M, Maeda K, Nitta N, Takahashi M, et al. Cross-sectional imaging in Crohn disease. *Radiographics.* 2004;24:689.

30. Hommes DW, van Deventer SJ. Endoscopy in inflammatory bowel diseases. *Gastroenterology.* 2004;126:1561.

31. Hanauer SB, Sandborn W. Practice Parameters Committee of the American College of Gastroenterology. Management of Crohn's disease in adults. *Am J Gastroenterol.* 2001;96:635.

32. Present DN, Rutgeerts P, Targan S, et al. Infliximab for the treatment of fistulas in patients with Crohn's disease. *N Engl J Med.* 1999;340:1398.

33. Mantzaris GJ, Petraki K, Archavlis E, et al. A prospective randomized controlled trial of intravenous ciprofloxacin as an adjunct to corticosteroids in acute, severe ulcerative colitis. *Scand J Gastroenterol.* 2001;36:971.

34. Steinhart AH, Feagan BG, Wong CJ, et al. Combined budesonide and antibiotic therapy for active Crohn's disease: a randomized controlled trial. *Gastroenterology.* 2002;123:33–40.

16

Mesenteric Ischemia

Rachel M. Gilmore
Michael C. Plewa

HIGH YIELD FACTS

- Early diagnosis of mesenteric ischemia is notoriously difficult; a very high level of clinical suspicion is required to avoid the high mortality associated with advanced mesenteric infarction and necrosis.
- The sensitivity of plain radiography for mesenteric ischemia is less than 30% which, combined with poor specificity, limits the usefulness of this tool in the diagnosis of acute mesenteric ischemia.[1,2]
- Noninvasive imaging of the bowel wall and vasculature with computed tomography (CT) and magnetic resonance imaging (MRI) continues to improve, but with a sensitivity of over 90% conventional mesenteric angiography remains the gold standard in diagnosis of acute mesenteric ischemia. [2,3]

EPIDEMIOLOGY

Acute mesenteric ischemia (AMI) is a devastating illness caused by the abrupt disruption of blood flow to a portion of the bowel. It accounts for 1% to 2% of all hospital admissions with abdominal pain.[4] Many patients go on to develop bowel infarction and transmural necrosis, which explains the high associated mortality rate of 60% to 80%.[5–7] Mortality from AMI has not shown any significant decline over the past number of decades despite advances in diagnostic tools.[8] Specific risk factors associated with the different types of AMI are listed in Table 16-1.

PATHOPHYSIOLOGY

The vascular supply of the small intestine is provided by the celiac axis and superior mesenteric artery. Superior mesenteric artery embolus (SMAE) accounts for 40% to 50% of cases of AMI. The majority of emboli arises from the left heart chambers and lodge in the SMA at a site of anatomic narrowing.[9] Superior mesenteric artery thrombosis (SMAT) accounts for approximately 15% of cases and usually occurs in patients with known atherosclerotic disease, at a site of significant luminal stenosis. Nonocclusive mesenteric ischemia (NOMI) causes 20% to 30% of cases of AMI and is due to severe vasoconstriction, typically in the setting of relatively low mesenteric blood flow. Superior mesenteric venous thrombosis (SMVT) is associated with hypercoagulable states, cirrhosis, or malignancy and causes 5% to 10% of cases of AMI.

CLINICAL FEATURES

Abdominal pain is described in 75% to 98% of cases and is typically greatly out of proportion to the severity of the clinical findings. The pain varies in location and generally commences as a colicky pain and later becomes more constant. Other patients may present with abdominal distension or gastrointestinal bleeding. Early in the course of the disease there may be no abnormal physical findings. As ischemia progresses to infarction, signs of peritonitis may develop. Bowel sounds may be diminished or absent, and 75% have occult blood present in the stool. Elderly patients, however, may present solely with altered mental status.[10]

DIAGNOSIS

The diagnosis is dependent on maintaining a high level of clinical suspicion, particularly in those patients with known risk factors for mesenteric ischemia. Laboratory studies are nonspecific. Typically, patients will have an elevated white cell count with neutrophilia.[11,12] An estimated 50% of patients will have metabolic acidosis,[13] and others will have elevated levels of phosphate, lactate, amylase, and alkaline phosphatase as the ischemia progresses to infarction. Unfortunately, a sensitive and specific biochemical marker of mesenteric ischemia which is detectable early in the course of the disease has yet to be identified.

Approximately 25% of patients with AMI have a normal abdominal x-ray,[14] although this test remains useful in excluding other causes of abdominal pain. Nonspecific x-ray findings include adynamic ileus. More specific findings in advanced disease include thickened bowel wall with thumb printing, pneumatosis intestinalis, and portal vein gas. Doppler ultrasonography may detect stenosis or absence of flow in the SMA or celiac plexus.[15] However, ultrasonography may be compromised by the

Table 16-1. Risk Factors for the Development of AMI

Embolus	Thrombus	NOMI
Atrial fibrillation	Prior arterial insufficiency	Cardiogenic shock
Prosthetic valve	Old age	Hypovolemic shock
RWMA	Low flow states	Pulmonary edema
Recent MI	Diabetes	CHF
	Hypercholesterolemia	Aortic regurgitation
	Hypertension	Vasoconstrictive drugs
	CHF	
	Vasculitis	

Abbreviations: CHF, congestive heart failure; MI, myocardial infarction; NOMI, nonocclusive mesenteric ischemia; RWMA, regional wall motion abnormalities.

presence of dilated, gas-filled bowel, which can impair visualization of even these relatively large vessels. Moreover, false-negative results for mesenteric ischemia may be reported in the context of NOMI, or with more peripheral emboli. Abdominal multidetector CT has a newly defined role in the diagnosis of mesenteric ischemia. See Figure 16-1. Sensitivity for AMI is over 90% and findings include mesenteric arterial or venous thrombus, mesentric venous gas, pneumatosis intestinalis, bowel-wall thickening, increased or decreased enhancement of the bowel wall, bowel dilatation, mesenteric or perienteric fat stranding, ascites, pneumoperitoneum, and solid organ infarction.[16,17] Abdominal CT exhibits excellent sensitivity in the diagnosis of mesenteric venous thrombosis, with studies showing sensitivity of between 90% and 100%[18,19]. Contrast enhanced CT is therefore the diagnostic test of choice in those suspected of having acute MVT.[18] Magnetic resonance angiography also has shown promise in the diagnosis of AMI[2]. Although certain cases will still require the use of standard angiography, multidetector row CT angiography has become the initial diagnostic modality of choice for AMI because of its high sensitivity and case of access.[16,17]

Conditions that may mimic the presentation of AMI include perforated viscus, bowel obstruction, pancreatitis, and indeed any cause of peritonitis. These diseases should be considered in the differential diagnosis.

EMERGENCY DEPARTMENT CARE AND DISPOSITION

Patients with AMI require aggressive fluid resuscitation while the underlying cause is being established and treated. Vasoconstrictive medications should be discontinued where possible. Patients should receive broad-spectrum antibiotics, and if possible, acid-base and electrolyte abnormalities should be corrected prior to surgery. Placement of a nasogastric tube may decrease intraluminal pressure and thereby improve intramural blood flow in nonocclusive mesenteric ischemia. Urinary catheterization facilitates accurate monitoring of urine output.

Definitive treatment depends on the specific cause of AMI. If an embolus is identified by angiography, conventional treatment involves emergent surgical embolectomy. Intravenous vasodilators may be administered postoperatively. Superior mesenteric artery thrombosis necessitates urgent surgical revascularization, thrombectomy, and resection of nonviable bowel segments. Local infusion of fibrinolytics for embolic/thrombotic AMI with successful restoration of blood flow has also been

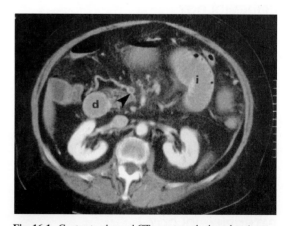

Fig. 16-1. Contrast-enhanced CT scan reveals thrombus (arrowhead) in superior mesenteric vein. Second portion of duodenum (d) and proximal jejunum (i) are dilated and fluid-filled. (Reproduced with permission from *Am J Roentgenol.* 2000;175:1601.)

described in a number of reports.[20,21] First line therapy for NOMI is intraarterial infusion of vasodilating agents, in conjunction with treatment of the underlying condition that led to mesenteric vasoconstriction. Papaverine is the most commonly used agent and is administered directly into the SMA at a rate of 30 to 60 mg/h, an approach which may significantly reduce mortality.[22] Mesenteric venous thrombosis may be treated with anticoagulant therapy in the absence of peritoneal signs. Heparin should be commenced immediately with an intravenous bolus of 5000 IU followed by a continuous infusion at 1000 IU/h and adjusted according to the partial thromboplastin time. Persistent signs of peritonitis regardless of the cause, mandates laparotomy and resection of the necrotic bowel segment.

PITFALLS

- No noninvasive diagnostic test reliably identifies early AMI when the jeopardized bowel segment is still salvageable. Intestinal viability dramatically decreases with duration of symptoms, falling from 100% viability with symptoms of less than 12 hours to 18% viability when symptoms have been present for more than 24 hours.

- Surgical risk in patients with AMI is high, due to severity of the disease and the frequent presence of significant cardiovascular comorbidity. Advances in percutaneous mesenteric revascularization techniques may improve outcomes in this context.

REFERENCES

1. Klein HM, Lensing R, Klosterhalfen B, et al. Diagnostic imaging of mesenteric infarction. *Radiology.* 1995;197:79.
2. Kim AY, Ha HK. Evaluation of suspected mesenteric ischemia: efficacy of radiologic studies. *Radiol Clin North Am.* 2003;41:327.
3. Taourel PG, Deneuville M, Pradel JA, et al. Acute mesenteric ischemia: diagnosis with contrast-enhanced CT. *Radiology.* 1996;199:632.
4. Schneider TA, Longo WE, Ure T, et al. Mesenteric ischemia. Acute arterial syndromes. *Dis Colon Rectum.* 1994;37:1163.
5. Lock G. Acute intestinal ischaemia. *Best Pract Res Clin Gastroenterol.* 2001;15:83.
6. Sitges-Serra A, Mas X, Roqueta F, et al. Mesenteric infarction: an analysis of 83 patients with prognostic studies in 44 cases undergoing a massive small-bowel resection. *Br J Surg.* 1988;75:544.
7. Stoney RJ, Cunningham CG. Acute mesenteric ischemia. *Surgery.* 1993;114:489.
8. Mamode N, Pickford I, Leiberman P. Failure to improve outcome in acute mesenteric ischaemia: Seven-year review. *Eur J Surg.* 1999;165:203.
9. Brandt L. Intestinal Ischemia. In: *Gastrointestinal and Liver Disease.* Philadelphia: WB Saunders; 2002:2321.
10. Finucane PM, Arunachalam T, O'Dowd J, et al. Acute mesenteric infarction in elderly patients. *J Am Geriatr Soc.* 1989;37:355.
11. Kaleya RN, Boley SJ. Acute mesenteric ischemia. *Crit Care Clin.* 1995;11:479.
12. Reinus JF, Brandt LJ, Boley SJ. Ischemic diseases of the bowel. *Gastroenterol Clin North Am.* 1990;19:319.
13. Tsai CJ, Kuo YC, Chen PC, et al. The spectrum of acute intestinal vascular failure: A collective review of 43 cases in Taiwan. *Br J Clin Pract.* 1990;44:603.
14. Smerud MJ, Johnson CD, Stephens DH. Diagnosis of bowel infarction: A comparison of plain films and CT scans in 23 cases. *AJR Am J Roentgenol.* 1990;154:99.
15. Harward TR, Smith S, Seeger JM. Detection of celiac axis and superior mesenteric artery occlusive disease with use of abdominal duplex scanning. *J Vasc Surg.* 1993;17:738.
16. Horton, KM, Fishman EK. Multidetector CT angiography in the diagnosis of mesenteric ischemia. *Radiol Clin North Am.* 2007;45:275.
17. Iannaccone R, Laghi A, Passariello R. Mltislice CT angiography of mesenteric vessels. *Abdom Imaging.* 2004;29:146.
18. Rhee RY, Gloviczki P. Mesenteric venous thrombosis. *Surg Clin North Am.* 1997;77:327.
19. Brandt LJ, Boley SJ. AGA technical review on intestinal ischemia. American Gastrointestinal Association. *Gastroenterology.* 2000;118:954v968.
20. Simo G, Echenagusia AJ, Camunez F, et al. Superior mesenteric arterial embolism: Local fibrinolytic treatment with urokinase. *Radiology.* 1997;204:775.
21. McBride KD, Gaines PA. Thrombolysis of a partially occluding superior mesenteric artery thromboembolus by infusion of streptokinase. *Cardiovasc Intervent Radiol.* 1994;17:164.
22. Ward D, Vernava AM, Kaminski DL, et al. Improved outcome by identification of high-risk nonocclusive mesenteric ischemia, aggressive reexploration, and delayed anastomosis. *Am J Surg.* 1995;170:577. discussion 580.

17

Abdominal Aortic Aneurysm

Bret A. Nicks

HIGH YIELD FACTS

- Approximately 30% of abdominal aortic aneurysms (AAAs) are misdiagnosed on initial evaluation.

- Only 25% of patients with ruptured AAAs present with pain, pulsatile mass and shock, with hypotension occurring in only 50% of presentations.

- Physical exam and abdominal palpation are not sufficient to rule out an AAA.

- A normal chest x-ray is present in 80% of thoracic aortic dissection cases.

- Ultrasound (US) at the bedside is nearly 100% sensitive for detecting AAA under adequate conditions.

- Acute decompensation can occur at any time with a ruptured AAA.

EPIDEMIOLOGY

An aortic aneurysm is a focal dilation of the aorta involving all three layers of the arterial wall. Abdominal aortic aneurysm is classically defined as a localized dilatation of the abdominal aorta greater than 1.5 times the normal diameter at the level of the renal arteries. The normal measurement at this level is approximately 2.0 cm (range 1.4 to 3.0 cm) in most individuals; a diameter greater than 3.0 cm is generally considered aneurysmal.[1] Although any portion of the infradiaphragmatic aorta could be termed an AAA, current convention limits this definition to the infrarenal aorta. Abdominal aortic aneurysms should not be confused with aortic dissections, where blood dissects through the media layer of the aortic wall creating an intimal flap or false lumen.

In the United States, the aortic aneurysm is the 13th leading cause of death with over 15,000 deaths annually; of these, 9000 are abdominal in origin.[2,3] The incidence of AAA has increased in the past two decades, due in part to the aging population, prevalence of smokers, and improved screening and diagnostic modalities. Abdominal aortic aneurysm, commonly associated with aging, is found in 5% to 7% of the U.S. population greater than the age of 60.[3-5] Abdominal aortic aneurysm occurs four to five times more commonly in men than women; prevalence 3% to 8% and 1% to 3%, respectively, with an average age of 65 at the time of diagnosis.[6,7] The disparity in these values is anticipated to decrease with the rising number of female smokers. Screening studies are increasingly common; however, most AAA identified do not require immediate surgical intervention. When AAAs are repaired electively, the overall mortality rate is 0.9% to 9%.[8] The overall mortality rate for patients with ruptured AAA is between 65% to 85%, with nearly half of the deaths associated with rupture prior to reaching surgery. Prance and coworkers suggested five preoperative risk factors to predict the mortality rate of ruptured abdominal aortic aneurysms: (1) age older than 76 years; (2) creatinine higher than 190 milli mol/L; (3) hemoglobin below 9g/dL; (4) loss of consciousness; and (5) electrocardiogram (ECG) evidence of ischemia. In their study, the mortality rate was 100% when the patient had three or more risk factors and decreased to 48%, 28%, and 18% when the risk factor number decreased to two, one, or zero, respectively.[9]

In aneurysms 4 to 5 cm in diameter, the risk of rupture approaches 25%. Abdominal aortic aneurysms most often occur in the segment of the aorta between the renal and inferior mesenteric arteries; approximately 5% involve the renal or visceral arteries.[3] Associated risk factors predisposing to aneurysmal formation include male sex, age, hypertension, chronic obstructive pulmonary disease, atherosclerotic disease, hyperlipidemia, family history, and tobacco smoking. The prevalence of AAA in tobacco smokers is four times greater than nonsmokers.[10] Smoking is the risk factor most strongly associated with AAA (odds ratio 5.07), and the excess prevalence associated with smoking accounted for 75% of all aneurysms that were ≥4.0 cm in diameter. Smoking also promotes the rate of aneurysm growth; as a result, smoking cessation is an essential component of the medical management of patients with an AAA.[5] Hypertension is also associated with abdominal aortic aneurysm but the effect is relatively small. The adjusted odds ratio for coronary disease in the Veterans Affairs study was 1.15 to 1.25, depending upon the definition of aortic aneurysm.[5] Family history increases the risk of having an aneurysm by fourfold; the highest risk is among brothers older than 60 years of age, in whom the prevalence was 12% to 18%.[5,11]

Aortic dissections, occurring with an incidence twice that of ruptured AAA, are rare in those under 40 years, with a peak between 50 to 70 years of age. Aortic dissections are noted to have an equal male:female ratio and have been associated with hypertension and congenital diseases such as Marfan syndrome and bicuspid aortic valves.

PATHOPHYSIOLOGY

Classically, AAAs have been attributed to weakening of the arterial wall as a result of atherosclerotic disease. It is now widely accepted that an AAA is the end result of a multifactorial process culminating in irreversible remodeling of the aortic wall connective tissue structure, not atherosclerotic induced occlusive disease. Recent evidence supports changes in the elastin matrix of the aortic wall with age, compensatory collagen synthesis, proteolysis, metalloproteinase changes, inflammatory infiltration, apoptosis of vascular smooth muscle cells, along with precipitation from infectious agents (e.g., syphilis, mycotic infections), and genetic predisposition (e.g., Marfan syndrome, Ehlers-Danlos syndrome).[3] The overall result is gradual imbalance between synthesis and destruction of the elastin and collagen matrix leading to permanent alteration of the vessel wall structure predisposing to aneurysmal formation.

The natural history of aneurysms is to expand and ultimately rupture. The most important factor determining the risk of aneurysmal rupture is the size. Although ruptures occur at any size, most ruptured AAAs have a diameter greater than 5 cm. However, the rate of increased size, underlying comorbidities, and luminal structural changes all affect the rupture profile more than size alone. Histographically, true aneurysms involve dilation of all three layers of the vessel wall, whereas false aneurysms are caused by the disruption of one or more layers of the vessel wall. Elastin and collagen are the primary determinants of the aortic wall structural properties. Aneurysmal tissues demonstrate fragmentation of the elastic fibers and a decreasing concentration of elastin until the point of rupture. This occurs primarily in the media, while collagen is predominant in the adventitia and assumes the structural support in the absence of adequate elastin. The alteration of elastin and collagen in the aortic wall is influenced by protease formation within the wall and lymphomonocystic infiltration. In a complex interplay of proteases, inflammatory mediators, and immune response, the catabolic conditions that lead to aneurysmal formation proliferate leading to potential rupture.[3]

Inflammatory aneurysms, once believed to be distinct entities, are currently considered one extreme in the spectrum of atherosclerotic aneurysms; these account for 3% to 10% of all AAAs. Clinical and imaging characteristics differentiate inflammatory from noninflammatory aneurysms. The familial pattern of AAA has long been recognized with a 15% to 19% incidence among first-degree relatives.[11] This observation suggests that one or more genes are related to AAA and atherosclerosis. The identification of these genes may enable the early detection and prevention of AAA in high-risk patients. The development of AAA is often associated with mural thrombus formation. Aneurysmal degeneration has been well studied and the role of adherent thrombus, although reducing wall stress, leads to local hypoxia of the media, thus enhancing the inflammatory process and subsequent rupture as described above.

Dissections develop from intimal tears caused by luminal abnormalities and shear forces. This results in blood splitting the aortic media and producing a false lumen that can progress in an antegrade or retrograde direction. Once created, the rupture can occur back into the lumen or externally into the pericardium or mediastinum. External rupture often results in fatal pericardial tamponade. The most common site of intimal tear is within 2 to 3 cm of the aortic valve, but it is also seen in the descending aorta distal to left subclavian artery. Dissection can result in occlusion of aortic branches; most commonly involved are renal, spinal, coronary, or iliac arteries.[12]

CLINICAL FEATURES

The majority of AAAs produce few if any symptoms and are often detected as an incidental finding on ultrasonography, abdominal computed tomography (CT), or magnetic resonance imaging (MRI) during unrelated medical assessments. Most aneurysms remain quiescent until rupture, and those aneurysms that produce symptoms are at increased risk for rupture. Frequent complaints of back, abdominal, chest, flank, buttock, leg, groin, or scrotal pain have been associated with AAA. With increasing AAA size, bowel loop compression may cause functional bowel obstruction and underlying nausea and vomiting. Retroperitoneal hematomas from a leaking posterior AAA will often compress the ureter and cause genitourinary complaints.

Classically, the rupture of an AAA is heralded by the triad of sudden-onset mid-abdominal or flank pain, a pulsatile abdominal mass, and shock. However, this triad is present in less than 25% of AAA rupture, with hypotension occurring in only 50% of initial presentations.[3] Most patients with a ruptured AAA complain of acute, severe, and constant pain in the abdomen, flank, or back that may radiate to the thigh, inguinal area, or scrotum but the mechanism is poorly understood. The symptoms of a ruptured or leaking aneurysm may mimic other acute conditions such as renal colic, diverticulitis, pancreatitis, inferior wall coronary ischemia, mesenteric ischemia, bowel obstruction, or biliary tract disease. In addition, elderly patients who present with hypotension from a leaking abdominal aortic aneurysm may have ECG changes consistent with coronary ischemia. If symptoms develop in someone with known AAA, the presumptive diagnosis is rupture until proven otherwise.

The physical examination for abdominal aortic aneurysm is frequently confounded by a variety of complaints, comorbidities, and findings. Examination may reveal a pulsatile aneurysm at or above the umbilicus; however, the sensitivity for detection ranges from 22% to 96%.[13] Approximately 30% of asymptomatic AAAs are discovered when a pulsatile abdominal mass is palpated on routine physical examination.[14] It is easier to detect large aneurysms and aneurysms in thin people. Even an experienced clinician may miss palpating an AAA in the presence of truncal obesity, abdominal distension, or tense abdominal musculature. The vascular examination should include auscultation of the abdomen since the presence of a bruit may indicate aortic or visceral arterial atherosclerotic disease or an aortocaval fistula. However, the absence of these physical findings does not rule out AAA as the causative agent. Any history of connective tissue disorders, aortic disease (familial or bicuspid), or Turner syndrome should raise suspicion in younger patients. Marfan syndrome alone is associated with a 100-fold increased risk of AAA or dissection. The patient with a ruptured AAA who survives long enough to reach the emergency room classically presents with abdominal or back pain, hypotension, and a pulsatile abdominal mass. Aneurysm rupture typically causes exsanguinating hemorrhage and profound, unstable hypotension. Hypovolemic shock is less likely with a contained retroperitoneal bleed or tamponade causing normotensive presentation with variable complaints. The survival rate of patients who experience a ruptured AAA is less than 10% in the prehospital setting and less than 50% within the hospital itself.[15,16]

The degree of shock relates to the location, size, and time from the rupture. An anterolateral wall rupture into the peritoneal cavity is often associated with death at the scene, while the patient arriving to the emergency department (ED) with variable levels of shock often have a posterolateral wall rupture or small tears. This initial event is systematically followed within hours by a larger rupture, emphasizing the importance of the initial assessment, correct diagnosis, medical transfer, and emergent surgical repair. While rapid identification is paramount for patient survival in all patients, surgical treatment of nonruptured abdominal aortic aneurysms relies on specific indications (age, size of aneurysm, current symptoms, progression of aneurismal size, comorbidities) and is deduced from the estimated risk of rupture, the estimated risk of surgery, and the estimated life expectancy of the patient. A commonly proposed management plan for asymptomatic AAA is provided (Figure 17.1).

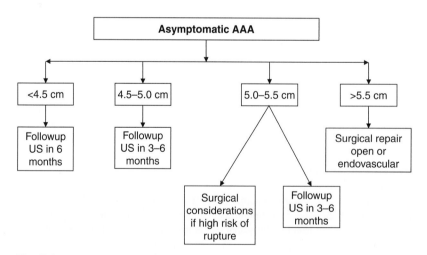

Fig. 17-1. Asymptomatic abdominal aortic aneurysm algorithm. Management plan for asymptomatic abdominal aortic aneurysm.

The classical description of aortic dissection symptoms is sudden onset of severe and tearing chest pain radiating to the back. But that is often not the case, which may explain why the diagnosis of aortic dissection is delayed or frequently made postmortem. Onset of symptoms is frequently associated with syncope. Physical examination may show reduced or absent peripheral pulses and a soft early diastolic murmur. If aortic branches are occluded, there may be clinical evidence of acute renal failure, paraplegia, acute limb ischemia, myocardial infarction, and cerebrovascular accident.

DIAGNOSIS AND DIFFERENTIAL

There are no specific laboratory tests utilized for diagnosing AAA. However, considering the breadth of the differential diagnoses and the potential need for acute resuscitation and operative management for ruptured AAA, several laboratory tests would be valuable. A complete blood count (CBC), type and cross-match, and coagulation studies are essential for the patient with acute AAA rupture. A base excess or lactate may prove helpful in guiding resuscitative efforts. Depending on the presenting symptoms, appropriate complaint specific assessments would be prudent. For those with chest pain, consider cardiac markers. Abdominal or flank complaints may warrant evaluation including urinalysis, amylase, lipase, and a complete metabolic panel. Although these may be prove helpful with the differential, if AAA is suspected, a surgical consult should not be delayed for completed laboratory assessment.

Considering that nearly 30% of those presenting with symptomatic AAAs were misdiagnosed initially, and physical exam is unreliable with a sensitivity of 68% and a specificity of 75%, further evaluation is often paramount for diagnostic confirmation.[13,17,18] Classically, the initial evaluation was assessed with standard abdominal plain films, which may show a curvilinear rim of calcification in the wall of the aneurysm, see Figure 17-2. However, plain films are not a reliable means of detection, as nearly one-third of patients will have a normal radiograph.[19]

Ultrasound at the bedside is nearly 100% sensitive for detecting AAA under adequate conditions.[7] It is rapid, readily available, nonionizing, requires no contrast, and can be repeated if needed.[7] The purpose of the study is to exclude or confirm the presence of AAA. It cannot reliably identify whether an AAA has ruptured or if the bleed is retroperitoneal. Improved outcome and substantially decreased time to diagnosis in patients with ruptured AAA has been demonstrated when bedside US

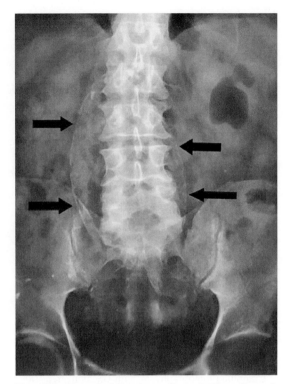

Fig. 17-2. Abdominal flat plate radiograph. The radiograph demonstrates a calcific aortic wall (arrows), identifying the aneurysm.

was used compared to traditional diagnostic methods.[20] Time to disposition for those requiring operative management decreased from 90 minutes to 12 minutes in one study. Similar to the unstable trauma patient, the hypotensive patient with abdominal or flank pain benefits tremendously from this technique. Technically, the anteroposterior diameter in the transverse plane is the most accurate when measuring outer wall to outer wall, see Figure 17-3, although anteroposterior and longitudinal images should also be obtained. The entire aorta from the xiphoid to the bifurcation should be visualized. The inferior vena cava (IVC) may be confused with the aorta, but the IVC is thin walled, and collapses except in the presence of right heart failure. However, if the clinical suspicion for AAA is high despite a negative US, further evaluation should be obtained. Potential problems with abdominal ultrasonography are that it is operator dependent and in approximately 1% to 2% of cases, the aorta cannot be imaged because of technical difficulty such as overlying bowel gas and obesity.[1]

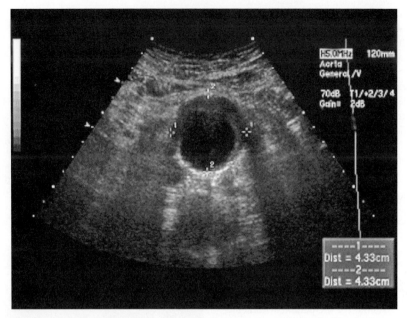

Fig. 17-3. Ultrasound of the Abdominal Aorta. Transverse image obtained of the distal aorta demonstrating an AAA with a luminal diameter of 4.3 cm.

Computed tomography, as with US, is nearly 100% sensitive for identifying AAAs, but also provides information regarding the entire aorta (size, rupture, leak volume), the extent of the AAA, retroperitoneal images, and details about thrombus formation within aneurysm, see Figure 17-4. Computed tomography scan provides additional information regarding other intraperitoneal disorders that may assist with diagnosis such as aortic dissection, see Figure 17-5. False positive CT scans, although rare, can occur when inflammatory soft tissue, loops of bowel, tumor, or lymph nodes are identified as blood adjacent to the aorta.[21] Disadvantages of CT scan

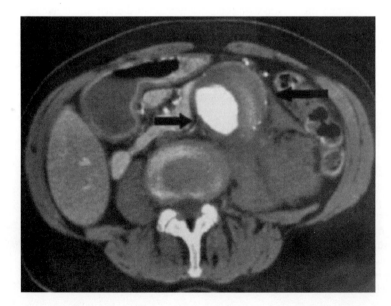

Fig. 17-4. Abdominal CT with infusion demonstrating aortic aneurysm. The arrows demarcate the contrast filled aortic lumen and the surrounding aneurysm.

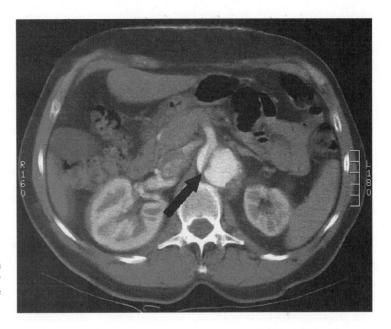

Fig. 17-5. Abdominal CT with infusion demonstrating aortic dissection. Arrow demonstrates luminal separation and evidence of an aortic dissection.

compared to US include greater cost, increased time, transport out of the ED in potentially critical patients, and the associated risks for contrast-induced nephropathy in this patient population. Magnetic resonance angiography (MRA) may be more accurate than CT, but more expensive, less available, and requires greater time for evaluation.[16,22] Hemodynamic deterioration in a patient with a diagnosed AAA should warrant surgical management regardless of the CT results. Differential diagnosis is listed in Table 17-1.

EMERGENCY DEPARTMENT CARE AND DISPOSITION

Treatment of AAA consists of both medical and surgical management. In the ED, a patient with a ruptured AAA will remain unstable until the aorta is cross clamped and repaired in the operating room. Acute resuscitation and consultation should be performed simultaneously in the acutely ruptured or leaking patient. However, the degree of shock varies according to the location and size of the rupture and the delay before the patient is examined.

Initial management should consist of two large bore IVs, and laboratory specimens including a type and cross-match for a minimum of 10 units of blood and any further testing as clinically indicated. Immediate surgical consultation is essential. After consultation, resuscitation and evaluation should be driven by the clinical presentation

and stability of the patient. Any patient with a ruptured AAA, if hemodynamically unstable, should be taken to the OR emergently. Attempts to stabilize the patient in the ED are commonly unsuccessful and waste valuable time. Although bedside US can often confirm the diagnosis, definitive diagnostic imaging should not delay operative evaluation in patients presenting with signs and symptoms causing high clinical suspicion for AAA. Laparotomy in

Table 17-1. Differential of Aortic Aneurysm

Aortic dissection
Gastrointestinal bleed
Renal colic
Biliary colic
Splenic infarction
Ectopic rupture
Inflammatory bowel disease
Appendicitis
Peptic ulcer disease
Mesenteric ischemia
Myocardial infarction
Sepsis
Ovarian torsion
Diverticulitis
Trauma
Testicular torsion

the latter scenario may not reveal a ruptured AAA, but may identify another surgical emergency.

Acute volume resuscitation in symptomatic and hypotensive patients remains an area of controversy. Although preoperative hypotension is the strongest predictor of mortality in ruptured AAA, it has been argued that permissive hypotension may slow AAA bleeding allowing clot formation.[16,23] Therefore, any increase in intravascular volume and subsequently the blood pressure may dislodge formed clots and worsen bleeding. Conversely, complications of prolonged hypotension such as renal failure, myocardial infarction, and cerebrovascular insults increase postoperative mortality. Regardless of perspective, perfusion of the vital organs and prevention of irreversible end organ damage should remain the resuscitative focus until emergent operative management is available. When interventions in a patient with severe decompensation or cardiac arrest fail and cannot be taken emergently to the OR, ED thoracotomy may be appropriate.

In patients who present to the ED with stable vital signs and acute onset of abdominal, chest, back, or groin pain with a clinical history concerning for AAA, additional time can be taken to confirm the diagnosis. If bedside US is negative or unavailable, a CT scan should be obtained if the patient remains stable and is monitored closely. The detailed evaluation of the CT scan will assist both with diagnosis and operative planning if indicated. If a patient becomes hypotensive at any point during this evaluation, operative intervention should occur immediately. Identification of a ruptured AAA requires emergent repair. However, with an intact AAA, surgical intervention may be delayed to optimize the preoperative plan and decrease mortality, necessitating intensive care monitoring.

Incidental, asymptomatic AAA are common findings in the ED. Since it is uncommon for asymptomatic AAAs smaller than 5 cm to rupture, many vascular surgeons have adopted this measurement as an indication for elective repair. However the rate of expansion, sex, life expectancy, and surgical risk may clarify the need for repair versus medical management. The cumulative evidence from studies that prospectively followed the size of AAAs suggests that larger aneurysms expand about 0.3 to 0.4 cm per year. Elective resection is considered for AAAs that exceed 5.5 cm in diameter or when a small aneurysm increases in diameter by more than 0.5 cm within a 6-month interval.[24–26] Other indications for surgery include aneurysms that are tender or are associated with abdominal or back pain, both of which are suggestive of recent aneurysm expansion, iliac or femoral artery aneurysms requiring treatment, and aneurysms that

occur in patients with severe coexistent occlusive disease or thrombotic or embolic complications. The question of how to manage asymptomatic 4 to 5.5 cm aneurysms has been addressed by the United States ADAM (Aneurysm Detection and Management); the trial consisted of 1136 patients (over 99% male), aged 50 to 79 years, with an aneurysm 4.0 to 5.4 cm in diameter. Patients were randomly assigned to surgery within 6 weeks or surveillance with US or CT every 6 months; elective surgery was performed when the aneurysm enlarged to more than 5.5 cm or became symptomatic. Operative mortality in this trial was only 2.7%. After a follow-up of 4.9 years, there was no difference in mortality between surgery and surveillance (25% versus 21.5%) or death related to the aneurysm itself (3% versus 2.6%).[5]

In general, patients with a ruptured AAA or an acutely symptomatic AAA require emergent or urgent surgical repair. An incidental, asymptomatic aneurysm must be referred for consideration of elective repair. Serial measurements and comorbid medical management will assist with optimal elective intervention. Patients with newly identified AAA should be referred for an outpatient workup only if it is clear that the presenting symptoms were unrelated to the AAA. Appropriate medical management of concurrent medical problems should also be addressed. At discharge, specific instructions should be given regarding seeking medical assistance for any of the signs and symptoms of AAA emergencies.

PITFALLS

- The lack of classic symptoms does not exclude the diagnosis.
- Remember the entire aorta is not visualized during routine examination.
- Never assume chest pain with ECG changes is isolated to the coronaries.
- Gastroenteritis is a diagnosis of exclusion.
- Acute symptoms of diverticulitis in the elderly should warrant AAA evaluation.

REFERENCES

1. Scott RAP, Ashton HA, Kay DN. Abdominal aortic aneurysm in 4237 screened patients: prevalence, development and management over 6 years. *Br J Surg.* 1991;78:1122.
2. Gillum RF. Epidemiology of aortic aneurysm in the United States. *J Clin Epidemiol.* 1995;48:1289.
3. Sakalihasan N, Limet R, Defawe OD. Abdominal aortic aneurysm. *Lancet* 2005;365:1577.

4. Fleming C, Whitlock EP, Beil TL, et al. Screening for abdominal aortic aneurysm: A Best-evidence systematic review for the US Preventive Services Task Force. *Ann Int Med.* 2005;142:203.

5. Lederle FA, Johnson GR, Wilson SE, et al. The aneurysm detection and management study screening program: validation cohort and final results. Aneurysm Detection and Management Veterans Affairs Cooperative Study Investigators. *Arch Intern Med.* 2000;160:1425.

6. Lederle FA, Johnson GR, Wilson SE. Abdominal aortic aneurysm in women. *J Vasc Surg.* 2001;34:122.

7. Tayal VS, Graf CD, Gibbs MA. Prospective study of accuracy and outcome of emergency ultrasound for AAA over two years. *Acad Emerg Med.* 2003;10:867.

8. Lederle Fa, Wilson SE, Johnson GR, et al. Immediate repair compared with surveillance of small abdominal aortic aneurysms. *N Engl J Med.* 2002;346:1437.

9. Prance SE, Wilson YG, Cosgrove CM, Walker AJ, Wilkins DC, Ashley S. Ruptured abdominal aortic aneurysms: selecting patients for surgery. *Eur J Vasc Endovasc Surg.* 1999;17:129.

10. Vardulaki KA, Walker NM, Day NE, et al. Quantifying the risks of hypertension, age, sex, and smoking in patients with abdominal aortic aneurysm. *Br J Surg.* 2000;87:195.

11. Salo JA, Soisalon-Soininen S, Bondestam S, et al. Familial occurrence of abdominal aortic aneurysm. *Ann Intern Med.* 1999;130:637.

12. Dmowski AT, Carey MJ. Aortic dissection. *Am J Emerg Med.* 1999;17:372.

13. Fink HA, Lederle FA, Roth CS, et al. The accuracy of physical examination to detect AAA. *Arch Intern Med.* 2000;160:833.

14. Simon G, Nordgren D, Connelly S, et al. Screening for abdominal aortic aneurysms in a hypertensive patient population. *Arch Intern Med.* 1996;156:2081.

15. Minino AM, Arias E, Kochanek KD, et al. Deaths: Final Data for 2000. *Natl Vital Stat Rep.* 2002;50:1.

16. Ernst CB. Abdominal aortic aneurysm. *N Engl J Med.* 1993;328:1167.

17. Rohrer MJ, Cutler BS, Wheeler HB. Long term survival and quality of life following ruptured AA. *Arch Surg.* 1988;123:1213.

18. Lederle FA, Simel DL. The rational clinical examination. Does this patient have an AAA? *JAMA.* 1999;281:77.

19. Loughran CF. A review of the plain abdominal radiograph in acute rupture of abdominal aortic aneurysms. *Clin Radiol.* 1986;37:383.

20. Plummer D, Clinton J, Matthew B. Emergency department ultrasound improves time to diagnosis and survival in ruptured AAA. *Acad Emerg Med.* 1998;5:417.

21. Siegal CL, Cohen RH. CT of abdominal aortic aneurysms, *AJR Am J Roentgenol.* 1994;163:17.

22. Petersen, MJ, Cambria, RP, Kaufman, JA, et al. Magnetic resonance angiography in the preoperative evaluation of abdominal aortic aneurysms. *J Vasc Surg.* 1995;21:891.

23. Johansson G, Swedenborg J. Ruptured AAA: A Study of incidence and mortality. *Br J Surg.* 1986;73:101.

24. Gadowski GR, Pilcher DB, Ricci MA. Abdominal aortic aneurysm expansion rate: effect of size and beta-adrenergic blockade. *J Vasc Surg.* 1994;19:727.

25. Flores J, Kunihara T, Shiiya N, et al. Importance of early repair of isolated abdominal aortic dissecting aneurysm. *Vasa.* 2005;34:118.

26. Chuter TA, Parodi JC, Lawrence-Brown M. Management of abdominal aortic aneurysm: a decade of progress. *J Endovasc Ther.* 2004;11(Suppl 2):II82.

18

Diverticulitis

Simon A. Mahler

HIGH YIELD FACTS

- Left lower quadrant pain has sensitivity of greater than 92% for sigmoid diverticulitis.
- Leukocytosis and fever may be absent in up to 31% and 43% of diverticulitis patients, respectively.
- Computed tomography (CT) is 93% to 100% sensitive and nearly 100% specific for diverticulitis.

EPIDEMIOLOGY

Diverticulitis is an increasingly common problem in the United States and other industrialized nations. It has been referred to as "a disease of western civilization," because an increased prevalence has been linked to decreased dietary fiber common to our fast food society.[1] The prevalence of diverticulosis among the general population in the United States has been estimated to be between 30% to 50%.[2] The incidence and prevalence of disease increases with age. The incidence is approximately 30% in patients over 50 years old and 66% for patients above the age of 85.[3,4] Most patients with diverticulosis remain asymptomatic with only 10% to 25% developing diverticulitis.[3,5,6]

Men and women above the age of 40 are equally affected by diverticular disease.[7] In "early" divericulitar disease (less then 40 years old) males appear to predominate.[8–10] Patients with "early" diverticulitis represent 5% to 7% of all cases and are often misdiagnosed, which in some studies has led to a higher complication rate.[9,10] In North Americans and Europeans 85% to 90% of cases of diverticulitis occur in the sigmoid colon.[6,18] Asians have an increased prevalence of right colonic diverticular disease.[7,11] The overall mortality from diverticular disease is low, but Caucasian patients with diverticulitis (death rate: 24–30/100,000) have a more than twofold greater death rate than Non-Caucasians (death rate: 10–12/100,000).[12]

Diverticular disease (including diverticulitis and diverticular hemorrhage) is the second most common cause for hospitalization and the 13th leading cause of death among gastrointestinal (GI) causes in the United States.[13] It is responsible for over 200,000 hospitalizations and an estimated cost of over $300 million.[14]

PATHOPHYSIOLOGY

Diverticular disease can be subdivided into three overlapping clinical and pathological entities: diverticulosis, diverticulitis (and its associated complications), and diverticular hemorrhage (see Figure 18-1). Diverticulosis refers to the presence of colonic diverticulae, which are predominately found in the sigmoid colon. Diverticulitis occurs when there is obstruction, inflammation, overgrowth of anaerobic and gram negative bacterial pathogens, and either microperforation or macroperforation of diverticulae.[5] Diverticular hemorrhage typically occurs in non-inflamed right colonic diverticulae.

The underlying cause of diverticulae formation is not completely understood.[15] The current theory is that decreased dietary fiber leads to decreased stool bulk and increased intralumenal pressure. The increased intralumenal pressure is thought to cause herniation of submucosa and mucosa of the bowel through its muscular layer forming an out-pouching lesion. Technically these lesions are "pseudo" or "false" diverticulae, rather than "true" diverticulae, because they do not include the muscular layer. The formation of diverticulae causes mechanical strain/stretch on vesa rectae, small blood vessels that supply the colon, which can result in vessel rupture and intraluminal hemorrhage.[6,7,16–18]

CLINICAL FEATURES

Diverticulitis classically presents with left lower quadrant pain and tenderness, fever, and elevated white count. Left lower quadrant pain is seen in 93% to 100% of patients, leukocytosis in 69% to 83%, and fever in greater than 57%.[5] The pain from diverticulitis may begin as generalized and vague but typically localizes quickly to the left lower quadrant causing severe, constant, sharp pain. Other associated symptoms may include nausea, vomiting, anorexia, constipation, diarrhea, dysuria, urinary frequency, and hematuria.[5–7] Elderly and immunocompromised patients are more likely to have atypical presentations and may present with only mild abdominal pain without fever or leukocytosis.[18–20]

The most common finding on physical exam in diverticulitis is left lower quadrant tenderness. However the

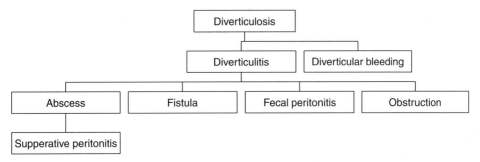

Fig. 18-1. Diverticular diseases.

severity of pain may vary depending on the degree of inflammation and presence or absence of an abscess or peritonitis. Peritoneal signs such as rebound tenderness and guarding indicate complicated diverticulitis with macroperforation and pyogenic or fecal peritonitis. Approximately 25% of patients will be positive for fecal occult blood.[7] Palpation of a mass in the left lower quadrant is less common but can be caused by colonic inflammation and/or abscess formation.

Fistula formation is a common complication of patients with a history of diverticulitis with a lifetime risk of 10% to 25 %.[19,21] Fecaluria, pneumaturia, and recurrent urinary tract infections (UTIs) in a patient with a history of diverticulitis indicate the presence of a colovesical fistula. Colovesical fistulas are the most

common type accounting for approximately 65% of diverticular fistulas.[22] Colovaginal fistulas are less common and are seen most often in elderly females with a prior hysterectomy.[23] Obstruction is a less frequent complication, typically affecting the small bowel due to adhesions from recurrent diverticular inflammation. However, colonic obstruction or stricture can also occur.[5]

Diverticulosis, without diverticulitis, is typically asymptomatic and often goes unrecognized. However, some patients with diverticulosis complain of mild left lower quadrant pain. Diverticulosis can also cause changes in bowel habits that resemble irritable bowel syndrome with alternating bouts of constipation and diarrhea. These patients will have only mild abdominal tenderness with the absence of fever and leukocytosis.[7]

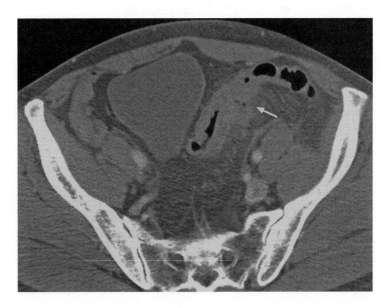

Fig. 18-2. Computed tomography. This CT demonstrates complicated diverticular disease with a diverticular abscess (arrow).

Diverticular bleeding is the most common cause of lower GI bleeding, responsible for 30% to 40% of all cases of hematochezia.[17] The risk of diverticular bleeding among patients with diverticulosis is approximately 17%.[24] The typical presentation is acute onset of painless hematochezia. Patients may have mild lower abdominal pain, tenesmus, and occasionally present with melena rather than hematochezia.[16,19] Approximately 3% to 5% of cases are severe enough to require transfusion.[25]

DIAGNOSIS AND DIFFERENTIAL

The diagnosis of diverticulitis is based on a suggestive history and physical exam along with characteristic changes seen on computed tomography (CT), see Figure 18-2. Although ultrasound (US) and contrast enemas can be used to evaluate for diverticulitis, CT is the most commonly used imaging modality. Computed tomography has a sensitivity of 93% to 100% and a specificity of 100% for the diagnosis of diverticulitis.[26–28] Helical CT with water soluble rectal contrast has achieved the highest sensitivity and specificity.[27] However, the diagnosis can be established in the vast majority of patients without the use of rectal contrast. Intravenous administration of contrast is recommended, if the patient's renal function will allow, in order to improve detection of pericolonic inflammation and abscesses.[29] Computed tomography diagnosis is based on the presence of diverticuli with colon wall thickening and pericolic fat inflammation (stranding). Pericolic or remote abscess formation, perforation with free air or fluid, and obstruction are important findings indicating complicated diverticulitis.[27–30] The ability to distinguish between complicated and uncomplicated diverticulitis allows the practitioner to determine the most appropriate treatment and disposition.

Computed tomography is more sensitive than contrast enema, is less invasive, and has the additional benefit of providing a higher alternate diagnosis rate due to its ability to identify extracolonic disease.[28–30] Some studies have shown that US can achieve sensitivities nearly equal to CT.[31] However, US is extremely operator dependent and not uniformly available. Diverticular fistulas can typically be diagnosed clinically, but contrast fistulagrams are useful for confirmation and defining anatomy.[23]

Not all patients require definitive imaging studies for diagnosis. Patients with a history of prior uncomplicated diverticulitis, a classic history, and a physical exam may be clinically diagnosed and treated presumptively as long as they are nontoxic, with normal vital signs, a benign abdominal examination, able to tolerate pills and fluids by mouth, and have access to close follow up.[5,6] Unfortunately, the clinical diagnosis of diverticulitis has a low sensitivity with misdiagnosis rates above 34%.[32,33]

There are no laboratory studies sensitive or specific enough to provide a definitive diagnosis of diverticulits. Leukocytosis is seen in 69% to 83% of patients with diverticulitis. A urinalysis may show pyuria or hematuria from ureteral inflammation caused by diverticulitis or may be abnormal due to fistula formation.[5] Amylase, lipase, and liver function tests may be useful when considering other diagnosis. Electrolytes and coagulation studies are frequently obtained. Plain films may be helpful if there is concern for obstruction or free air.[17,19]

Any significant lower GI bleed including diverticular bleeding deserves a complete blood count, coagulation studies, electrocardiogram (ECG), and a type and crossmatch for possible transfusion. A nasogastric tube can help differentiate a massive upper GI bleed from a lower GI cause and anoscopy can rule out a rectal source such as hemorrhoids or an anal fissure. Colonoscopy by a gastroenterologist is the diagnostic procedure of choice and can be used to control bleeding as well.[16]

The differential diagnosis of diverticulitis is summarized in Table 18-1.

Table 18-1. Differential Diagnosis for Diverticulitis

Ulcerative colitis
Crohn disease
Ischemic colitis
Appendicitis
Colon carcinoma
Mesenteric ischemia
Intestinal obstruction
Ruptured aortic aneurysm
Sigmoid volvulus
Intussusception
Cystitis and pyelonephritis
Nephrolithiasis
Pelvic inflammatory disease
Ectopic pregnancy
Ovarian cyst/torsion
Cholecystitis
Pancreatitis
Perforated peptic ulcer
Gastroenteritis
Irritable bowel syndrome

EMERGENCY DEPARTMENT CARE AND DISPOSITION

The treatment of diverticulitis differs between complicated and uncomplicated diverticulitis. Patients with complicated diverticulitis, with an abscess or phlegmon, free perforation (peritonitis), or obstruction, require attention to their airway, breathing, and circulation (ABCs), fluid resuscitation, IV antibiotics, opiate analgesia, and immediate surgical consultation. Patients with true peritoneal signs on exam, or radiographic evidence of free perforation (free air or free fluid) will require emergent surgery. Patients with an abscess, but without perforation may be treated with IV antibiotics and CT guided percutaneous abscess drainage instead of surgery. Antibiotic choice should target gram-negative rods and anaerobes (Table 18-2). Patients with diverticular fistulas also require surgical consultation for eventual operative repair.[5,6,17,19]

Most patients with uncomplicated diverticulitis without abscess, phlegmon, perforation, or obstruction can be treated medically. Nontoxic patients with normal vital signs, benign abdominal examination, the ability to tolerate pills and fluids by mouth, and access to close follow up may be treated as outpatients. A typical outpatient regiment would include a course of antibiotics (Table 18-2)[34] and opiate analgesics with close follow up. Any patient with intractable pain, inability to tolerate orals, dehydration,

abnormal vital signs, or unreliable follow up should be admitted.[5,6,17,19] Patients with recurrent symptoms should be given consideration for admission and surgical referral. Typically any patient with two episodes of sigmoid diverticulitis becomes a candidate for an elective sigmoid resection.[5] Approximately 20% to 30% of patients with diverticulitis will require surgical intervention.[3,6] Special consideration for admission should be given to the elderly and the immunocompromised, especially those on steroids, because of their tendency to present atypically and their increased risk of complications and mortality.

Dietary modification has been the primary means of preventing diverticular disease and future exacerbations. High fiber diets have been shown to reduce symptoms in patients with diverticular disease but many of these studies do not have control groups or enrolled small numbers of patients.[7,17,35] It is also common practice to warn patients that seeds and nuts may get trapped in diverticula causing diverticulitis. However, there is little evidence to support such warnings.[17]

For an emergency or primary care physician the treatment of diverticular bleeding is no different than any other type of lower GI bleed. Attention to ABCs should be the first priority along with establishing adequate IV access (at least two large bore IVs), and appropriate monitoring. A nasogastric tube should be inserted to evaluate for a massive upper GI bleed.[19] Unstable patients

Table 18-2. Recommended Antimicrobial Therapy for Diverticulitis

Mild disease Outpatient	Ciprofloxacin 500 mg PO BID + Metronidazole 500 mg PO QID for 7–10 days. or
	Trimethoprim/sulfamethoxazole DS 1 tablet PO BID + Metronidazole 500 mg PO QID for 7–10 days. or
	Amoxicillin clavulanate 875 mg PO BID for 7–10 days
Moderate disease Inpatient	Ampicillin sulbactam 3 g IV Q 6 hours or
	Piperacillin tazobactam 3.375 g IV Q 6 hours or
	Ciprofloxacin 400 mg IV Q 12 hours + Metronidazole 500 mg IV Q 6 hours.
Severe disease/ICU	Imipenem ciliastin 500 mg IV Q 6 hours or
	Meropenem 1 g IV Q 8 hours or
	Ampicillin 2 g IV Q 6 hours + Ciprofloxacin 400 mg IV Q 12 hours + Metronidazole 500 mg IV Q 6 hours.
Severe disease and penicillin allergic	Aztreonam 2 g IV q 6 + Metronidazole 500 mg IV Q 6 hours.

Abbreviations: BID, two times per day; ICU, intensive care unit; IV, intravenous; PO, by mouth; QID, four times per day should be aggressively resuscitated with crystalloid and blood and admitted to an intensive care unit setting. Gastroenterology should be consulted for colonoscopy; however, if brisk bleeding precludes endoscopy and the bleeding cannot be controlled by angiographic therapies, then general surgery should be consulted for operative control.[16,17,19] Fortunately approximately 80% of diverticular bleeding will stop spontaneously without intervention.[36] The risk of rebleeding after a single episode is 25%, but after two episodes the risk increases to 50%.[25] All patients with significant lower GI bleeding, even if the bleeding has resolved, warrant admission to a monitored setting.

PITFALLS

• Failure to recognize that elderly and immunocompromised patients with diverticulitis are more likely to present atypically, with mild pain, absence of fever, and without leukocytosis. These patients, despite the lack of signs and symptoms, have an increased risk of complications and mortality.

• Failure to consider diverticulitis in patients under 40 years of age.

• Failing to use CT in patients with suspected diverticulitis to differentiate between complicated and uncomplicated diverticulitis and to exclude other intraabdominal processes in the differential diagnosis.

• Underestimating the significance of a lower GI bleed and failing to recognize the high rate of rebleeding in diverticular disease can lead to an inappropriate floor admission or discharge.

REFERENCES

1. Painter NS. Diverticular disease of the colon: the first of Western diseases shown to be due to a deficiency of dietary fiber. *S Afr Med J.* 1982;61:1016.
2. Konvolinka CW. Acute diverticulitis under the age 40. *Am J Surg.* 1994;167:562.
3. Parks TG. Natural history of diverticular disease of the colon: a review of 521 cases. *BMJ.* 1969;4:639.
4. Welch CE, Allen AW, Donaldson, GA. An appraisal of resection of the colon for diverticulitis of the sigmoid. *Ann Surg.* 1953;138:332.
5. Wong DW. The Standards Task Force American Society of Colon and Rectal Surgeons: practice parameters for sigmoid diverticlitis-supporting documentation. *Dis Colon Rectum.* 1995;38:126.
6. Ferzoco LB, Raptopoulos V, Silen W. Acute diverticulitis. *N Engl J Med.* 1998;338:1521.
7. Deckman RC, Cheskin LJ. Diverticular disease in the elderly. *J Am Geria Soc.* 1993;40:986.
8. West SD, Robinson EK, Delu AN. Diverticulitis in the younger patient. *Am J Surg.* 2003;186:743.
9. Freischlag J, Bennion RS, Thompson JE. Complications of diverticular disease of the colon in young people. *Dis Colon Rectum.* 1986;29:639.
10. Cunningham MA, Davis JW, Kaups KL. Medical versus surgical management of diverticulitis in patients under age 40. *Am J Surg.* 1997;174:733.
11. Wong SK, Ho YH, Leong AP, et al. Clinical behavior of complicated right-sided and left sided diverticulosis. *Dis Colon Rectum.* 1997;40:344.
12. Mendeloff AI, Dunn JP. Nonspecific inflammatory bowel diseases. In: *Digestive Diseases.* American Public Health Association. Harvard University Press, Cambridge, Massachusetts, 1971;132–34:57.
13. Russo MW, Wei JT, Thiny MT, et al. Digestive and liver statistics 2004. *Gastroenterology.* 2004;126:1448.
14. Salem L, Veenstra DL, Sullivan SD, et al. The timing of elective colectomy in diverticulitis: a decision analysis. *J Am Coll Surg.* 2004;199:69.
15. Almy TP, Howell DA. Diverticular disease of the colon. *N Engl J Med* 1980;302:324.
16. Vernava AM, Moore BA, Longo WE, et al. Lower gastrointestinal bleeding. *Dis Colon Rectum.* 1997;40:846.
17. Stollman NH, Raskin JB. Diverticular disease of the colon. *J Clin Gastroenterol.* 1999;29:241.
18. Esses D, Brinbaum A, Bijur P, et al. Ability of CT to alter decision making in elderly patients with acute abdominal pain. *Am J Emerg Med.* 2004;22:270.
19. Farrell RJ, Farrell JJ, Morrin MM. Gastrointestinal disorders in the elderly. *Gastroenterol Clin North Am.* 2001;30:475.
20. Perkins JD, Shield CF, Chang FC, et al. Acute diverticulitis: Comparison of treatment in immunocompromised and non-immunocompromised patients. *Am J Surg.* 1984;148:745.
21. Whiteway J, Morson B. Pathology of the ageing: Civerticular disease. *Clin Gastroenterol.* 1985;14:829.
22. Pontari MA, McMillen MA, Garvey RH, et al. Diagnosis and treatment of enterovesical fistulae. *Am Surg.* 1992; 58:258.
23. Tancer ML, Veridiano NP. Genital fistulas caused by diverticular disease of the sigmoid colon. *Am J Ob Gyn.* 1996;174:1547.
24. Rushford AJ. The significance of bleeding as a symptom in diverticulitis. *J R Soc Med.* 1956;49:577.
25. McGuire JJ, Haynes BW. Massive hemorrhage from diverticulosis of the colon: guidelines for therapy based on bleeding patterns observed in fifty cases. *Ann Surg.* 1972;175:847.
26. Rao PM, Rhea JT, Novelline RA, et al. Helical CT with only colonic contrast material for diagnosing diverticulitis: prospective evaluation of 150 patients. *AJR Am J Roentgenol.* 1998;170:1445.
27. Cho KC, Morehouse HT, Alterman DD, et al. Sigmoid diverticulitis: Diagnostic role of CT—comparison with barium enema studies. *Radiology.* 1990;176:111.

28. Ambrosetti P, Grossholz M, Becker C, et al. Computed tomography in acute left colonic diverticulitis. *Br J Surg.* 1997;84:532–34.

29. Urban BA, Fishman EK. Tailored helical CT evaluation of acute abdomen. *Radiographics.* 2000;20:725–49.

30. Hunlick DH, Megibow AJ, Balthazar EJ, et al. Computed tomography in the evaluation of diverticulitis. *Radiology.* 1984;152:491–95.

31. Pradel JA, Adell JF, Taourel P, et al. Acute colonic diverticulitis: Prospective comparative evaluation with US and CT. *Radiology.* 1997;205:503–12.

32. Wexner SD, Dailer TH. The initial management of left lower quadrant peritonitis. *Dis Colon Rectum.* 1986; 29:635–638.

33. Brengman ML, Otchy DP. Timing of computed tomography in acute diverticulitis. *Dis Colon Rectum.* 1998;41:1023–28.

34. Gilbert DN, Moellering RC, Eliopoulos GM, et al. The Sanford Guide To Antimicrobial Therapy. 36th ed. Antimicrobial Therapy Inc, Sperryville, VA 2006.

35. Brodribb AJ. Treatment of symptomatic diverticular disease with a high-fibre diet. *Lancet* 1977;1:664–66.

36. Bokhari M, Vernava AM, Ure T, et al. Diverticular hemorrhage in the elderly: Is it well tolerated? *Dis Colon Rectum.* 1996;39:191–95.

19

Alcoholic Hepatitis

Thomas A. Brunell

HIGH YIELD FACTS

- Alcoholic hepatitis (AH) has a highly variable clinical presentation and patients may be mildly or severely affected.
- There are no single emergency department (ED) tests for AH and clinical suspicion is necessary to make the diagnosis.
- Emergency department management is primarily supportive.
- Alcoholic hepatitis, unlike fatty liver (steatosis), is probably not reversible by abstinence.
- Use of corticosteroids as a treatment modality is promising, but is still not part of current ED management.
- Patients may be immunocompromised.

EPIDEMIOLOGY

Alcohol is a primary cause of end-stage liver disease in the United States. There are well over ten million alcoholics in the United States alone and over two million people with alcohol related liver diseases.[1,2] It has been estimated that up to 1% of all health care dollars is spent on alcohol related liver diseases.[3] Whether a patient encounter is the result of trauma, domestic violence, psychiatric conditions, transplant surgery, or hepatic dysfunction in general, the emergency physician faces the complications of alcohol abuse on a daily basis.

Although the number of alcoholics whose liver undergoes fatty change (steatosis) may approach 90%, the disease state progresses to AH in only a small fraction—from 10% to 35%.[4–6] Due to the continuum of the severity of illness, mortality estimates are wide ranging: One study quotes mortality measurements as ranging from "0 to 100%."[5] Therefore, in the acute setting, the disease state may manifest itself as anything from mild to premorbid.

PATHOPHYSIOLOGY

Alcohol affects the liver through a myriad of mechanisms. It is generally accepted, however, that most hepatocellular damage is mediated through acetaldehyde—alcohol's principal metabolic end-product. As yet, it is unclear whether one particular type of spirit is more or less likely to induce liver damage and lead to hepatitis. Consensus appears to be that consumption of greater than 60 to 80 g/dL per day for males and greater than 20 to 40 g/dL per day for females places that individual at risk for liver damage and hepatitis.[7–9] This amount represents between two and six "drinks" per day for a man, and one to four "drinks" a day for a woman (one "drink" is equivalent to 12 ounces of beer, 5 ounces of wine, or $1^1/_2$ ounces of an 80 proof spirit).[10]

The disease state of AH may be thought of as an intermediate state between fatty liver change and cirrhosis. Although it is possible for a patient to progress to cirrhosis and liver failure without having progressed through a stage of AH, it is likely that a preponderance of cases first develop AH prior to cirrhosis. It may be that many cases of AH are subclinical, or that the patient never seeks medical attention prior to severe progression of the disease.

Alcoholic hepatitis is characterized by parenchymal necrosis, infiltration of polymorphonuclear lymphocytes into hepatic structures (especially Mallory bodies), and collagen deposits within the liver.[4,5] This results both in hepatocellular dysfunction and decreased blood flow to the liver. There is undoubtedly a large interplay between immune factors, underlying nutritional state, genetic predisposition (including sex), and environmental factors (especially tobacco use). Other factors, such as concomitant infection with hepatitis B and C, influence the progression of fatty change into hepatitis. Although it is still unknown who among heavy users of alcohol will progress to AH, it is likely that infection with the hepatitis C virus places the patient at the most risk for more severe disease.[11–13]

CLINICAL FEATURES

The presentation of AH is greatly varied; symptoms may be as subtle as mild abdominal pain or as pronounced as acute jaundice and shock. In addition to generalized abdominal pain; nausea, vomiting, diarrhea, and malaise are common complaints. Aside from a history of alcohol consumption, there is no set constellation of symptoms that isolate the diagnosis.

Physical findings may include hyperpyrexia, anorexia, tachycardia, right upper quadrant tenderness, hepatomegaly, diffuse abdominal tenderness, orthostatic hypotension, or overt jaundice. Depending on the age and history of alcohol abuse, the patient may have spider angioma, ascites, altered mentation, gynecomastia, and other signs and symptoms of liver failure (Chapter 21).

DIAGNOSIS AND DIFFERENTIAL

The alcoholic patient represents a particularly difficult challenge to emergency physicians. The intoxicated patient may be difficult to examine and interview. These patients are easily stereotyped, often quickly and inappropriately medicated or sedated, and may be relegated to the hallway or psychiatric area of the ED prior to a complete history or physical exam.

The differential diagnosis for AH is broad. Within it must be considered the large number of alcohol-related maladies. These include esophagitis, gastritis, pancreatitis, esophageal varices, both perforated and nonperforated ulcers, cholecystitis, cholangitis, hepatic failure, renal failure, withdrawal syndromes, as well as toxic ingestions such as toxic alcohols or coingestion of other medications. In patients with fever or altered mentation, the diagnoses of sepsis, encephalitis, and meningitis should be considered. Unlike many patients that are encountered in the ED, the alcoholic patient is likely to exhibit multiple disorders simultaneously.

There is no single ED test to validate AH. Laboratory investigation is dictated by clinical presentation. Alcoholic hepatitis will result in an elevation of serum transaminases. Aspartate aminotransferase (AST) may be more elevated than alanine aminotransferase (ALT). If either exceeds 8 times the normal range, another diagnosis (such as viral hepatitis) should be considered.[14]Total bilirubin and prothrombin time (PT) may be used to provide a measure of hepatic dysfunction. As with ALT and AST, marked elevation of either of these measures requires consideration of other clinical entities more severe than AH (e.g., hepatic failure, Chapter 21). A serum ammonia should be sent when there is suspicion for hepatic encephalopathy. Serum electrolytes may be altered due to either nausea or vomiting. Blood urea nitrogen (BUN) and creatinine should be sent to evaluate renal function. Serum glucose may be altered from a variety of causes and should be checked when the patient arrives (as point of care testing). Serum glucose levels should then be followed serially. A complete blood count is helpful for evaluating sepsis and immunocompetency: white blood count, hemoglobin and hematocrit, and platelets. Mean corpuscular volume (MCV) may be high in patients with underlying nutritional deficiencies.[15] If the patient is febrile, blood cultures should be obtained from at least two separate sites. A serum lipase should be sent when pancreatitis is suspected. Urinalysis is useful for evaluation of infection, hydration status, and renal function. Although of limited utility in the ED, drawing other hepatic studies (e.g., anti-HAV IgM and HBcAb-IgM), if not previously done, may be helpful for the patient's continued care. Ultrasonography and computed tomography(CT)-imaging of the abdomen and biliary system is usually not necessary for AH. However, these may be useful in patients with severely altered vital signs for ruling out other more potentially life-threatening diagnoses.[16]

EMERGENCY DEPARTMENT CARE AND DISPOSITION

Supportive care is the most useful management modality for patients with suspected AH. Establish intravenous (IV) access and administer IV fluids. If the patient has near-normal renal function, then IV fluid administration may be titrated to urine output (1–2 mL/kg of patient's ideal body weight). If thiamine is to be given, administer it prior to the administration of glucose to avoid precipitating the Wernicke-Korsakoff syndrome.[15] Heavy alcohol users are often magnesium depleted and repletion of 1 to 2 g of magnesium intramuscularly (IM) or IV may be helpful, but its benefit has yet to be proven.[15,17] Administration of benzodiazepines for withdrawal symptoms may be necessary. Neuroleptic agents are problematic as they may mask withdrawal symptoms and precipitate seizures.

Suspicion or evidence of infection warrants broad-spectrum antibiotic therapy. Alcoholic hepatitis patients are likely to be immunocompromised from a variety of factors. Infection remains the most common cause of morbidity and mortality in patients with AH.[18] Evidence of hemodynamic instability, such as hypotension and tachycardia, are predictors of severe infection. These patients have significantly higher mortality rates and warrant admission to intensive care.[5]

There are a variety of newer therapies currently being examined for the treatment of severe, acute AH. Most promising among them is the early use of corticosteroids. If there is a role for these agents, it will be for the more severely ill patient, but this remains a controversial and unproven modality. Therefore, corticosteroids should be given only in consultation with an intensivist or gastroenterologist. Because of this, these agents have little or no role for the AH patient in the ED.[5,19,20] The most effective treatment for AH is cessation of alcohol consumption, whichconfers maximum benefit to the patient with regard to long-term prognosis.[4,5] For the patient with mild disease, follow-up with a gastroenterologist and alcohol detoxification may suffice. It is often hard to determine the severity of a patient's alcoholism by ED history and physical alone; therefore, it is difficult to predict which patients are at high risk for withdrawal syndromes and delirium tremens. It is wise to recommend medical detoxification to any patient who is clinically well enough for discharge. Most patients who present to the ED with suspected AH, however, will be admitted and closely monitored for signs of withdrawal. It is always good practice to discuss this possibility with the admitting service as the signs of withdrawal may be slow in manifesting and may be mistaken for other clinical entities, especially psychiatric disorders.

PITFALLS

- Maintain a high clinical suspicion for severe disease in any alcoholic patient presenting to the ED with suspected AH.

- The alcoholic patient requires a thorough history and physical exam. Failure to do so has many times resulted in the delay of diagnosing severe disease.

- Anticipate the potential for alcohol withdrawal and delirium tremens. Often the alcoholic patient resists cessation and becomes exquisitely ill prior to stopping alcohol intake.

- Suspect an infectious etiology in any alcoholic patient presenting in withdrawal. Have a low threshold for lumbar puncture in the febrile patient in withdrawal.

- It is prudent to consider a broad differential diagnosis. Be very cautious about limiting your diagnosis to AH prior to ruling out other etiologies.

- The alcoholic patient is at risk for multiple simultaneous severe disorders.

- Patients with AH and unstable vital signs have a high likelihood of a bad outcome. These patients require admission to intensive care.

REFERENCES

1. Mandayam, S. Epidemiology of alcoholic liver disease. *Semin Liver Dis.* 2004;4:217.
2. Maher JJ, Alcoholic liver disease. In: Feldman M. Sleisenger M. Fordtran J. *Gastrointestinal and liver disease.* Philadelphia: Elsevier; 2002:1375.
3. Sandler RS, Everhart JE, Donowitz M, et al. The burden of selected digestive diseases in the United States. *Gastroenterology.* 2002;122:1500.
4. Hall PD. Pathological spectrum of alcoholic liver disease. *Alcohol Alcohol Suppl.* 1994;2:303.
5. O'Shea RS. Treatment of alcoholic hepatitis. *Clin Liver Dis.* 2005;9:113.
6. Stickel F, Hoehn B, Schuppan D, Seitz HK. Review article: nutritional therapy in alcoholic liver disease. *Aliment Pharmacol Ther.* 2003;18:357.
7. Day CP. Alcoholic liver disease: Dose and threshold—new thoughts on an old topic. *Gut.* 1997;41:857.
8. Becker U, Deis A, Sorensen TIA, et al. Prediction of risk of liver disease by alcohol intake, sex, and age: A prospective population study. *Hepatology.* 1996;23:1025.
9. Orrego H, Blendis LM, Blake JE, et al. Reliability of assessment of alcohol intake based on personal interviews in a liver clinic. *Lancet.* 1979;2:1354.
10. Becker U, Deis A, Sorensen TIA, et al. Prediction of risk of liver disease by alcohol intake, sex, and age: a prospective population study. *Hepatology.* 1996;23:1025.
11. Maddrey WC. Alcohol-induced liver disease. *Clin Liver Dis.* 2005;4:115.
12. Willner, IR, Reuben, A. Alcohol and the liver. *Curr Opin Gastroenterol.* 2005;21:323.
13. Peters MG, Terrault NA. Alcohol use and hepatitis C. *Hepatology.* 2002;36(Suppl 1):S220.
14. Sorbi D, Boynton J, Lindor KD. The ratio of aspartate aminotransferase to alanine aminotransferase: potential value in differentiating nonalcoholic steatohepatitis from alcoholic liver disease. *Am J Gastroenterol.* 1999;94:1018.
15. Leevy CM, Moroianu SA. Nutritional aspects of alcoholic liver disease. Clin *Liver Dis.* 2005;9:67.
16. Rubens, DJ. Hepatobiliary imaging and its pitfalls. *Radiol Clin N Am.* 2004;42:257.
17. Wilson AV. A double-blind, placebo-controlled trial of magnesium sulfate in the ethanol withdrawal syndrome. *Alcohol Clin Exp Resp.* 1984;8:542.
18. Menon KV, Gores GJ, ShahVH. Pathogenesis, diagnosis, and treatment of alcoholic liver disease. *Mayo Clin Proc.* 2001;76:1021.
19. Imperiale TF, McCullough AJ. Do corticosteroids reduce mortality from alcoholic hepatitis? *Ann Intern Med.* 1990; 113:299.
20. Mathurin P, Mendenhall CL, Carithers RL, et al. Corticosteroids improve short term survival in patients with severe alcoholic hepatitis (AH): individual data analysis of the last three randomized placebo controlled double blind trials of corticosteroids in severe AH. *J Hepatol.* 2002;36:480.

20

Viral Hepatitis

Esther H. Chen
Bruce Y. Lee

HIGH YIELD FACTS

- Risk factors for viral hepatitis include poor hygienic conditions, intravenous drug use, men who have sex with men, blood product recipients, and health-care work.

- As hepatitis is endemic in parts of Africa, Central and South America, the Middle East, and Southeast Asia, a patient's travel history or country of origin may reveal a potential etiology.

- There are a wide variety of presentations of hepatitis, ranging from no symptoms to minor viral illness symptoms, fulminant hepatitis, cirrhosis, or hepatocellular carcinoma.

- Emergency treatment is largely supportive, including fluid resuscitation, pain control, antiemetics, and correction of electrolyte and coagulation abnormalities.

EPIDEMIOLOGY

Viral hepatitis infection should not be overlooked as a potential cause of acute abdominal pain. Each year in the United States alone, over 7000 new cases of hepatitis A virus (HAV) infections occur, over 7000 people are newly infected with hepatitis B virus (HBV), and over 1000 people are newly infected with hepatitis C virus (HCV).[1] Worldwide, an estimated 350 million people are chronic carriers of HBV infection.

Since the prevalence of viral hepatitis varies around the world, a patient's country of origin and travel history may affect the likelihood of hepatitis being the cause of the patient's symptoms. Hepatitis A virus is most common in areas without adequate sanitation, sewage, and water purification systems. In many African, Central and South American, Mid Eastern, and Southeast Asian countries, over 90% of the population is seropositive for anti-HAV antibody; Southern and Eastern European countries have higher HAV seroprevalences than Northern Europe countries.[2]

Hepatitis B virus should be heavily considered in patients from sub-Saharan Africa, Southeast Asia, and the Amazon basin, where 70% to 95% of the population have had HBV infections and 8% are chronic carriers.[3] Hepatitis B virus infection rates are lower in Eastern and Southern Europe, the Middle East, Japan, and parts of South America, where 10% to 60% of the population are infected and 2% to 7% are chronic carriers. The prevalence is lower in North America, Northern and Western Europe, and Australia, where 5% to 7% of the population are infected and 0.5% to 2% are chronic carriers.[3] The geographic distribution of HCV is similar to that of HBV, with the prevalence of HCV infection ranging from 1.8% in the United States to 25% in Egypt.[4] Hepatitis D virus (HDV) can only infect patients already infected (superinfection) or concurrently infected (coinfection) by HBV. Approximately 5% of HBV carriers or 15 million people are infected by HDV. Hepatitis D virus is most prevalent in Italy, Eastern Europe, the Amazon Basin, Columbia, Venezuela, Western Asia, and parts of the Pacific Islands. Hepatitis E virus (HEV) is most prevalent (2% to 15%) in the Indian subcontinent, Southeast and Central Asia, the Middle East, Africa, and Mexico. In the United States, Hispanic Americans, African Americans, and Native Americans appear to have higher rates of viral hepatitis infection than non-Hispanic whites. Hepatitis C virus infection is especially high among Native Americans, with incidence rates more than 6 times higher than white Americans.[5]

In addition to geography, certain medical conditions, medical interventions, and habits can predispose patients to contracting viral hepatitis, such as preexisting liver disease, IV drug use, hemodialysis, men who have sex with men, and blood product transfusions. Poor hygienic conditions (at work or home) and ingesting improperly prepared food are risk factors for HAV and HEV. Health-care workers who are exposed to blood and other body fluids are also at higher risk.

PATHOPHYSIOLOGY

Both HAV and HEV are transmitted through the ingestion of fecal material containing the virus, which can occur during close personal contact or drinking and eating contaminated materials,[6] although 45% to 50% of

HAV infected people have no identifiable source of infection.[7] Acute HAV infection occurs after an incubation period of 4 weeks and remains asymptomatic in most children less than 6 years old (70%). In contrast, 70% of older children and adults will be jaundiced, usually lasting less than 2 months, although only 10% to 15% of symptomatic patients will progress to fulminant disease.[8] Acute HEV infection occurs after an incubation period of 3 to 8 weeks, and although jaundice may persist for several weeks, most recover fully and never progress to chronic infection.[9]

Hepatitis B virus is primarily transmitted through sexual or close physical contact with infected individuals, parenteral inoculation (e.g., injection drug use, occupational needle stick injuries), and perinatally from mother to child, although over one-third of acutely infected patients report no risk factors. After an incubation period of 1 to 4 months, symptoms from acute infections develop in 30% to 50% of infected adults, but chronic infection rates vary with age, ranging from 90% in infected neonates to 30% in young children, and 5% in adults.[10] Approximately 2% of patients with chronic infection develop liver cirrhosis each year.[11]

Hepatitis C virus is transmitted parenterally, usually through injection drug use and, prior to 1992, blood transfusion. In 15% to 30% of acute infections, symptoms will resolve in 3 to 6 months. However, up to 85% of patients will become chronically infected, with more than 20% of patients progressing to cirrhosis.[11]

Similar to HBV, HDV is spread through parenteral or sexual exposure to blood or body fluids, although sexual transmission of HDV may be less efficient than that of HBV. Following HBV–HDV coinfection, symptoms usually occur 2 to 5 weeks later and are accompanied by a biphasic increase (i.e., a peak followed by a decrease, then a second peak) in serum aminotransferase activity that is rarely seen in acute HBV infection alone. Although HDV coinfection may make fulminant hepatitis more likely, it usually does not affect the long-term progression and natural course of HBV infection. By contrast, HDV superinfections of HBV may result in fulminant hepatitis and are usually not self-limited, as 90% of patients develop chronic progressive liver disease.[12]

CLINICAL FEATURES

Patients with acute viral hepatitis infection may be asymptomatic, exhibit minor symptoms of abdominal pain and vomiting, or present with fulminant hepatitis. Some may have persistent subclinical infection whereas others will rapidly progress to cirrhosis and hepatocellular carcinoma (Table 20-1).

Prodromal Phase

Like other viral illnesses, early symptoms are nonspecific, including abdominal pain, generalized malaise, fatigue, anorexia, nausea, vomiting, myalgias, arthralgias, and headache.[13] Smokers may suddenly develop distaste for cigarettes. Fever is more likely to develop in HAV or HEV infections. Prodromal symptoms often will intensify as aminotransferase levels peak.

Table 20-1. Clinical Features of Viral Hepatitis

	Transmission	Jaundice	Fulminant Hepatitis	Chronic Infection	Mortality
HAV	Fecal-oral	Adults 30% Children <5%	<1%	None	0.1–2.7%
HBV	Percutaneous, sexual, perinatal	5–20%	<1%	<5%	1–3%
HCV	Percutaneous, sexual, perinatal	5–10%	Rare	80–90%	1–2%
HDV	Percutaneous, sexual	Unknown	2–7.5%	70–90% with superinfection	<1% coinfection
HEV	Fecal-oral	Common	<1%*	None	0.5–4%
HGV	Percutaneous	Unknown	Unknown	Unknown	Unknown

*Fulminant hepatitis is 30% in pregnancy with HEV.
Abbreviations: HAV, hepatitis A virus; HBV, hepatitis B virus; HCV, hepatitis C virus; HDV, hepatitis D virus; HEV, hepatitis E virus; HGV, hepatitis G virus.

Clinical Jaundice

Within weeks of the prodromal symptoms, jaundice develops in 90% of HAV infections,[13] 30% to 50% of HBV infections,[14] and 25% of HCV infections.[15] Other symptoms of hepatic cholestasis (i.e., pruritus, dark urine, clay-colored stools) frequently occur as well. Children infected with HAV are less likely to develop jaundice than adults.[13] Exam findings may include liver tenderness, splenomegaly, and posterior cervical lymphadenopathy.[13]

Fulminant Hepatitis

Fulminant hepatitis is a life-threatening complication, manifested by hepatic encephalopathy and coagulation abnormalities that develops in less than 1% of HAV, HBV, and HEV infections, and is very rare in HCV infections. HEV-infected pregnant patients are more likely (up to 30%) to develop fulminant hepatitis.[16] Patients with symptoms of acute hepatitis and a prolonged prothrombin time (PT) (international normalized ratio [INR] >1.5) may progress toward hepatic failure.

Extrahepatic Manifestations

Extrahepatic manifestations of hepatitis, such as arthralgias and arthritis, vasculitis, dermatologic lesions, and glomerulonephritis may be important clues in establishing the diagnosis.[17] In fact, acute abdominal pain can result from polyarteritis nodosa causing ischemia to the bowel or gallbladder, which can be seen in both HBV and HCV.[18] Extrahepatic symptoms are very rare in HAV, more common in HBV (approximately 25%), and rare in HCV (approximately 1%–2%). A serum sickness-like syndrome, polyneuropathy, or Guillain-Barré can be seen in HBV[18] and corneal ulcers, non-Hodgkin lymphoma, or diabetes mellitus can be seen in HCV.[19]

Chronic Hepatitis

While HAV and HEV infections usually are self-limited, some HBV infections (less than 5%), most HCV infections (80%–90%), and HBV–HDV coinfections (80%–90%) may progress to chronic hepatitis.[11,12]

DIAGNOSIS AND DIFFERENTIAL

Since prodromal symptoms are fairly nonspecific, it is easy to miss a diagnosis of viral hepatitis. Furthermore, the diagnosis of viral hepatitis is often presumed at an emergency visit and the specific viral pathogen identified after discharge. Elevated alanine transaminase (ALT) and aspartate transaminase (AST) levels strongly suggest hepatocellular injury; elevated alkaline phosphatase and bilirubin imply hepatic cholestasis; and elevated PT and decreased serum albumin levels occur when the liver is not functioning properly and unable to normally manufacture proteins.[20] Acute viral hepatitis can result in AST and ALT elevations ranging from less than 5 times normal to greater than 15 times normal. Alanine transaminase predominant elevations (ALT>AST) are seen in viral infections whereas AST predominant elevations (AST>ALT) are characteristic of alcohol-induced liver injury.

Patients with elevated liver enzymes and appropriate risk factors should be screened for viral hepatitis. Acute HAV-infected individuals will have positive immunoglobulin-M (IgM) HAV antibody detected by either radioimmunoassay (RIA) or enzyme-linked immunoassay (EIA). Acute HBV infection is characterized by elevated HBV surface antigen (HBsAg) levels followed by elevated HBV core antibodies, mainly IgM type,[21] but chronic and past infections may also be determined by viral serology (Table 20-2). The assay for HCV infection (EIA or recombinant EIA for anti-HCV antibody) does not distinguish acute from chronic or resolved infection, but active viral infection may be detected by an HCV-RNA polymerase chain reaction (PCR) assay.[7] Similarly, EIA or recombinant EIA assays for anti-HDV IgM (acute infection) and IgG (chronic infection) are available, as well as EIA and Western blot assays for anti-HEV antibody.[16] Liver biopsy may help identify other causes of hepatitis or hepatic failure but are rarely indicated in acute viral hepatitis.

Table 20-2. Interpretation of Serologic Tests for Hepatitis B Virus

Interpretation	HBsAg	Anti-HBs	Anti-HBc IgM	Anti-HBc IgG
Immunity (vaccination)	Negative	Positive	Negative	Negative
Immunity (natural infection)	Negative	Positive	Negative	Positive
Acute infection	Positive	Negative	Positive	Positive
Chronic infection	Positive	Negative	Negative	Positive

Abbreviations: HBsAg, hepatitis B virus surface antigen; Anti-HBs, hepatitis B virus surface antibody; Anti-HBc, hepatitis B virus core antibody.

The differential diagnosis of viral hepatitis includes other conditions that can cause right upper quadrant pain, such as nonviral liver diseases (e.g., alcoholic, autoimmune, or drug-induced hepatitis, or Wilson disease), gallbladder diseases, lower lobe pneumonia, pancreatitis, Fitz-Hugh-Curtis, as well as conditions that cause nausea, vomiting, and fatigue, including gastroenteritis and other viral syndromes (e.g., Epstein-Barr virus, Rotavirus).

EMERGENCY DEPARTMENT CARE AND DISPOSITION

Treatment is primarily supportive, such as fluid resuscitation for volume loss, correction of electrolyte imbalances, administration of antiemetic agents, and pain control. Medications that are primarily metabolized by the liver and alcoholic consumption should be discontinued in patients with significantly depressed liver function.

Hospital admission is indicated for patients with intractable vomiting, severe volume depletion, significant electrolyte imbalances requiring in-hospital monitoring, and altered sensorium or prolonged PT indicating fulminant disease. Patients with reliable health-care follow-up may be managed as outpatients and specifically instructed to practice good personal hygiene, use barrier protection during sexual contact, and not to share toiletries or utensils.

Because viral hepatitis is a communicable disease, emergency physicians are required to report new cases to the public health department and provide immunoprophylaxis to close personal contacts of infected patients.

PITFALLS

- Patients with nonviral liver disease should still be screened for viral hepatitis given a typical presentation, since viral hepatitis frequently afflicts patients with other types of liver disease.

- Avoid administering medications that are metabolized by the liver until you have ruled out hepatitis or other liver disease.

- Absence of obvious risk factors does not exclude viral hepatitis.

- Discharged patients should receive appropriate instructions (e.g., good personal hygiene, barrier protections during sex) to avoid transmission to other people.

- Hepatitis should be reported to public health authorities.

REFERENCES

1. Hopkins RS, Jajosky RA, Hall PA, et al. Summary of notifiable diseases—United States, 2003. *MMWR Morb Mortal Wkly Rep.* 2005;52:1.
2. Jacobsen KH, Koopman JS. Declining hepatitis A seroprevalence: a global review and analysis. *Epidemiol Infect.* 2004;132:1005.
3. Hou J, Liu Z, Gu F. Epidemiology and prevention of hepatitis B virus infection. *Int J Med Sci.* 2005;2:50.
4. Thomson BJ, Finch RG. Hepatitis C virus infection. *Clin Microbiol Infect.* 2005;11:86.
5. Rawls RA, Vega KJ. Viral hepatitis in minority America. *J Clin Gastroenterol.* 2005;39:144.
6. Wasley A, Samandari T, Bell BP. Incidence of hepatitis A in the United States in the era of vaccination. *JAMA.* 2005; 294:194.
7. Weinbaum C, Lyerla R, Margolis HS. Prevention and control of infections with hepatitis viruses in correctional settings. Centers for Disease Control and Prevention. *MMWR Recomm Rep.* 2003;52(RR-1):1–36; quiz CE31-34.
8. Glikson M, Galun E, Oren R, et al. Relapsing hepatitis A. Review of 14 cases and literature survey. *Medicine (Baltimore).* 1992;71:14.
9. Emerson SU, Purcell RH. Running like water—the omnipresence of hepatitis E. *N Engl J Med.* 2004;351:2367.
10. Hyams KC. Risks of chronicity following acute hepatitis B virus infection: a review. *Clin Infect Dis.* 1995;20:992.
11. Lin OS, Keeffe EB. Current treatment strategies for chronic hepatitis B and C. *Annu Rev Med.* 2001;52:29.
12. Rosina F, Cozzolongo R. Interferon in HDV infection. *Antiviral Res.* 1994;24:165.
13. Lednar WM, Lemon SM, Kirkpatrick JW, et al. Frequency of illness associated with epidemic hepatitis A virus infections in adults. *Am J Epidemiol.* 1985;122:226.
14. Pan CQ, Zhang JX. Natural history and clinical consequences of hepatitis B virus infection. *Int J Med Sci.* 2005; 2:36.
15. Alter HJ, Seeff LB. Recovery, persistence, and sequelae in hepatitis C virus infection: a perspective on long-term outcome. *Semin Liver Dis.* 2000;20:17.
16. Mast EE, Krawczynski K. Hepatitis E: an overview. *Annu Rev Med.* 1996;47:257.
17. Schiff ER. Atypical clinical manifestations of hepatitis A. *Vaccine.* 1992;10(Suppl 1):S18.
18. Willson RA. Extrahepatic manifestations of chronic viral hepatitis. *Am J Gastroenterol.* 1997;92:3.
19. Zignego AL, Brechot C. Extrahepatic manifestations of HCV infection: facts and controversies. *J Hepatol.* 1999;31:369.
20. Green RM, Flamm S. AGA technical review on the evaluation of liver chemistry tests. *Gastroenterology.* 2002; 123:1367.
21. Hoofnagle JH, Schafer DF. Serologic markers of hepatitis B virus infection. *Semin Liver Dis.* 1986;6:1.

21

Cirrhosis and Liver Failure

Susan P. Torrey

This chapter covers cirrhosis in general, the complications of portal hypertension, and liver failure from both chronic and acute liver disease.

CIRRHOSIS
High Yield Facts

> - Most cirrhosis is due to chronic alcoholic liver disease or chronic viral infection.
> - Portal hypertension is responsible for the development of ascites, renal dysfunction, and gastrointestinal (GI) bleeding from esophageal varices.
> - Synthetic dysfunction associated with cirrhosis accounts for acquired coagulopathies, such as vitamin K-associated prolongation of the prothrombin time (PT)/ international normalized ratio (INR).

Epidemiology

The overall prevalence of cirrhosis in the United States is estimated at 360 per 100,000, the vast majority of whom have either alcoholic liver disease or chronic viral infection.[1] Alcoholic liver disease is directly attributable to chronic ingestion of large quantities of alcohol. It has been estimated that liver disease is associated with the daily consumption of 50 grams, or 3 to 4 drinks, for 10 to 15 years in women, or 5 to 6 drinks a day in men.[2] Cirrhosis following viral infection is most often due to hepatitis C in the United States, while hepatitis B continues to have a significant impact in developing nations. Following infection with hepatitis C, approximately 25% of patients will eventually develop cirrhosis, with the average rate of progression estimated at 30 years.[1] Other less common causes of cirrhosis include metabolic diseases (e.g., Wilson disease and hemochromatosis) and biliary disorders (e.g., primary biliary cirrhosis) (Table 21-1).

Pathophysiology

Cirrhosis develops after chronic injury to the liver from a variety of causes. It is characterized by destruction of hepatocytes and changes in normal hepatic architecture as it is replaced by fibrotic tissue and regenerative nodules. Cirrhosis has been divided into three main categories: Laënnec, postnecrotic, and biliary. Laënnec cirrhosis is a diffuse process involving the entire organ and typically follows chronic alcohol use. Postnecrotic cirrhosis is non-homogenous with areas of fibrosis alternating with more normal tissue. It is usually a consequence of chronic hepatitis (viral, drug induced, or metabolic). Biliary cirrhosis occurs because of chronic extrahepatic biliary obstruction or primarily as an autoimmune intrahepatic duct inflammation and scarring.

Clinical Features

Clinical features of cirrhosis are related to progressive loss of hepatocellular function or to the fibrotic changes leading to impaired portal blood flow and portal hypertension. These two processes eventually lead to the sequelae of cirrhosis (e.g., ascites, variceal bleeding, and hepatic encephalopathy), which lead to the diagnosis in many patients. Prior to the development of the complications of portal hypertension, up to 40% of patients with cirrhosis are asymptomatic.[1]

Physical exam of a cirrhotic patient may reveal muscle wasting, thinning of skin with ecchymoses, spider angiomata, and palmar erythema, and in men, gynecomastia and testicular atrophy. The liver span may be small or large, depending on the amount of concurrent inflammatory change. A palpable left lobe of the liver in the epigastrium has been shown to be predictive of cirrhosis with a sensitivity of 86% and a specificity of 67%.[3] Splenomegaly and distension of abdominal wall veins (caput medusa) are further signs of cirrhosis associated with significant portal hypertension.

Diagnosis and Differential

The "gold standard" for the diagnosis of cirrhosis remains a liver biopsy. In many cases, however, the clinical diagnosis is easily made by a combination of history and physical exam, particularly when portal hypertension brings the patient to medical attention.

Table 21-1. Causes of Cirrhosis

Autoimmune hepatitis
Alcohol-induced liver disease
Drug- or toxin-induced liver injury
    (amiodarone, carbon tetrachloride, methotrexate)
Viral hepatitis (B, C, or D)
Metabolic disease
    α_1-Antitrypsin deficiency
    Hemochromatosis
    Wilson disease
Nonalcoholic steatohepatitis (fatty liver)
Vascular derangements
    Chronic right-sided heart failure
    Budd-Chiari syndrome
    Long-standing portal vein thrombosis
Biliary disorders
    Primary biliary cirrhosis
    Cystic fibrosis
    Sarcoidosis
Primary sclerosing cholangitis

Emergency Department Care and Disposition

The management of the complications of cirrhosis are covered below. Well-compensated cirrhosis, without evidence of any of its complications, can be managed as an outpatient, but all patients with this diagnosis require ongoing follow-up with an internist or a gastroenterologist. Abstinence from alcohol is absolutely necessary for cirrhotics of any cause. Any drug metabolized by the liver may precipitate complications in the fragile cirrhotic patient; commonly sedative or narcotic drugs are implicated.

ASCITES
High-Yield Facts

- Ascites is the most common complication of cirrhosis and portends a poor prognosis.
- Large volume paracentesis can be safely performed with attention to colloid replacement.
- Serum-ascites gradient is a sensitive method of diagnosing ascites due to portal hypertension.

Epidemiology

Ascites is the most common complication of cirrhosis, and its presence is associated with poor long-term survival (30%–40% survival at 5 years).[4] Approximately 50% of patients with compensated cirrhosis will develop ascites within 10 years.[5] Ascites may be further complicated by spontaneous bacterial peritonitis or the hepatorenal syndrome, either of which is associated with a substantial increase in mortality.[6]

Pathophysiology

Increased hepatic resistance to portal flow causes the development of portal hypertension, collateral-vein formation, and shunting of blood to the systemic circulation. As cirrhosis progresses, increasing portal hypertension causes the local production of vasodilators, primarily nitric oxide, leading to splanchnic arterial vasodilation. The combination of portal hypertension and splanchnic vasodilation alters intestinal capillary pressure and permeability, allowing the accumulation of retained fluid within the abdominal cavity.[4] In advanced stages, splanchnic vasodilation is significant enough to decrease systemic arterial pressure, which activates homeostatic mechanisms including vasoconstriction of renal vasculature and antinatriuretic factors. This leads to impairment of renal excretion of free water causing dilutional hyponatremia, while renal vasoconstriction eventually precipitates the hepatorenal syndrome.[7]

Clinical Features

Increasing abdominal girth is a common presentation of ascites; however, a more severe symptom is shortness of breath due to limitation of diaphragmatic movement. Physical exam may confirm the suspicion of ascites with percussion dullness of the flank and shifting dullness with partial decubitus positioning. If clinically indicated, ultrasound of the abdomen remains a very sensitive method of diagnosing fluid within the abdominal cavity.

Diagnosis and Differential

The most common cause of ascites is chronic parenchymal liver disease, accounting for 84% of cases.[5] Other causes of ascites that must be considered include malignancy, tuberculosis, and heart failure. The new presentation of ascites to the emergency department is an indication for urgent diagnosis of the cause of the ascites.

Diagnostic paracentesis can be safely performed in patients with clinically evident ascites. If the diagnosis of cirrhosis is unconfirmed, serum and ascites albumin levels should be obtained for calculation of the serum-ascites albumin gradient (simply calculated as the difference in serum minus ascites albumin). A serum-ascites gradient ≤1.1 g/dL is nearly 100% accurate in detecting portal hypertension and chronic liver disease as the cause of ascites.[8] All ascites should also be sent in a EDTA blood tube for cell count, and in sterile, no-additive (usually red-top) tubes for chemistries, Gram stain, and culture. In addition to albumin, other appropriate chemistries include glucose (low glucose indicates infection or gut perforation), LDH (increased presence indicates infection or tumor production), and amylase (increase often indicates complicated pancreatitis).

Occasionally large volume, symptomatic, or refractory ascites will require removal of a significant amount of ascites. While this produces early benefits and is well tolerated by cirrhotic patients, it is occasionally followed by a disorder known as paracentesis-induced circulatory dysfunction,[9] characterized by a high-rate of recurrence of ascites, development of hepatorenal syndrome, or dilutional hyponatremia in 20% of patients. Plasma expanders are effective in preventing this complication, and current recommendations include the infusion of albumin if more than 5 L of ascites is removed (8 g of albumin per liter of ascites removed);[10] however, survival is not affected.

Emergency Department Care and Disposition

Initial outpatient treatment of ascites includes fluid and sodium restriction. If ascites becomes less responsive to these conservative measures, sequential use of diuretics is appropriate, first with spironolactone, then with the addition of furosemide. Once refractory ascites develops, options include repeated large volume paracentesis or the use of transjugular intrahepatic portosystemic shunts (TIPS).[11] While the use of TIPS has been shown to control large volume ascites better than repeat paracentesis, patient survival is not improved. The only sure way to cure ascites is liver transplantation with a survival rate of 70% to 80% at 5 years.[12]

Pitfalls

- Large volume paracentesis can be associated with complications from paracentesis-associated circulatory dysfunction.
- While TIPS may control refractory ascites, its use does not improve survival.

- Ascites associated with cirrhosis is an indication for liver transplant.

SPONTANEOUS BACTERIAL PERITONITIS
High Yield Facts

- Spontaneous bacterial peritonitis (SBP) must be considered when cirrhotic patients with ascites present with acute symptoms, particularly abdominal pain.
- Paracentesis is diagnostic of SBP if >250 granulocytes/mm^3 are detected.
- The current treatment recommendation for SBP is cefotaxime.

Epidemiology

Ten percent to 20% of cirrhotic patients who are hospitalized have SBP.[5] Factors that independently predispose to the development of SBP include severe liver disease, acute GI bleeding, urinary tract infection (UTI), and the presence of intravascular catheters.[13] The one-year survival of patients who survive an episode of SBP is 30% to 50%, and this complication remains an important indication for liver transplantation.[14]

Pathophysiology

Once ascites develops from portal hypertension, several additional factors put the patient with advanced liver disease at increased risk of developing SBP. These include intestinal bacterial overgrowth, increased intestinal permeability and bacterial translocation, and alterations of the immune system.

Clinical Features

The presentation of SBP can be subtle, but may include abdominal pain, increased ascites volume, fever, and hepatic encephalopathy. Physical exam may also be unimpressive with minimal tenderness, but ascites and other stigmata of cirrhosis will be present. In the past, SBP was considered an infrequent complication of cirrhosis, probably because of infrequent paracentesis (often due to unfounded concerns about complications).[13]

Thus, diagnostic paracentesis should be performed whenever a cirrhotic patient presents with abdominal pain, fever, increasing ascites, or other signs of clinical deterioration.[2]

Diagnosis and Differential

Diagnostic paracentesis for volumes sufficient to identify infection can safely be accomplished and should be considered an appropriate emergency department procedure. Fluid should be sent for cell count, gram stain, and culture. Spontaneous bacterial peritonitis is diagnosed if ascitic fluid has ≥250 neutophils/mm[3]. Fluid should be inoculated into blood culture bottles at the bedside as this has been shown to improve diagnostic yield over delayed inoculation in the lab.[15] Ninety percent of cases of SBP are monomicrobial, with *Escherichia coli* most common, followed by *Klebsiella* series, and other gram-negative organisms. Gram-positive organisms occur in 25% of cases.

Secondary peritonitis from intestinal perforation should also be considered in any patient with neutrophilic ascites. Again, classic peritoneal signs will not be present in the patient with ascites. This diagnosis should be considered if 2 of the following 3 criteria are met: total protein >1 g/dL, glucose <50 mg/dL, and LDH > upper limit of normal for serum.[13,16] In addition, the presence of multiple organisms suggests this diagnosis. Empirical treatment for suspected secondary peritonitis includes cefotaxime and metronidazole. Further evaluation with abdominal computed tomography (CT) to rule out perforation or intraabdominal abscess and surgical consultation is appropriate.

Emergency Department Care and Disposition

Spontaneous bacterial peritonitis can be treated with cefotaxime (2 gm IV every 8 hours) for 5 to 7 days. While 75% to 90% of patients will respond to third-generation cephalosporins, mortality remains high (between 20% and 40%).[5]

Pitfalls

- Failure to consider the diagnosis of SBP in a cirrhotic patient will contribute to substantial morbidity and mortality.

VARICEAL BLEEDING

The management of variceal bleeding is covered in Chapter 12.

HEPATIC FAILURE AND ENCEPHALOPATHY
High Yield Facts

- Acute hepatic failure differs clinically, prognostically, and therapeutically from an exacerbation of chronic liver failure, but the priorities for the management of both entities are similar.

- Spontaneous bacterial peritonitis, pneumonia, UTI, bacteremia, or other bacterial infection complicates the hospital course of 80% of patients in fulminant hepatic failure (FHF), and these infections account for 25% of deaths.

- Patients with FHF who demonstrate clinical signs of significant, increased intracranial pressure, such as abnormal posturing or unreactive pupils, should receive mannitol and careful hyperventilation.

Pathophysiology

Ammonia, a substance liberated from the intestinal flora and known to accumulate in hepatic failure, is a key factor in the development of hepatic encephalopathy.[17] However, ammonia accumulation causes an excitable state rather than neural inhibition, and the severity of hepatic coma does not always correlate with blood ammonia levels. It has been shown that a systemic inflammatory response is an essential component initiating hepatic encephalopathy.[18] Infection generally plays a role in this inflammatory response.[19]

Viral hepatitis has traditionally been regarded as the most common cause of FHF worldwide. In the United States, drug related hepatotoxicity accounts for over 50% of acute liver failure, including acetaminophen (40%) and idiosyncratic drugs (12%), including cocaine and MDMA (ecstasy).[20] Less common causes include fatty degeneration of pregnancy, Reye syndrome, heat stroke, *Amanita phalloides* mushroom poisoning, and metastatic cancer to the liver.

Clinical Features

The presentation of FHF is, to some degree, dependent on the specific etiologic agent, but the majority of patients have altered mentation, coagulopathy with clinical bleeding, jaundice (especially in children), motor dysfunction, and fetor hepaticus, a sweetish, musty, or pungent odor on the breath. Patients may have bradycardia, papilledema, and hypertension in association with cerebral edema, or they may present with a signs indistinguishable from sepsis including tachycardia and hypotension.

Fulminant hepatic failure may present with rapid deterioration of mental status, with progression over several hours from slowed response times to frank coma. Patients with cirrhosis commonly present with euphoria, depression, or muscular incoordination, or may demonstrate more obvious mental status changes. Physical findings may include hepatomegaly, spider nevi, ascites, and jaundice. Asterixis, a flapping tremor best seen with the patient's arms outstretched and wrists hyperextended, is a classic symptom but is not present in all cases. The factors most commonly precipitating hepatic encephalopathy in cirrhotics are GI bleeding, use of tranquilizing drugs or alcohol, overuse of diuretics, and infection.

Cerebral edema is a universal feature of acute hepatic failure and the most common cause of death in untreated cases. Early warning signs include systemic hypertension and increased muscle tone, which progresses to decerebrate posturing and eventual respiratory arrest if left untreated. Hypoglycemia may be profound and recurrent. More than 50% of patients demonstrate clinical evidence of coagulopathy, usually in the form of GI, nasopharyngeal, or bronchial tree bleeding. Hypotension secondary to decreased systemic vascular resistance may occur in the absence of hemorrhage. Hypoxia and noncardiogenic pulmonary edema are common. Prerenal azotemia, acute tubular necrosis, or renal failure of unknown cause may occur. Hypokalemia and hypocalcemia are common.

SBP, pneumonia, UTI, bacteremia, or other bacterial infection complicates the hospital course of 80% of patients in FHF, and these infections account for 25% of deaths.[19]

Diagnosis and Differential

The diagnosis of hepatic encephalopathy is largely clinical; no single laboratory test can confirm the diagnosis with certainty. Hypoxemia and hypoglycemia should be ruled out. A serum ammonia level should be measured and symptomatic patients with elevated levels are likely to have hepatic encephalopathy[21]; however, patients may be encephalopathic before an elevation in the serum ammonia is observed. Serum aminotransferases, bilirubin, serologic tests, and serum amino acid levels may aid in diagnosis but do not alter management acutely. Abdominal and pelvic computed tomography may be required to rule out surgical causes of abdominal pain.

In the patient without chronic liver disease, the differential diagnosis of hepatic encephalopathy includes viral hepatitis, fatty degeneration of pregnancy, Reye syndrome, and hepatotoxic ingestions such as acetaminophen, isoniazid, rifampin, *A. phalloides* mushrooms, carbon tetrachloride, or MDMA (ecstasy). There are few clinical features that help to differentiate hepatic encephalopathy from other causes of acute mental status change, with the exception of fetor hepaticus, which frequently goes unrecognized.

Patients with hepatic cirrhosis may have chronic jaundice and may sustain acute mental status changes for reasons other than hepatic encephalopathy. Because alcoholic patients are at greater risk for accidents as well as for bleeding, subdural hematoma must be ruled out in cirrhotics with an altered sensorium.

Emergency Department Care and Disposition

Hepatic encephalopathy in acute hepatic failure develops more rapidly than with chronic liver disease and is almost always complicated by cerebral edema, with possible central herniation of the brain. Immediate attention should be given to securing a patent airway and initiating artificial ventilation if the patient is comatose or lacks an active gag reflex. Propofol, 1 to 2.5 mg/kg intravenously (or 40 mg every 10 seconds until desired effect), may be better tolerated and is considered the sedative agent of choice in acute liver failure for its protective effects from intracranial hypertension.[22] Fluid resuscitation should be aggressive in hypotensive or bleeding patients. Dopamine (2 to 20 microgram/kg/min) is recommended for persistent hypotension, but norepinephrine (0.5 to 30 microgram/min) may be required.

Patients with a blood glucose level below 100 mg/100 dL should receive 50% dextrose and thiamine intravenously, followed by an infusion of 10% or 20% dextrose solution. Patients who demonstrate clinical signs of significant, increased intracranial pressure, such as abnormal posturing or unreactive pupils, should receive mannitol 0.5 g/kg intravenously over 10 minutes.[23] Hyperventilation is also recommended for brief periods but PaCO$_2$ should not be reduced below 25 mm Hg.[24] Proven or suspected infection should be treated promptly, using cultures to modify empiric therapy. The responsible organisms are usually gram-negative; cefotaxime (1 to 2 g intravenously) or a similar broad-spectrum cephalosporin is recommended.

Lactulose accelerates recovery from hepatic coma and can be given as a syrup, 50 cc every 1 to 2 hours until results are obtained, or it can be given as an enema, 300 cc in a liter of saline. Oral neomycin, 2 to 4 g/d divided q 6 hours, also has been shown to be effective, but should be withheld if an aminoglycoside is being considered for treatment of a coexisting infection. Metronidazole, 800 mg/d divided q 12 hours, is an alternative.[23] Flumazenil has been shown to improve the short-term recovery from hepatic encephalopathy in patients with an exacerbation of chronic liver disease, but has not been shown to improve survival.[25]

Decisions concerning liver support measures are best made by a gastroenterology consultant. In many cases of severe acute hepatic failure, transplantation is the only means of increasing the chance of survival. Patients with GI bleeding, SBP, and hepatic encephalopathy should be admitted to the hospital. For severe cases, consideration should be given to transporting the patient to a facility capable of critical care and liver transplantation, provided intensive care transport is available.

Pitfalls

- The diagnosis of hepatic encephalopathy cannot be ruled out on the basis of a normal serum ammonia level.

- Failing to consider a hepatotoxic drug as the cause of the patient's symptoms.

- One bolus of 50% dextrose may not be adequate therapy because of depleted glycogen stores; maintenance infusions of D_{10} or D_{20} should be administered.

- It is essential that the emergency physician attempt to identify causes of coma other than hepatic encephalopathy in patients with cirrhosis.

REFERENCES

1. Friedman SL, Schiano TD. Cirrhosis and its sequelae. In Goldman L, Ausiello D (eds.): *Cecil Textbook of Medicine*. 22nd ed. Philadelphia: Saunders, 2004.
2. Becker U, Deis A, Sorensen TIA, et al. Prediction of risk of liver disease by alcohol intake, sex, and age: A prospective population study, *Hepatology*. 1996;23:1025.
3. McCormick PA, Nolan N. Palpable epigastric liver as a physical sign of cirrhosis: a prospective study. *Eur J Gastroenterol Hepatol*. 2004;16:1331.
4. Gines P, Cardenas A, Arroyo V, et al. Management of cirrhosis and ascites. *N Engl J Med*. 2004;350:1646.
5. Menon KVN, Kamath PS. Managing the complications of cirrhosis. *Mayo Clin Proc*. 2000;75:501.
6. Gines P, Arroyo V. Hepatorenal syndrome. *J Am Soc Nephrol*. 1999;10:1833.
7. Gentilini P, Vizzutti F, Gentilini A, et al. Ascites and hepatorenal syndrome. *Eur J Gastroenterol Hepatol*. 2001;13:313.
8. Runyon BA, Montano AA, Akriviadis EA, et al. The serum-ascites albumin gradient is superior to the exudates-transudate concept in the differential diagnosis of ascites. *Ann Intern Med*. 1992;117:215.
9. Sola-Vera J, Such J. Understanding the mechanisms of paracentesis-induced circulatory dysfunction. *Eur J Gastroenterol Hepatol*. 2004;16:295.
10. Sanyal AJ, Genning C, Reddy KR, et al. The North American Study for the treatment of refractory ascites. *Gastroenterology*. 2003;124:634.
11. LeBrec D, Vinel JP, Dupas JL. Complications of portal hypertension in adults: a French consensus. *Eur J Gastroenterol Hepatol*. 2004;17:403.
12. Such J, Runyon BA. Spontaneous bacterial peritonitis. *Clin Infect Dis*. 1998;27:669.
13. Kramer L, Druml W. Ascites and intraabdominal infection. *Curr Opin Crit Care*. 2004;10:146.
14. Runyon BA, Antillon MR, Akriviadis EA, et al. Bedside inoculation of blood culture bottles with ascitic fluid is superior to delayed inoculation in the detection of spontaneous bacterial peritonitis. *J Clin Microbiol*. 1990;28:2811.
15. Nietsch HH. Management of portal hypertension. *J Clin Gastroenterol*. 2005;39:232.
16. Lecleire S, DiFiore F, Merle V, et al. Acute upper gastrointestinal bleeding in patients with liver cirrhosis and in non-cirrhotic patients. *J Clin Gastroenterol*. 2005;39:321.
17. Vaquero J, Chung C, Cahill ME, et al. Pathogenesis of hepatic encephalopathy in acute liver failure. *Semin Liver Dis*. 2003;23:259.
18. Rolando N, Wade J, Davalos M, et al. The systemic inflammatory response syndrome in acute liver failure. *Hepatology*. 2000;32:734.
19. Rolando N, Harvey F, Brahm J, et al. Prospective study of bacterial infection in acute liver failure: an analysis of fifty patients. *Hepatology*. 1990;11:49.
20. Ostapowicz G, Rontan RJ, Schiodt FV, et al. Results of a prospective study of acute liver failure at 17 tertiary care centers in the United States. *Ann Intern Med*. 2002;137:947.
21. Ong JP, Aggarway A, Krieger D, et al. Correlation between ammonia levels and the severity of hepatic encephalopathy. *Am J Med*. 2003;114:188.
22. Wijdicks EFM, Nyberg SL. Propofol to control intracranial pressure in fulminant hepatic failure. *Transplant Proc*. 2002;34:1220.
23. Riordan SM, Williams R. Treatment of hepatic encephalopathy. *N Engl J Med*. 1997;337:473.
24. Stauss G, Hansen BA, Knudsen, et al. Hyperventilation restores cerebral blood flow autoregulation in patients with acute liver failure. *J Hepatol*. 1998;28:199.
25. Lock BG, Pandit K. Is Flumazenil an effective treatment for hepatic encephalopathy? *Ann Emerg Med*. 2006;47:286.

22

Cholecystitis and Biliary Colic

William P. Scruggs
John Christian Fox

HIGH YIELD FACTS

- Biliary pain typically resolves within 5 to 6 hours. Persistent pain warrants investigation for acute cholecystitis even without fever or abnormal laboratory values.
- Ultrasound (US) is the initial imaging study for acute cholecystitis, but cholescintigraphy is the "gold standard" imaging modality. It should be considered in patients with a negative US and a high clinical suspicion.
- Sensitivity of computed tomography (CT) scanning for acute cholecystitis varies between studies, ranging as high as 92% and as low as 39%.

EPIDEMIOLOGY

The Third National Health and Nutrition Examination Survey (NHANES III) estimates that 7.9% of men and 16.6% of women in the United States have gallbladder disease resulting in 700,000 office visits, 800,000 hospital admissions, and 600,000 cholecystectomies each year.[1,2] The associated annual costs total 5200 lives and $5.8 billion.[3,4] Cholecystitis, the most common emergent surgical condition of the gallbladder, is diagnosed in up to 10% of total patients and 21% of elderly patients presenting to the emergency department (ED) with acute abdominal pain.[5–7]

Gallstones are strongly associated with cholecystitis and are present in 90% to 95% of cases. Age and sex are the primary risk factors for gallstone development. By the age of 60, 33% of women and 25% of men have gallstones or have had their gallbladder removed.[1] Females are more likely to be affected in all age groups. However, the rate of development equalizes as both sexes approach age 60.[1,8–10]

Race is also a factor in gallstone development. Mexican American females are more likely to have gallstones

than Caucasian (9%) or African American women (8%). American Indians are particularly prone to gallbladder disease with a prevalence of 64% in women and 30% of men over the age of 46.[4,11] Patients who are symptomatic at diagnosis (most consistent with the ED population) have a higher complication rate. Up to 3% percent will develop worsening symptoms each year and 11% may develop acute cholecystitis.[12]

PATHOPHYSIOLOGY

Gallstones are identified as cholesterol or pigmented stones. In the west, approximately 75% are cholesterol based.[13] Cholesterol stone formation is multifactorial and involves the concentration of cholesterol in the bile and bile acids, the balance of stone promoters and inhibitors, and prolonged retention of bile within the gallbladder. Diet, obesity, increased cholesterol intake, rapid weight loss, and estrogens increase the concentration of cholesterol in bile by increasing the amount of cholesterol secreted in bile. The concentration of bile acids diminishes with age as production slows and chronic ileal diseases also decrease this concentration by inhibiting proper bile acid reabsorption in the small intestines.[14]

Pigmented stones make up 20% to 25% of all gallstones in patients from western countries. Black pigment stones form in the setting of chronic hemolysis as bilirubin becomes saturated in the bile and forms a calcium salt that is extremely insoluble. Brown pigment stones occur in only 5% of cases and form in the setting of chronic anaerobic infection. They are more likely to form in the hepatic ducts than other types of stones and are associated with parasitic infections in the biliary tree.[13]

Acute cholecystitis occurs with prolonged obstruction of the cystic duct, generally by gallstones, and distension of the gallbladder, increased wall tension, wall inflammation, and edema result. The initial inflammation is most often chemically mediated, as bile cultures are positive in only 52% of cases.[15] Prostaglandins play an important role via contraction of the gallbladder wall as well as increasing mucin production. In severe cases, distension and edema may cause ischemia of the gallbladder wall leading to necrosis and perforation.

CLINICAL FEATURES

Biliary pain is most often severe, steady pain located in the upper abdomen lasting 15 minutes to 5 hours.[16] Radiation of the pain to the right scapular region from the epigastrium or right upper quadrant is significant for biliary pain versus other causes of abdominal pain.[17] Dyspeptic symptoms such as nausea, vomiting, bloating, belching, acid regurgitation, and heartburn are not more common in patients with gallstones.[18,19] Conversely, heartburn along with upper abdominal pain suggests gallstones are less likely.[17] Fatty food intolerance, a classic association, is not supported in the literature.[19–21] There is a circadian periodicity to biliary pain with symptoms commonly occurring between 8:00 P.M. and 4:00 A.M. and generally occurring at approximately the same time for a given patient.[22,23]

There is no single, presenting symptom that allows for the differentiation between biliary colic and acute chole-cystitis.[24] Prior biliary pain is reported in 75% of those with acute cholecystitis.[25] Upper abdominal pain is present in 88%.[26] Theoretically, acute cholecystitis patients should have more right upper quadrant complaints, as the visceral pain from initial distension of the gallbladder will migrate from the epigastrium to the right upper quadrant as inflammation ensues and focal peritoneal signs develop. However, that assertion is not supported in the literature.[26] Anorexia, nausea, and vomiting are only slightly more likely to occur with acute cholecystitis.[24] The duration of pain is probably helpful in the diagnosis of cholecystitis as 84% of biliary pain resolves within 5 hours.[27] More persistent pain is concerning for cholecystitis.

On physical examination right upper quadrant tenderness is usually demonstrated, but epigastric tenderness is found in 14%, diffuse tenderness in 2%, and tenderness localized to another portion of the abdomen is found in 2%.[26] Murphy sign, the arrest of inspiration on deep palpation of the right upper quadrant, is present in 90% of patients with acute cholecystitis and appears to help predict acute cholecystitis with an odds ratio of 2.3 to 2.8.[24,26,28] Fever is typically quoted in surgical texts as common in acute cholecystitis, but it is not well studied. If present, however, fever with upper abdominal pain is a marker for acute cholecystitis, but up to 90% of patients may not be febrile at the time of presentation.[26,29] Jaundice occurs in a minority of patients when Mirizzi syndrome develops. Mirizzi syndrome occurs when obstruction of the cystic duct by a gallstone compresses the hepatic duct causing jaundice. A palpable gallbladder is present on superficial examination in 30% to 40% of patients, but guarding caused by deep palpation may obscure this finding.[30]

Complications of acute cholecystitis are related to delays in diagnosis and treatment by both patients and physicians and increase the risk of sepsis and death if not rapidly diagnosed and treated. Gallbladder perforation occurs in 6% of patients with acute cholecystitis and is more common in diabetics and the elderly,[31] and related mortality may be as high as 30%. Gangrenous cholecystitis occurs when vascular compromise is superimposed on an inflamed gallbladder wall. The complication is present in up to 30% of acute cholecystitis cases and the majority of patients are elderly and/or diabetic. Morbidity and mortality for gangrenous cholecystitis are three times that of acute cholecystitis and emergent surgery is indicated, but only 50% of cases are diagnosed preoperatively.[32,33] Cholecystoenteric fistula is a rare complication that is formed when the inflamed gallbladder erodes into the duodenum or colon. Gallstone ileus or obstruction may occur when a stone passes through a fistula and lodges in the small intestines, and clinicians should consider this diagnosis when elderly patients present with unexplained small bowel obstruction. Ascending cholangitis is a true emergency caused by obstruction of the common bile duct with superimposed infection of the biliary tract. It classically presents with fever, jaundice, and right upper quadrant pain (Charcot triad). Reynaud pentad, which includes the signs and symptoms of Charcot triad along with altered mental status and hypotension, may be present in those patients with more severe cases. Choledocolithiasis is obstruction of the common bile duct without evidence of infection.

Acalculous cholecystitis comprises 10% of all cases of acute cholecystitis. Risk factors include total parenteral nutrition, human immunodeficiency virus (HIV)infection, mechanical ventilation, major infection, or critical illness due to trauma, major burns, or sepsis. Because these risk factors are generally not seen in outpatients, classic teaching suggests that acute acalculous cholecystitis is not likely to be diagnosed in the emergency department (ED). However, recent literature suggests age and atherosclerotic disease are also risk factors, and patients may present more frequently to the ED than previously thought.[34]

DIAGNOSIS AND DIFFERENTIAL

The final diagnosis of acute cholecystitis begins with history and physical and may be further elucidated with laboratory evaluation, but relies heavily on diagnostic imaging. No single clinical feature or combination of clinical features or laboratory values can rule in or rule out acute cholecystitis.[24] Leukocytosis is predictive for the disease with a likelihood ratio of 2.26. However, the sensitivity is only 63% and specificity only 57%.[28] The presence or absence of the combination of fever and leukocytosis offers no predictive value.[24] Elevated total bilirubin and alkaline phosphatase are slightly predictive of positive US diagnosis.[28]

Ultrasound is the initial imaging study for the diagnosis of acute cholecystitis.[35] Adjusting for verification bias, sensitivity is 88% and specificity is 80%.[36] Ultrasound does not expose the patient to radiation and is much more accurate than plain film radiographs or CT. Furthermore, the modality is faster and more generally more readily available than cholescintigraphy or MRI. Findings include gallstones (Figure 22-1), thickened gallbladder wall (Figure 22-2), pericholecystic fluid, and sonographic Murphy sign. Sonographic Murphy sign is elicited when the point of maximal tenderness is demonstrated when the gallbladder is centered on US examination. The sensitivity of the sonographic Murphy sign is reported from 75 % to 86% with a positive predictive value of 92% when combined with the finding of gallstones.[37-39] Acalculous cholecystitis is shown in Figure 22-3.

A growing body of literature supports emergency physician use of bedside US for the diagnosis of cholelithiasis and acute cholecystitis.[39-42] Sensitivity for the diagnosis of gallstones is 86 % to 96% and specificity of 78 % to 98%. Sensitivity for the diagnosis of acute cholecystitis is 91%.[40] Furthermore, use of bedside US by emergency physicians for gallbladder decreases the length of stay in the ED and decreases the number of return visits in those with newly diagnosed symptomatic gallstones.[42,43]

Cholescintigraphy, most commonly in the form of the HIDA scan, is the gold standard imaging study for acute cholecystitis.[35] Scintigraphy utilizes intravenous (IV) contrast material excreted into the bile via the liver and taken up by the gallbladder through the cystic duct. Cystic duct obstruction is confirmed when no contrast material is found within 4 hours. Intravenous morphine administration may speed the process. Sensitivity and specificity of scintigraphy for acute cholecystitis is 97% and 90%, respectively.[36] Elevated bilirubin levels and severe systemic illness can cause false positives. When clinical suspicion is high and US is negative, scintigraphy is indicated.

Plain films are not recommended for acute cholecystitis, but may help rule out gastrointestinal perforation and obstruction. Pneumobilia, air within the gallbladder and/or biliary system, may be present in gangrenous cholecystitis. Computed tomography is helpful for ruling out other abdominal pathology, but demonstrates sensitivity as low as 39% and specificity of 93% for acute cholecystitis. Addition of CT to US for the diagnosis of acute cholecystitis has not been shown to be helpful.[44]

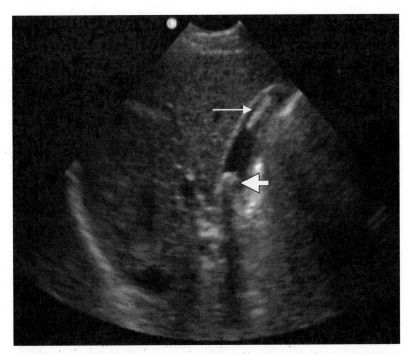

Fig. 22-1. Ultrasound demonstration of gallstone. The figure demonstrated two gallstones, one in the neck of the gallbladder (larger arrow). Smaller arrow depicts a gallstone in the gallbladder.

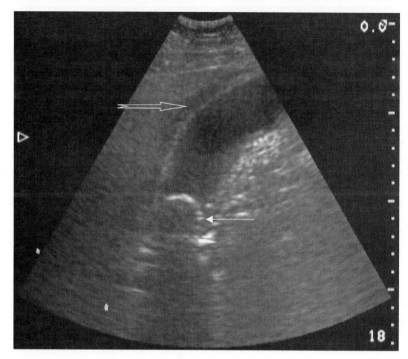

Fig. 22-2. Ultrasound image of acute calculous cholecystitis. The figure finds a large stone at the neck of the gallbladder as well as a markedly thickened gallbladder wall (transparent arrow). Simple arrow depicts a large gallstone.

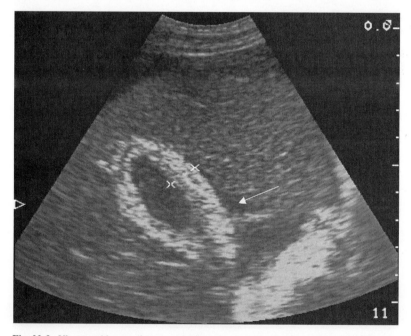

Fig. 22-3. Ultrasound image of acute acalculous cholecystitis. Note the thickened gallbladder wall (calipers), pericholecystic fluid (arrow), and lack of gallstones.

A more recent study suggests that the sensitivity of CT may be higher—as high as 92%.[45] Magnetic resonance imaging (MRI) is very accurate for demonstrating cystic duct obstruction, but it is limited by poor availability, prolonged examination time, and expense.

The differential diagnosis of acute cholecystitis is broad and includes acute hepatitis, pancreatitis, peptic ulcer disease, gastritis, gastroesophageal reflux disease, pyelonephritis, and nephrolithiasis. Appendicitis can rarely present with right upper quadrant pain, particularly in pregnancy and children. Females may present with Fitz-Hugh-Curtis disease or, rarely, ectopic pregnancy. Acute coronary disease such as myocardial infarction must be considered. Pneumonia, pleural effusion, and empyema should be ruled out, especially in the very young, the very old, and immunocompromised individuals.

EMERGENCY DEPARTMENT CARE AND DISPOSITION

Patients with acute cholecystitis are potentially very ill and clinicians must first address hemodynamic and respiratory compromise. Intravenous fluid boluses should be administered for those with signs of sepsis syndrome. Patients who are less ill but in whom acute cholecystitis is part of the differential should be kept NPO and maintenance fluids started. Clinicians should consider antiemetics for those with nausea and/or vomiting. Prochlorperazine 5 to 10 mg IV or promethazine 12.5 to 25 mg IV may be used but care must be taken not to oversedate patients, particularly if used concurrently with narcotics. Nasogastric decompression is not necessary unless intractable vomiting or severe ileus is present.

Adequate doses of parenteral analgesia should be administered as needed. Intravenous morphine 0.1 mg/kg or hydromorphone 0.015 mg/kg may be necessary. Fentanyl 1 μg/kg is useful if clinicians prefer a shorter duration of action while the diagnosis is still in question. The classic use of meperidine rather than morphine for biliary related pain is not supported in the literature.[46,47] In fact, morphine offers several advantages over meperidine including longer duration of action, less of a "drug high," no accumulation of normeperidine (the toxic metabolite of meperidine), and less induction of nausea.[48]

Less used for biliary pain, but potentially as effective, are nonsteroidal antiinflammatory drugs (NSAIDs). Intravenous (30 mg) and intramuscular (60 mg) ketorolac are as effective for biliary pain as meperidine 50 mg.[49,50] There are limited data to suggest that NSAIDs may

decrease the rate of progression of biliary pain to acute cholecystitis.[51]

Gram-negative organisms, namely *Escherichia coli*, *Enterococcus*, and *Klebsiella*, are the most common organisms isolated from the bile in cholecystitis patients. The risk of positive biliary culture is much greater for patients who are diabetic or over the age of 60. The presence of any combination of fever, leukocytosis, and hyperbilirubinemia also demonstrates an increased risk of bactrobilia.[15,52]

Newer, more expensive beta-lactams have not been shown to be more effective than older agents such as cefazolin.[15,53] However, for patients demonstrating signs of sepsis syndrome, risk factors for positive bile cultures, or evidence of complications (gangrenous cholecystitis, ascending cholecystitis, or perforation), broader coverage of gram-positive organisms and anaerobes is necessary. Such coverage is obtained with piperacillin/tazobactam 3.375 gm IV or ampicillin/sulbactam 3 gm IV. Broad combination therapy is obtained with ampicillin 2 gm IV, gentamicin 2 mg/kg IV, and metronidazole 500 mg IV. Ciprofloxacin 400 mg IV and metronidazole 500 mg IV may be used when a penicillin allergy is present.

All patients with acute cholecystitis should be admitted. Recent surgical literature finds no benefit to the traditional practice of "cooling off" a patient with medical therapy and delaying surgery by 8 to 12 weeks and the trend is toward cholecystectomy on initial admission.[54] Up to 25% of patients treated conservatively will return with further biliary complications within 3 months and no benefit to morbidity or mortality is realized.[55] Emergency surgery is necessary in approximately 20% of patients and is indicated for patients with peritonitis, deteriorating condition, or gangrenous cholecystitis.[56] If the patient is too unstable for surgery, then percutaneous cholecystostomy may be a temporizing option.

The diagnosis of biliary pain is made when patients present with classic upper abdominal pain without evidence of infection or biliary obstruction that resolves within 6 hours after only moderate amounts of analgesia. These patients may be discharged home with surgical follow-up, oral analgesics, and detailed instructions regarding the need to seek emergent medical care. The diagnosis of gallstones is not necessarily a requirement for surgical referral. Biliary dyskinesia is the presence of biliary pain without apparent gallstones or other structural abnormalities. It is a diagnosis of exclusion that is usually made and treated in outpatient surgical practice and may require cholecystectomy to alleviate symptoms.

PITFALLS

- Failure to maintain a broad differential, including cardiopulmonary and lower abdominal disease, in patients with apparent biliary pathology.

- Failure to obtain surgical consultation and consider admission for patients with persistent abdominal pain, tenderness, evidence of infection, or biliary obstruction in the face of normal initial diagnostic testing and imaging.

- Failure to consider acute cholecystitis and ascending cholangitis for undifferentiated critically ill patients, particularly diabetics and the elderly.

REFERENCES

1. Everhart JE, Khare M, Hill M, et al. Prevalence and ethnic differences in gallbladder disease in the United States. *Gastroenterology.* 1999;117:632.
2. Go V, Everhart JE. Gallstones. In *Digestive Diseases in the United States: Epidemiology and Impact.* US Department of Health and Human Services. National Institute of Diabetes and Digestive and Kidney Diseases. 1994;NIH Publication no. 94-1447.
3. Sandler RS, Everhardt JE, Donowitz M, et al. The burden of selected digestive diseases in the United States. *Gastroenterology.* 2002;122:1500.
4. Diehl AK. Epidemiology and natural history of gallstone disease. *Gastroenterol Clin North Am.* 1991;20:1.
5. Powers RD, Guertler AT. Abdominal pain in the ED: Stability and change over 20 years. *Am J Emerg Med.* 1995;13:301.
6. de Dombal FT. The OMGE acute abdominal pain survey: Progress report, 1986. *Scand J Gastroenterol Suppl.* 1988;144:35.
7. Telfer S, Fenyo G, Holt PR, et al. Acute abdominal pain in patients over 50 years of age. *Scand J Gastroenterol Suppl.* 1988;144:47.
8. Barbara L, Sama C, Morselli Labate AM, et al. A population study on the prevalence of gallstone disease: The Sirmione Study. *Hepatology.* 1987;7:913.
9. Jensen KH, Jorgensen T. Incidence of gallstones in a Danish population. *Gastroenterology.* 1991;100:790.
10. Bateson MC. Gallstones and cholecystectomy in modern Britain. *Postgrad Med J.* 2000;76:700.
11. Everhart JE, Yeh F, Lee ET, et al. Prevalence of gallbladder disease in American Indian populations: findings from the Strong Heart Study. *Hepatology.* 2002;35:1507.
12. Friedman GD. Natural history of asymptomatic and symptomatic gallstones. *Am J Surg.* 1993;165:399.
13. Carey MC. Pathogenesis of gallstones. *Am J Surg.* 1993;165:410.
14. Paumgartner G, Sauerbruch T. Gallstones: pathogenesis. *Lancet.* 1991;338:1117.
15. Kanafani ZA, Mehio-Sibai A, Araj GF, et al. Antibiotic use in acute cholecystitis: Practice patterns in the absence of evidence-based guidelines. *J Infect.* 2005;51:128.
16. Berger MY, Olde Hartman TC, Bohnen AM. Abdominal symptoms: Do they disappear after cholecystectomy? *Surg Endosc.* 2003;17:1723.
17. Festi D, Sottili S, Colecchia A, et al. Clinical manifestations of gallstone disease: Evidence from the multicenter Italian study on cholelithiasis (MICOL). *Hepatology.* 1999;30:839.
18. Thijs C, Knipschild P. Abdominal symptoms and food intolerance related to gallstones. *J Clin Gastroenterol.* 1998;27:223.
19. Kraag N, Thijs C, Knipschild P. Dyspepsia—how noisy are gallstones? A meta-analysis of epidemiologic studies of biliary pain, dyspeptic symptoms, and food intolerance. *Scand J Gastroenterol.* 1995;30:411.
20. Glambek I, Arnesjo B, Soreide O. Correlation between gallstones and abdominal symptoms in a random population: Results from a screening study. *Scand J Gastroenterol.* 1989;24:277.
21. Berger MY, Van der Velden JJ, Lijmer G, et al. Abdominal symptoms: do they predict gallstones? A systematic review. *Scand J Gastroenterol.* 2000;35:70.
22. Rigas B, Totosis J, McDougall CJ, et al. The circadian rhythm of biliary colic. *J Clin Gastroenterol.* 1990;12:409.
23. Minoli G, Imperiale G, Spinzi GC, et al. Circadian periodicity and other clinical features of biliary pain. *J Clin Gastroenterol.* 1991;13:546.
24. Trowbridge RL, Rutkowski NK, Shojania KG. Does this patient have acute cholecystitis? *JAMA.* 2003;289:80.
25. Raine PA, Gunn AA. Acute cholecystitis. *Br J Surg.* 1975;62:697.
26. Singer AJ, McCracken G, Henry MC, et al. Correlation among clinical, laboratory, and hepatobiliary scanning findings in patients with suspected acute cholecystitis. *Ann Emerg Med.* 1996;28:267.
27. Diehl AK. Symptoms of gallstone disease. *Baillieres Clin Gastroenterol.* 1992;6:635.
28. Mills LD, Mills T, Foster B. Association of clinical and laboratory variables with ultrasound findings in right upper quadrant abdominal pain. *South Med J.* 2005;98:155.
29. Lorberhoym M, Simon J, Horne T. The role of morphine-augmented cholescintigraphy and real-time ultrasound in detecting gallbladder disease. *J Nucl Med Technol.* 1999;27:294.
30. Ahmad M, Cheung, RC, Keeffe EB, et al. Differential diagnosis of gallstone-induced complications. *South Med J.* 2000;93:261.
31. Menakuru SR, Kaman L, Behera A, et al. Current management of gall bladder perforations. *ANZ J Surg.* 2004;74:843.
32. Fagan SP, Awad SS, Rahwan K, et al. Prognostic factors for the development of gangrenous cholecystitis. *Am J Surg.* 2003;186:481.
33. Contini S, Corradi D, Busi N, et al. Can gangrenous cholecystitis be prevented? A plea against a "wait and see" attitude. *J Clin Gastroenterol.* 2004;38:710.

34. Ryu JK, Ryu KH, Kim KH. Clinical features of acute acalculous cholecystitis. *J Clin Gastroenterol.* 2003;36:166.

35. Bree RL, Ralls PW, Balfe DM, et al. Evaluation of patients with acute right upper quadrant pain. American College of Radiology. ACR Appropriateness Criteria. *Radiology.* 2000; 215(Suppl):153.

36. Shea JA, Berlin JA, Escarce JJ, et al. Revised estimates of diagnostic test sensitivity and specificity in suspected biliary tract disease. *Arch Intern Med.* 1994;154:2573.

37. Ralls PW, Quinn MF, Boswell WD Jr, et al. Real-time sonography in suspected acute cholecystitis: Prospective evaluation of primary and secondary signs. *Radiology.* 1985;155:767.

38. Bree RL. Further observations on the usefulness of the sonographic Murphy sign in the evaluation of suspected acute cholecystitis. *J Clin Ultrasound.* 1995;23:169.

39. Kendall JL, Shimp RJ. Performance and interpretation of focused right upper quadrant ultrasound by emergency physicians. *J Emerg Med.* 2001;21:7.

40. Rosen CL, Brown DF, Chang Y, et al. Ultrasonography by emergency physicians in patients with suspected cholecystitis. *Am J Emerg Med.* 2001;19:32.

41. Durston W, Carl ML, Guerra W, et al. Comparison of quality and cost-effectiveness in the evaluation of symptomatic cholelithiasis with different approaches to ultrasound availability in the ED. *Am J Emerg Med.* 2001;19:260.

42. Schlager D, Lazzareschi G, Whitten D, et al. A prospective study of ultrasonography in the ED by emergency physicians. *Am J Emerg Med.* 1994;2:185.

43. Blaivas M, Harwood RA, Lambert MJ. Decreasing length of stay with emergency ultrasound examination of the gallbladder. *Acad Emerg Med.* 1999;6:1020.

44. Harvey RT, Miller WT, Jr. Acute biliary disease: Initial CT and follow-up US versus initial US and follow-up CT. *Radiology.* 1999;213:831.

45. Bennett GL, Rusinek H, Lisi V, et al. CT findings in acute gangrenous Cholecystitis. *AJR Am J Roentgenol.* 2002; 178;275.

46. Thompson DR. Narcotic analgesic effects on the sphincter of Oddi: a review of the data and therapeutic implications in treating pancreatitis. *Am J Gastroenterol.* 2001;96:1266.

47. Lee F, Cundiff D. Meperidine vs. morphine in pancreatitis and cholecystitis. *Arch Intern Med.* 1998;158:2399.

48. Hansen GR. The drug-seeking patient in the emergency room. *Emerg Med Clin North Am.* 2005;23:349.

49. Henderson SO, Swadron S, Newton E. Comparison of intravenous ketorolac and meperidine in the treatment of biliary colic. *J Emerg Med.* 2002;23:237.

50. Dula DJ, Anderson R, Wood GC. A prospective study comparing i.m. ketorolac with i.m. meperidine in the treatment of acute biliary colic. *J Emerg Med.* 2001;20:121.

51. Akriviadis EA, Hatzigavriel M, Kapnias D, et al. Treatment of biliary colic with diclofenac: a randomized, double-blind, placebo-controlled study. *Gastroenterology.* 1997;113:225.

52. Thompson JE, Jr, Bennion RS, Doty JE, et al. Predictive factors for bactibilia in acute cholecystitis. *Arch Surg.* 1990;125:261.

53. Westphal JF, Brogard JM. Biliary tract infections: A guide to drug treatment. *Drugs.* 1999;57:81.

54. Lo CM, Liu CL, Fan ST, et al. Prospective randomized study of early versus delayed laparoscopic cholecystectomy for acute cholecystitis. *Ann Surg.* 1998;227:461.

55. Yusoff IF, Barkun JS, Barkun AN. Diagnosis and management of cholecystitis and cholangitis. *Gastroenterol Clin North Am.* 2003;32:1145.

56. Indar AA, Beckingham IJ. Acute cholecystitis. *BMJ.* 2002;325:639.

23

Pancreatitis

David M. Cline

HIGH YIELD FACTS

- Despite advances in the diagnosis of pancreatitis, 10% of cases will be missed by laboratory or radiographic confirmation in the absence of clinical data.
- Using a cutoff of two times the upper limit of normal, lipase is approximately 90% sensitive and specific for the diagnosis of pancreatitis if the patient is tested within 24 hours of symptom onset. Sensitivity and specificity falls as time from onset of symptoms increases.
- Contrast enhanced, computed tomography (CT) scanning of the abdomen is only 78% sensitive and 86% specific for the diagnosis of pancreatitis, but may be used to predict a complicated course.

EPIDEMIOLOGY

In the United States, approximately 210,000 patients are admitted every year with acute pancreatitis[1] and 20% of these meet criteria for severe acute pancreatitis. In the United States cholelithiasis or alcohol abuse account for 90% of all cases of acute pancreatitis.[2] The list of other factors associated with acute pancreatitis is extensive as listed in Tables 23-1 and 23-2.

The incidence of pancreatitis varies between 5 to 50 per 100,000 in industrialized countries.[3,4] In mild pancreatitis, the death rate is less than 1%, while in severe acute pancreatitis, the death rate is 10% for sterile, and 25% with infected pancreatic necrosis.[5]

Criteria for severe acute pancreatitis (SAP) that can be assessed on admission to the emergency department (ED) include: (1) organ failure with 1 or more of the following: shock (systolic blood pressure <90 mmHg, pulmonary insufficiency (PaO2 <60 mmHg), renal failure (serum creatinine level >2 mg/dL or gastrointestinal tract bleeding (>500 mL in 24 hours); and (2) local complications such as necrosis, pseudocyst, or abscess (as determined by contrast computed tomography).[6] Only 5 of the 11 Ranson criteria can be calculated at admission, and the Acute Physiology and Chronic Health Evaluation scoring for pancreatitis is more reliable at 48 hours than on admission.[7]

Alcohol is the most important etiology of chronic pancreatic accounting for 70% to 80% of cases; the risk of chronic pancreatitis increases with duration and amount of alcohol consumed, not the type of alcohol.[8] Other important causes of chronic pancreatitis include idiopathic (10%–20%), hereditary, tropical, obstructive, hyperparathyroidism, and pancreas divisum (a congenital anomaly). Only 5% to 10% of heavy drinkers develop pancreatitis.

PATHOPHYSIOLOGY

The pathogenesis of pancreatitis varies with its different etiologies,[8,9] but the final common pathway is premature activation of proteolytic enzymes such as trypsin and zymogen, either in the ducts or cells, resulting in autodigestion of the pancreas.[9] Pancreatic digestion from activated proteolytic enzymes leads to edema, interstitial hemorrhage, vascular damage, coagulation, and cellular necrosis. Acute pancreatitis can also cause a generalized systemic inflammatory response that may lead to shock, acute respiratory distress syndrome (ARDS), and multisystem organ failure.[9]

CLINICAL FEATURES

A reliable standard for the diagnosis of pancreatitis does not exist, especially for its milder forms.[10] Therefore, studies that list sensitivity and specificity data for pancreatitis must be interpreted with caution. The classic presentation is acute, sharp, constant (noncolic-like) abdominal pain in the upper abdomen (60% to 78%) but may be generalized (11% to 35%).[11,12] In approximately 40% of cases the pain radiates to the back or flanks.[11,12] The pain increases rapidly initially, but the onset is less sudden than perforated viscous. Intensity varies greatly but may be severe. The pain may be partially relieved by sitting up or lying curled on the right or left side.[10] Nausea with vomiting is the second most common symptom; the vomitous comprises primarily gastric and duodenal contents and is not feculent.[10]

On physical examination, the abdomen is usually distended (approximately 82% of cases),[11] and may be particularly full in the epigastrium. Tenderness is classically more pronounced over the upper abdomen, but may be

Table 23-1. Causes of Acute Pancreatitis*

Biliary tract disease	Pancreatic tumors
Ethanol abuse	Vasculitis
Drugs (see Table 23-2)	Pregnancy
Hyperlipidemia	Mycoplasma
Abdominal surgery	Organ transplantation
Trauma (including ERCP)	End stage renal disease
Cardiopulmonary bypass	Hypercalcemia
Scorpion bites	Penetrating ulcer
Ascariasis	Idiopathic
Viral infection including mumps, coxsackie B, HIV	

*Other less common etiologies exist.
Abbreviations: ERCP, endoscopic retrograde cholangiopancreatography; HIV, human immunodeficiency virus.

generalized. Moderate muscle spasm is usual, but true rigidity is infrequent (based on two case series of over 400 patients).[11,12] Cullen sign, a bluish discoloration around the umbilicus, and Grey Turner sign, a bluish discoloration in the left flank, are signs of hemorrhagic pancreatitis found in less than 1% of patients.[10] Patients may also present with hypertension (20%) or tachycardia, tachypnea, and hypotension.[11,12]

Complications including ARDS, myocardial depression, disseminated intravascular coagulation, or renal failure, may be life-threatening. Blood loss, refractory hypotension, and respiratory failure may accompany more severe forms. Unfortunately, severity of illness and eventual complications are difficult to predict at the time of initial presentation for most patients.

Table 23-2. Drugs Associated with Pancreatitis*

5'-Aminosalicylic acid	Hydrochlorothiazide
6-Mercaptopurine	Methydopa
Acetaminophen (overdose)	Metolazone
Azathioprine	Metronidazole
Asparaginase	Estrogens
Corticosteroids	Pentamidine
Cimetadine	Piroxicam
Cyclosporin	Sulphasalazine
Didazosine	Sulphonamide
Erythromycin	Tetracyclines
Furosemide	

*Most common drugs, other drugs may be associated.

DIAGNOSIS AND DIFFERENTIAL

The diagnosis is made by a suggestive history and physical exam, associated with elevated pancreatic enzymes.[2,13] Amylase is primarily found in the pancreas and salivary glands; however, low levels can also be found in the fallopian tubes, ovaries, testes, adipose tissue, small bowel, lung, thyroid, skeletal muscle, and certain neoplasms, making this a relatively nonspecific test. Amylase greater than three times the upper limit of normal has a sensitivity of 80% to 90% and a specificity of 75% for acute pancreatitis.[13] Lipase is more specific than amylase for acute pancreatitis and is the preferred test. At a cutoff of two times the upper limit of normal, lipase is 90% sensitive and specific if the patient is tested within 24 hours of symptom onset.[13,14] As time progresses from the onset of symptoms, sensitivity and specificity of lipase and amylase falls,[14] yet the patient may be more critical ill. There is no benefit to ordering both amylase and lipase.[15] Leukocytosis may be present, and an elevated alkaline phosphatase suggests biliary disease. Hypotension, tachycardia >130 beats per minute, PO_2 <60 mmHg, oliguria, increasing blood urea nitrogen (BUN) or creatinine, or hypocalcemia are indicators of a potentially complicated course.[16] An elevated glucose >150 at admission may predict severe complications in the subset of gallstone pancreatitis.[17]

Plain radiographs of the abdomen are usually not helpful. Calcification is suggestive of chronic pancreatitis (seen in up to 9%), ileus (as much as 40% of severe cases) or a sentinel loop (4%) may be present, but are not diagnostic.[2,11] Ultrasonography is helpful in the identification of gallstones or dilatation of the biliary tree, but sensitivity ranges from 33% to 66% for the diagnosis of pancreatitis.[18,19] Computed tomography is the study of choice for visualizing the pancreas, confirmation of inflammation, and the identification of phlegmons, abscesses, or pseudocysts,[20] (Figure 23-1). The sensitivity of CT for pancreatitis is 78% (52%–93%, 95% confidence interval), and the specificity is 86% (63%–96%, 95% confidence interval).[21] It cannot be used to rule out acute pancreatitis, missing as many as 30% of patients,[22] but CT negative patients generally have a benign course,[10] and CT scanning provides an estimate of the severity of illness.[22]

Endoscopic retrograde cholangiopancreatography (ERCP) is rarely used in the ED, but can be useful when the etiology remains unclear after initial evaluation. Magnetic resonance imaging (MRI) in suspected pancreatitis yields a sensitivity of 83% (58%–96%, 95% confidence interval) and a specificity of 91% (68%–98%, 95% confidence interval).[21]

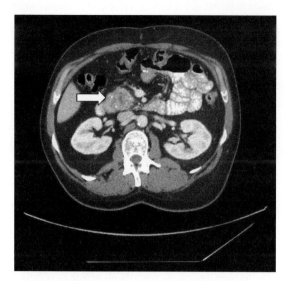

Fig. 23-1. CT findings of acute pancreatitis without necrosis. The figure demonstrates an enlarged and homogeneously enhanced pancreatic gland (arrow).

Differential diagnosis of pancreatitis includes left lower lobe pneumonia, rupture of a pseudocyst, gallbladder disease, peritonitis, peptic ulcer disease, small bowel obstruction, renal colic, dissecting aortic aneurysm, diabetic ketoacidosis, and gastroenteritis.

EMERGENCY DEPARTMENT CARE AND DISPOSITION

Treatment of acute pancreatitis primarily involves fluid resuscitation, pain control, and prevention of vomiting in patients with mild disease,[2] with intensive support including antibiotics in selected patients with severe acute pancreatitis.[6] Fluid resuscitation begins with normal saline to maintain blood pressure and adequate urine output.[2] Inotropic support with dopamine 2 to 20 μg/kg/min is indicated in patients with persistent hypotension despite adequate fluid resuscitation. Oxygen should be administered to maintain a pulse oximetry of greater than 95%. A nasogastric tube may be used if the patient is distended with persistent vomiting; however, no studies have demonstrated that its presence alters the course of the illness. Parenteral analgesia should be given as needed for patient comfort. Intravenous narcotics such as morphine 0.1 mg/kg are often required. Antiemetics, such as promethazine 12.5 to 25 mg IV may be helpful to reduce vomiting.[2] Enteral feeding is associated with fewer infectious complications, lower cost, and should be

instituted when feasible.[6] Prophylactic antibiotics for patients with pancreatic necrosis evident on CT scan have been recommended[6] but results of randomized controlled trials are conflicting.[23] Imipenem[24] and cefuroxime[25] have been recommended.

Urgent decompression by endoscopic sphincterotomy of the ampulla of Vater is indicated in persistent biliary obstruction.[2] Patients with mild pancreatitis, no evidence of systemic complications, and a low likelihood of biliary tract disease may be managed as outpatients if they are able to tolerate oral fluids and their pain is well controlled. Patients with significant systemic complications, shock, or extensive pancreatic necrosis will necessitate an intensive care setting. Surgical management is recommended in the case of infected necrosis of the pancreas.[26]

Patients with severe disease as evidenced by abnormal vital signs, evidence of organ dysfunction (pulmonary, renal, or active gastrointestinal bleeding) should be admitted to an intensive care setting. Milder forms of disease should be admitted based on their comorbidities, severity of pain, and ability to retain fluids. Otherwise healthy patients with controlled pain and vomiting may be considered for discharge with clear follow-up plans.

PITFALLS

- No single diagnostic test rules out pancreatitis, specifically including amylase, lipase, and CT scanning.[10]

- Although complications cannot always be predicted at the time of admission, failure to assess for hemorrhage in a patient with signs of blood loss, respiratory failure in a patient with reduced pulse oximetry, or pancreatic necrosis in a patient with a concerning abdominal exam may lead to floor admission with inadequate monitoring or underresuscitation of a patient needing intensive support.

REFERENCES

1. Russo MW, Wei JT, Thiny MT, et al. Digestive and liver disease statistics. *Gastroenterology*. 2004;126:1448.
2. Mergener K, Baillic J. Fortnightly review: Acute pancreatitis. *BMJ*. 1998;316:44.
3. Andersson R, Andersson B, Haraldsen, et al. Incidence, management, and recurrence rate of acute pancreatitis. *Scand J Gastroenterol*. 2004;39:1.
4. Go VLW, Everhart JE. Pancreatitis. In: *Digestive Diseases in the United States: Epidemiology and Impact*. Everhart, JE (ed.). US Department of Health and Human Services, Public Health Service, National Institutes of Health,

National Institute of Diabetes and Digestive and Kidney Diseases. Washington, DC. US Government Printing Office, NIH Publication no. 94-1447;1994:693.

5. Dervenis C, Johnson CD, Bassi C, et al. Diagnosis, objective assessment of severity, and management of acute pancreatitis. *Int J Pancreatol.* 1999;25:195.

6. Swaroop VS, Chari ST, Clain JE. Severe acute pancreatitis. *JAMA.* 2004;291:2865.

7. Khan AA, Parekh D, Cho Y, et al. Improved prediction of outcome in patients with severe acute pancreatitis by the APACHE II score at 48 hours after hospital admission compared with the APACHE II score at admission. Acute Physiology and Chronic Health Evaluation. *Arch Surg.* 2002;137:1136.

8. Stevens T, Conwell DL, Zuccaro G. Pathogenesis of chronic pancreatitis: An evidence-based review of past theories and recent developments. *Am J Gastroenterol.* 2004;99:2256.

9. Karne S, Baillic J. Etiopathogenesis of acute pancreatitis. *Surg Clin North Am.* 1999;79:699.

10. Ranson JC. Diagnostic standards for acute pancreatitis. *World J Surg.* 1997;21:136.

11. Albo R, Silen W, Goldman L. A critical clinical analysis of acute pancreatitis. *Arch Surg.* 1963;86:1032.

12. Paxton JR, Payne JH. Acute pancreatitis: a statistical review of 307 established case of acute pancreatitis. *Surg Gynecol Obstet.* 1948;86:69.

13. Vissers RJ, Abu-Laban RB, McHugh DF. Amylase and lipase in the emergency department evaluation of acute pancreatitis. *J Emerg Med.* 1999;17:1027.

14. Keim V, Teich N, Fiedler F, et al. A comparison of lipase and amylase in the diagnosis of acute pancreatitis in patient with abdominal pain. *Pancreas.* 1998;16:45.

15. Vissers RJ, Dagnone J, Abu-Laban R, Walls RM. Serum amylase offers no additional benefit to serum lipase in the ED diagnosis of acute pancreatitis. *Acad Emerg Med.* 1998;4:396.

16. De Bernadinis M, Violi V, Roncuroni L, et al. Discriminant power and information content of Ranson's prognostic signs in acute pancreatitis: a meta-analytic study. *Crit Care Med.* 1999;27:2272.

17. Meek K, Toosie K, Stabile BE, et al. Simplified admission criterion for predicting severe complications of gallstone pancreatitis. *Arch Surg.* 2000;135:1048.

18. McKay AJ, Imrie CW, O'Neill J, Duncan JG. Is an early ultrasound scan of value in acute pancreatitis. *Br J Surg.* 1982;69:369.

19. Jeffery RB: Sonography in acute pancreatitis. *Radiol Clin North Am.* 1989;27:5.

20. Balthazar EM. CT diagnosis and staging of acute pancreatitis. *Radiol Clin North Am.* 1989;27:19.

21. Arvanitakis M, Delhaye M, De Maertelaere V, et al. Computed tomography and magnetic resonance imaging in the assessment of acute pancreatitis. *Gastroenterology.* 2004;126:715.

22. Balthazar EM. Acute pancreatitis: Assessment of severity with clinical CT evaluation. *Radiology.* 2002;223:603.

23. Isenmann R, Rnzi M, Kron M, et al. Prophylactic antibiotic treatment in patients with predicted severe acute pancreatitis. *Gastroenterology.* 2004;126:997.

24. Ho HS, Frey CF. The role of antibiotic prophylaxis in severe acute pancreatitis. *Arch Surg.* 1997;132:487.

25. Sainio V, Kemppainen E, Puolakkainen P, et al. Early antibiotic treatment in acute necrotizing pancreatitis. *Lancet.* 1995; 346:663.

26. Connor S, Neoptolemos JP. Surgery for pancreatic necrosis: "Whom, when, and what." *World J Gastroenterol.* 2004; 10:1697.

24

Complications of Surgical Procedures

Christopher J. Fullagar

The complications of abdominal surgeries can reach far beyond the gastrointestinal (GI) system. Essentially every organ system can be affected by complications of abdominal surgery. While some complications are common to any surgery, others are fairly unique to a particular procedure. This chapter will first address complications of abdominal surgery by system. Complications of specific procedures and devices will follow.

HIGH YIELD FACTS

- Use the mnemonic of the "five Ws" to recall the common sources of postoperative fever: wind, water, wound, walking, and wonder drug (Table 24-1).
- When postoperative bariatric surgery patients become tachycardic, even in the absence of other signs and symptoms, consider intrabdominal abscess, anastomotic leak, and PE.[1]
- If a Foley catheter is used to temporarily replace a jejunostomy tube (rather than a gastrostomy tube), the balloon should not be inflated.

GENERAL COMPLICATIONS

Epidemiology

The incidence of nosocomial infection has been cited as being between about 6% and 14%. The most frequent type of nosocomial infection is surgical site infection.[2] In a study examining 5572 nonobstetric procedures among members of a health maintenance organization, 84% occurred after hospital discharge and 63% were managed outside the surgical facility.[3] This high incidence of complications occurring after hospital discharge has a significant impact on the emergency department (ED).

Pathophysiology

Postoperative fever is a common presenting complaint in the ED. The etiology of the fever depends on many variables such as the nature of the procedure, the duration of the surgery, and the patient's comorbidities (often classified as the American Society of Anesthesiology [ASA] score).[4] The likelihood of a particular etiology of fever also varies with the time that has passed since the surgery. Fever in the early postoperative period (up to about 48 hours) is rarely secondary to infection. Subsequently, the likelihood of an infectious etiology of fever increases. After about 96-hours postoperative, a fever is considered very likely to represent infection. When considering the etiologies of postoperative fever, the mnemonic of the five Ws is commonly recalled. Wind (atelectasis, pneumonia), water (urinary tract infections [UTIs]), wound, walking (deep venous thrombosis [DVT], pulmonary embolism [PE]), and wonder drug (pseudomembranous colitis, drug fever).

Clinical Features

During the early postoperative period, fever is typically secondary to atelectasis. Preexisting fever at the time of surgery may persist for up to 72 hours after surgery. During this early phase the rare infectious etiology of fever may be secondary to pulmonary aspiration or uncommon breaks in sterile technique. Streptococcal (necrotizing fasciitis) and clostridial wound infections may also be seen in the first 1 to 3 days after surgery.[4] Urinary tract infections are typically seen 3 to 5 days postoperative, DVT at about 5 days, and wound infections in about 7 to 10 days. Pseudomembranous colitis accounts for late fever occurring at about 6 weeks.

In addition to fever, other general postoperative complications include problems of wound closure and drug treatment. Aside from wound infection and necrotizing fasciitis, wound closure complications include dehiscence as well as hematoma and seroma formation.

Hematomas manifest with pain and swelling and may initially be difficult to differentiate from infection. Uncomplicated hematomas may be evacuated in the ED by releasing a few sutures over the incision site. If there is evidence of infection or if hemostasis cannot be maintained, surgical consultation is warranted. Hematomas that are associated with vascular procedures or that are in an area adjacent to major vascular structures (such as the neck) require particular caution. In these areas profound bleeding may follow release of sutures and exploration.

A seroma typically manifests as a painless swelling. Aspiration is both diagnostic and therapeutic. The aspirated

Table 24-1. Common Sources of Postoperative Fever

Mnemonic Clue	Complication	Typical Time Course*
Wind	Atelectasis	1 to 72 hours postsurgery
	Pneumonia	3 or more days postsurgery
	Aspiration	6 to 72 hours
Water	Urinary tract infection	3 or more days postsurgery
Wound	Wound cellulitis	7-10 days (or more) postsurgery
	Abdominal abscess	7-10 days (or more) postsurgery
Walking	Deep vein thrombosis	5-7 days (or more) postsurgery
	Pulmonary embolism	5-7 days (or more) postsurgery
Wonder drug	Pseudomembranous colitis	1 to 6 weeks postsurgery
	Drug fever	1 to 6 weeks postsurgery

*Use time course as a general guideline; exceptions occur.

fluid should be clear and free of purulence. After the fluid is removed, the patient should be made aware of the possibility of reaccumulation and the potential need for repeat aspiration.

Diagnosis and Differential

A thorough examination will guide your workup of postoperative fever. Recollection of the typical sources of postoperative fever is important. Physical examination warrants special attention to these areas. Diagnostic testing should then be used to confirm the source. Do not rely on the presence of an elevated white blood cell count to initiate your workup. Leukocytosis is an unreliable indicator of clinically significant infection.

Emergency Department Care and Disposition

Care and disposition depends on the underlying etiology of the complication and the patient's clinical condition. The patient's surgeon should be informed of postoperative complications that occur, and as indicated by diagnostic uncertainty, asked to examine the patient or to intervene surgically when required.

PULMONARY COMPLICATIONS

Epidemiology

Cardiopulmonary complications of abdominal surgery account for significant postoperative morbidity and mortality. While early studies focused on the cardiac complications, later research revealed that pulmonary complications occurred more frequently. The incidence of pulmonary complications after surgery is between about 3% and 10%.[5,6] Preoperative and intraoperative interventions, including optimizing control of chronic obstructive pulmonary disease (COPD) and minimizing the length of surgery, can decrease the risk of postoperative pulmonary complications.[7,8]

Pathophysiology

Atelectasis is often seen in the postoperative patient, especially in those who have undergone thoracic or upper abdominal surgery. Patients who are unable to sufficiently clear their secretions, such as those with inadequate pain control, are predisposed to atelectasis. Incentive spirometry can be used to reduce the incidence of atelectasis after surgery.

Clinical Features

Patients with atelectasis may present with postoperative fever or mild hypoxia. Hypercarbia, however, is not common. Atelectasis is an early postoperative complication that can typically be managed as an outpatient with pain management and pulmonary toilet. Patients with respiratory compromise or severe symptoms may require admission for more aggressive management. Pneumonia becomes more likely as the duration since surgery increases (typically 24 to 96 hours postoperative).

Patients with pneumonia may present similarly to those with atelectasis. Chest pain, productive cough, and tachypnea may also be present. Shoulder discomfort may represent referred pain from an ipsilateral pulmonary process.

Pneumothorax and PE should also be considered in the evaluation of postoperative chest pain. Presentation may be similar to that of atelectasis or pneumonia. The clinical presentation of patients with PEs is often nonspecific and may mimic many other processes.

Diagnosis and Differential

A chest radiograph is helpful in the diagnosis of postoperative pulmonary complications. The presence of densities or consolidation indicates atelectasis or pneumonia. If pneumonia is suspected sputum and blood cultures should be obtained; however, pneumonia in the postoperative patient is often polymicrobial. Expiratory chest radiographs are most helpful in identifying those patients with pneumothorax.

When considering PE, serum D-dimer concentration, lower extremity Doppler, ventilation-perfusion scans, or spiral computer tomography (CT) scans may be helpful. Diagnosis of PE is complicated by the poor sensitivity of noninvasive tests. Although pulmonary angiography is considered the gold standard, concern regarding the complications of the procedure has made many physicians apprehensive about using the test regularly. Although some studies have reported that the incidence of complications is low, they are not negligible. Patients who are severely ill with acute pulmonary hypertension are at the greatest risk for complications from pulmonary angiography.[9]

Emergency Department Care and Disposition

Care and disposition of those with pulmonary infection is often based on the patient's clinical condition. Comorbidities, especially underlying lung disease, may impact antibiotic choice and the decision to admit or discharge. Patients who are suspected of having PE are often admitted for anticoagulation therapy.

VASCULAR COMPLICATIONS

Clinical Features

Superficial thrombophlebitis and DVT are frequent complications of surgical procedures. Both may occur in the upper or lower extremities. Pain and swelling are common initial symptoms, especially in the calves. As the course progresses, erythema and warmth may develop. The patient may present with a palpable cord. Homans sign (maintenance of the relaxed foot in an abnormally flexed position) is not considered to be clinically predictive of DVT. Pain on passive dorsiflexion of the foot is often misrepresented as Homans sign; however, this too has been shown to have no clinical predictive value for DVT.

Diagnosis and Differential

When vascular complications are suspected color-flow Doppler ultrasonography is often the diagnostic tool of choice. A normal study should be repeated in 5 to 7 days.[10] Reevaluation may be required sooner if the patient's symptoms continue to progress.

Consideration must also be given to the presence of infection (such as cellulitis or suppurative thrombophlebitis) and pulmonary embolus. Other processes that may have similar presentations include ruptured Baker cyst, venous insufficiency, and trauma.

Emergency Department Care and Disposition

Suppurative thrombophlebitis often requires surgical resection of the vein concurrent with appropriate antibiotic therapy.[11] Uncomplicated superficial thrombophlebitis is treated conservatively with heat and elevation provided there is no associated infection or DVT. If DVT is present (or if the great saphenous vein is involved above the level of the knee) treatment should involve anticoagulation. Outpatient low molecular weight heparin or hospitalization and full-dose anticoagulation with intravenous (IV) unfractionated heparin should be considered.

GASTROINTESTINAL COMPLICATIONS
Epidemiology

General complications of abdominal surgeries that affect the GI tract include obstruction, intraabdominal abscess, pancreatitis, cholecystitis, and the formation of fistulas. Postoperative intestinal obstruction is most often caused by adhesions and may occur far into the postoperative period. Adhesiolysis accounted for over 300,000 hospitalizations in 1994.[12] Despite increasing use of less invasive techniques such as laparoscopy the incidence of hospitalization for adhesiolysis has not decreased.[13] Thus, it appears that small bowel obstruction secondary to adhesion formation will continue to be a common postoperative complication seen in the ED.

Clinical Features

Obstruction, both functional (ileus) and mechanical, typically presents with abdominal pain, vomiting, and obstipation. The pain associated with obstruction is usually diffuse and peritoneal signs, such as rebound tenderness, are usually lacking. As the small bowel dilates, blood flow to the bowel can be compromised and necrosis and sepsis may ensue. Abscess should be considered in patients who exhibit signs of sepsis such as fever, chills, hypotension, and tachycardia.

Acute pancreatitis is typically associated with direct manipulation of the pancreatic duct as occurs in gastric resection and procedures involving the biliary tract. In addition, acute pancreatitis is a known complication of endoscopic retrograde cholangeopancreatography (ERCP). Although symptoms range in severity, patients typically present with upper abdominal pain and vomiting. In many cases the pain reaches maximum intensity in about 10 to 20 minutes of onset and is persistent. On examination, signs may range from moderate epigastric tenderness to shock and coma. Rarely, ecchymotic discoloration in the flank (Grey-Turner sign) or the periumbilical region (Cullen sign) may be present and is associated with hemorrhage.

Biliary colic, as well as calculous and acalculous cholecystitis may occur in patients after abdominal surgery. Although some theories have been proposed, it is not well understood exactly why this occurs postoperatively. Patients with biliary colic typically present with right upper quadrant pain, nausea, and vomiting. Radiation to the flank or tip of the right scapula has also been described, especially with cholecystitis. Patients with cholecystitis may also present with fever and tachycardia. Cholangitis must be considered particularly when the patient presents with sepsis. The triad of right upper quadrant pain, fever, and jaundice, described by Charcot, is seen in approximately 70% of patients with cholangitis. Reynolds pentad includes Charcot triad plus the presence of altered mental status and shock.

Diagnosis and Differential

Abdominal radiographs are often helpful in confirming the diagnosis of intestinal obstruction. An upright chest x-ray may be useful in determining the presence of free air under the diaphragm. If the diagnosis is in question, or if additional information is needed, a CT scan may be helpful. The CT may provide additional information such as the exact location, severity, and etiology of the obstruction. If the diagnosis of obstruction is uncertain, the CT may reveal other etiologies of the patient's complaints.

A serum lipase level is often useful in the workup of a patient with suspected postoperative pancreatitis. An elevation in the serum amylase is considered more nonspecific as it may be seen in many other processes. Radiographically, plain films of the abdomen may demonstrate a sentinel loop (localized ileus in the area of the pancreas). Computed tomography scanning is recommended to evaluate for abscess or pancreatic fluid collection. The CT may also reveal a perforated viscous, a process which may present similarly to acute pancreatitis with abdominal pain and elevated serum lipase.

Ultrasound is most helpful when evaluating for acute cholecystitis in the postoperative setting. Ultrasound may reveal the presence of gallstones, gallbladder wall thickening, pericholecystic fluid, or a positive sonographic Murphy sign. Although serologic tests are often obtained in patients with suspected cholecystitis, it is important to remember that leukocytosis and elevations in the liver function tests may not be seen in some patients with the disease.

Emergency Department Care and Disposition

Although both operative and nonoperative modalities exist for the treatment of intestinal obstruction, surgical consultation should guide management in the postoperative setting. Initial treatment including gastric decompression with nasogastric suction, bowel rest, and IV hydration should be considered. Pain relief, typically with parenteral opioids, and correction of electrolyte abnormalities are also priorities. Patients who exhibit features of sepsis should be cultured and prompt administration of broad-spectrum antibiotics along with appropriate fluid resuscitation should be considered. Definitive treatment of intraabdominal abscess typically involves operative intervention.

Uncomplicated acute pancreatitis usually responds to nasogastric suction, bowel rest, and fluid hydration. Pain management and antiemetics are often required. Complications of acute pancreatitis must be considered and most of these patients are admitted.

Aside from supportive measures, the treatment for acute cholecystitis typically includes broad-spectrum parenteral antibiotics and cholecystectomy.

GENITOURINARY COMPLICATIONS

Clinical Features

Urinary tract infection is a common cause of postoperative fever. Instrumentation and bladder catheterization increases the risk for a UTI. Patients may present with dysuria, frequency, urgency, and suprapubic pain. Hematuria is seen in those with hemorrhagic cystitis. Upper tract infections, such as pyelonephritis, should be considered especially when fever, flank pain, and nausea are present.

Postoperative urinary retention is often transient and is thought to occur secondary to catecholamine stimulation as happens, for example, in states of increased pain. A loss of coordination of the trigone and detrussor muscles creates the inability to urinate. Patients will usually complain of a constant dull discomfort in the suprapubic area. As the process progresses, urgency and pain ensue. Certain patients, such as those who have undergone deep rectal dissection, may have difficulty sensing the fullness.

Postoperative acute renal failure (ARF) occurs when there is a reduction of renal function that results in accumulation of nitrogenous wastes. Acute renal failure may be oligouric or nonoligouric depending on the actual rate of urine production. Acute renal failure is further classified as prerenal, renal, or postrenal. Clinical features are secondary to the rapid decline in renal function. Volume depletion is a common prerenal cause of ARF.

Diagnosis and Differential

The diagnosis of UTI can be confirmed by urinalysis, for which cultures should be sent. Further testing may be warranted if there is evidence of upper tract infection. Urinary retention can be diagnosed by measuring postvoid residual. Catheterization can be both diagnostic and therapeutic.

The diagnosis of ARF is made by noting an increase in serum urea and creatinine. Urine output should be carefully monitored. Urine osmolality, urine electrolytes, and comparison between the plasma and urine creatinine, urea, and osmolality can help in determining whether the failure is prerenal, renal, or postrenal.

Emergency Department Care and Disposition

Most patients presenting with uncomplicated UTI can be treated with appropriate oral antibiotics as an outpatient. Admission may be required for those requiring parenteral antibiotic treatment such as patients with significant comorbidities and patients with signs of a systemic infection.

Patients who have undergone catheter bladder drainage for urinary retention do not always require ongoing catheterization. It is reasonable to discontinue bladder catheterization in those with normal renal function and without anatomic obstruction. If continued catheterization is required, prophylactic antibiotic treatment may be considered.

The treatment of those with ARF depends largely upon the etiology. A fluid bolus should be considered for those with a suspected prerenal etiology such as dehydration or hemorrhage. A blood transfusion may be required for hemorrhage. Those with postrenal urethral obstruction may benefit from catheter placement. Secondary electrolyte abnormalities must also be addressed.

COMPLICATIONS SPECIFIC TO ANASTOMOSIS

Clinical Features

Anastomotic leaks, with extravasation of bacteria-laden fluid, are of particular concern to emergency physicians. The signs of anastomotic complications are often initially nonspecific, such as fever, malaise, general failure to thrive, and possibly abdominal discomfort, yet the patient's course can quickly deteriorate resulting in septic shock and death. Abscess, fistula formation, and wound dehiscence may complicate recovery.

Diagnosis and Differential

Postoperative patients having undergone anastomosis and presenting with the aforementioned signs and symptoms should undergo CT scanning. Findings of a large amount of free fluid or free air in the peritoneal space, an abscess cavity with air-fluid levels, or localized large fluid collections are worrisome for anastomotic leak.

Emergency Department Care and Disposition

Appropriate antibiotic coverage and prompt surgical consultation should be considered when this diagnosis is suspected. Even with immediate reoperation morbidity and mortality remains high.

COMPLICATIONS SPECIFIC TO GASTRIC SURGERY

Epidemiology

The incidence of gastric surgery for morbid obesity has risen significantly. In 1996, 6868 bariatric procedures were reported; by 2001, the number had risen to 45,473.[14] Major complications occur in about 10% of patients undergoing bariatric surgery.[14] The most consistent risk factors for bariatric surgical complications include male gender and body size.[1,15] Age has also been cited as a potential risk factor but its reliability is variable.

Pathophysiology

Complications of bariatric surgery include anastomotic leaks, PE, DVT, inadequate weight loss, fascial dehiscence, staple line disruption, bowel obstruction, respiratory complications, gallbladder disease (3% – 30%), and portal vein injury. Anastomotic leaks, including staple line disruptions, typically occur up to 7 to 10 days postoperative. Common indicators including abdominal pain may be minimal or absent especially in very large patients. Pulmonary embolus carries a high mortality rate but is a rare complication occurring in only 1% to 2% of patients.

Specific postgastrectomy syndromes include dumping syndrome, alkaline reflux gastritis, afferent loop syndrome, and postvagotomy diarrhea. Dumping syndrome occurs when there is a disruption of the normal pyloric function, such as when the pylorus is removed. Current theory suggests that symptoms are secondary to hyperosmolar gastric contents passing rapidly into the proximal intestine. Late dumping syndrome is thought to be a result of overstimulation of insulin production from large quantities of carbohydrates that are rapidly absorbed from the proximal intestine. There is a surge of insulin that results in hypoglycemia occurring 2 to 4 hours after eating. This stimulates catecholamine release from the adrenal glands. Alkaline reflux gastritis is thought to be secondary to reflux of bile. The pain is described as burning, is exacerbated by eating, and is unrelieved by vomiting. Afferent loop syndrome occurs when the limb is obstructed, often secondary to "kinking," resulting in an accumulation of pancreatic and hepatobiliary secretion within the limb, with ensuing distension.

Clinical Features

By virtue of their often profound obesity, bariatric surgery patients may not manifest typical signs and symptoms of complications that are often seen in other patients. Even in the face of significant intraabdominal pathology these patients frequently lack fever, leukocytosis, and even severe abdominal pain. In fact, the only consistent and reliable sign of a considerable complication may be "significant tachycardia" described as a heart rate above 120.[1] Patients presenting with PE may be virtually indistinguishable from those presenting with anastomotic leak. Therefore, the diagnosis of PE must be simultaneously considered especially in light of the 20% to 30% mortality rate among patients who develop PE in this setting.

Symptoms of early dumping syndrome occur as a result of extracellular fluid shift. Patients develop a sense of fullness and crampy abdominal pain about 20 to 30 minutes after eating. A resultant autonomic response may then lead to palpitations, tachycardia, diaphoresis, and flushing. The hypoglycemia and chatecholamine surge associated with late dumping syndrome is responsible for the symptoms that occur about 2 to 3 hours after eating. The presentation may be very similar to hypoglycemic shock seen in patients with diabetes mellitus. Diaphoresis, tremulousness, and lightheadedness are common. Tachycardia and altered mental status have been described in more severe cases. Patients with afferent loop syndrome typically describe epigastric pain occurring 1 to 2 hours after eating. The pain, which may be severe, is often relieved with vomiting.

Diagnosis and Differential

The diagnosis of complications of bariatric surgery is mostly clinical. Radiologic studies are often impractical or of limited utility because of the patient's large size. Furthermore, CT and UGI series do not rule out one of the most worrisome complications, anastomotic leak. Waiting for laboratory confirmation of intraabdominal pathology is discouraged as these patients do not have significant reserve and can decompensate quickly.

Emergency Department Care and Disposition

The suggested approach to a patient who has undergone bariatric surgery with a high clinical suspicion of a complication is early surgical intervention. With the limited utility of diagnostic studies and the patient's limited physical reserves these patients are often quickly taken back to the operating room.

The immediate management of patients with dumping syndrome, alkaline reflux gastritis, afferent loop syndrome, and postvagotomy diarrhea is often supportive. These patients can typically be discharged with outpatient workup and surgical referral. Ideally, outpatient treatment should be coordinated with the patient's surgeon prior to the patient's discharge from the ED.

COMPLICATIONS SPECIFIC TO BILIARY TRACT SURGERY AND OTHER LAPAROSCOPIC SURGERIES

Laparoscopic cholecystectomy was introduced in the United States from France in 1988. By 1992, 80% of the general surgeons in the United States reported having adopted the procedure.[16] The laparoscopic technique has been applied to numerous other surgeries including herniorraphy, appendectomy, and fundoplication. Colon resection and hysterectomy can also be performed laparoscopically. For cholecystectomy, laparoscopic surgery appears to be as safe as the open procedure for selected patients with the exception of an increased risk of bile duct injury.[16]

Clinical Features

Patients often present with nonspecific complaints of abdominal pain. The presence of high fever and peritoneal signs warrant thorough investigation. The clinician should also be mindful of the secondary effects of laparoscopy. For example, increased intraabdominal pressure can ultimately result in decreased cardiac output. This can lead to significant complications such as myocardial infarction especially in patients with preexisting cardiac disease. Vascular function does not immediately return to normal and consequences of vascular compromise can persist well into the postoperative period.

Diagnosis and Differential

Laboratory workup of the patient with suspected complications of laparoscopic surgery should generally include a complete blood count (CBC), serum electrolytes, liver function testing, and a serum lipase. A CT scan may reveal bile collection or abscess. ERCP can identify the location of a suspected bile duct stricture or injury. Retained stones may be removed endoscopically. An upright chest x-ray can evaluate for pneumoperitoneum. The persistence of pneumoperitoneum secondary to the lapraroscopic procedure itself (not thought to be associated with perforated viscus) has been reported up to 14 days postoperative; however, most resolve within 1 to 2 days.[17] A persistent pneumoperitoneum may indicate a perforated viscus. Workup for other secondary complications, such as PE and myocardial infarction, should be initiated if clinically indicated.

COMPLICATIONS SPECIFIC TO STOMA

The ileostomy and colostomy are the two most common types of stomas encountered in the ED. The stoma should be pink and nontender. Inadequate blood flow can result in necrosis of the stoma and typically would occur soon after surgery. Local skin breakdown is often secondary to a poorly fitting appliance. Good skin care and replacement of the appliance with a properly fitting device is indicated. Prolapse of the stoma can also occur. Examination of the tissue for viability is required. If the tissue is pink and nontender, reduction can be attempted. Surgical consultation should be obtained.

COMPLICATIONS SPECIFIC TO GASTROINTESTINAL DEVICES

Placement of the nasogastric (NG) tube occurs frequently in the ED. Although less common, orogastric lavage tubes may also be placed in the ED and were once regularly used in the treatment of the overdose patient; however, the use of orogastric tubes is far less common today. Complications involving transabdominal feeding tubes such as the gastrostomy (G), jejunostomy (J), and the gastrojejunostomy (GJ) tubes are seen in the ED.

One of the most common complications of NG tube placement is improper placement. Many common methods of verification, such as auscultation, are unreliable. Radiographic confirmation of proper placement should be obtained especially before administration of medications. Charcoal has a particular tendency to cause a potentially fatal pneumonitis if instilled into the lungs. The presence of a properly placed endotracheal tube with the balloon inflated does prevent tracheal placement of the NG tube in all cases. An orogastric route should be taken in patients with observed or suspected craniofacial trauma to prevent introduction of the NG tube into the cranium. Other complications of NG tube placement include epistaxis or pharyngeal trauma. Bleeding may be significant especially in those with coagulopathy or who are on anticoagulants. Care should be taken when placing a gastric tube in a trauma patient to minimize cervical spine movement during placement. Chronic NG tube placement may result in gastric erosion and bleeding. Reported complications include esophageal tears and inability to remove the tube secondary to esophageal spasm. Placement of small bore nasointestinal tubes are more commonly subject to displacement and lumenal obstruction than NG tubes. Other complications of small bore nasointestinal tubes are similar to those seen with NG tubes.

Displacement and obstruction of a transabdominal feeding tube frequently results in an ED visit. Care should be taken to determine the type and size of the tube. Patient history or old records are often helpful as physical examination is often unreliable unless the patient presents with a dislodged tube in hand. If the tube is displaced, a replacement tube of the same type or Foley catheter should be placed promptly to prevent closure of the stoma. Even if the type of tube is unknown, the stoma should be promptly stented. If a Foley catheter is used to replace a J-tube, the balloon should not be inflated as bowel obstruction or tissue injury can result.[18] If significant resistance is met, a smaller tube should be attempted. Serious infection can occur; however, local nonpurulent drainage is not uncommon and is typically treated with good skin care.

Granuloma formation around the transabdominal feeding tube site can lead to bleeding due to tissue friability. Silver nitrate has been used to mitigate this complication.

PITFALLS

- Fever and elevated white blood cell count are not reliable indicators for infection in surgical patients. Among peritoneal infections, 35% may present without leukocytosis, 55% may present without fever, and 23% may present without either diagnostic symptom.[19]

- Failure to replace a displaced transabdominal feeding tube in a timely manner can result in closure of the tract.

- Before instilling a medication, such as charcoal, through an NG tube, radiographic confirmation should be obtained. Assessment of tube placement by auscultation is unreliable and if the NG tube is in the airway, a fatal pneumonitis can result.

REFERENCES

1. Livingston EH. Complications of bariatric surgery. *Surg Clin N Am.* 2005;85:853.
2. Vazquez-Aragon P, Lizan-Garcia M, Cascales-Sanchez P, et al. Nosocomial infection and related risk factors in a general surgery service: A prospective study. *J Infect.* 2002;46:17.
3. Sands K, Vineyard G, Platt R. Surgical site infections occurring after hospital discharge. *J Infect Dis.* 1996; 173:963.
4. Anonymous. National nosocomial infections surveillance (NNIS) system report, data summary from January 1992–June 2001, issued August 2001. *Am J Infect Control.* 2001; 29:404.
5. Lawrence VA, Hilsenbeck SG, Mulrow CD, et al. Incidence and hospital stay for cardiac and pulmonary complications after abdominal surgery. *J Gen Intern Med.* 1995;10:671.
6. McAlister FA, Bertsch K, Man J, et al. Incidence and risk factors for pulmonary complications after nonthoracic surgery. 2005;171:514.
7. Garibaldi RA, Britt MR, Coleman ML, et al. Risk factors for postoperative pneumonia. *Am J Med.* 1981;70:677.
8. Celli BR. Perioperative respiratory care of the patient undergoing upper abdominal surgery. *Clin Chest Med.* 1993;14:253.
9. Hofmann LV, Lee DS, Gupta A, et al. Safety and hemodynamic effects of pulmonary angiography in patients with pulmonary hypertension. *AJR Am J Roentgenol.* 2004; 183:779.
10. Birdwell BG, Raskob GE, Whitsett TL, et al. The clinical validity of normal compression ultrasonography in outpatients suspected of having deep venous thrombosis. *Ann Intern Med.* 1998;128:1.
11. Mermel LA, Farr BM, Sherertz RJ, et al. Guidelines for the management of intravascular catheter related infections. *Clin Infect Dis.* 2001;32:1249.
12. Ray NF, Denton WG, Thamer M, et al. Abdominal adhesiolysis: Inpatient care and expenditures in the United States in 1994. *J Am Coll Surg.* 1998;186:1.
13. Duron JJ, Hay JM, Msika S, et al. Prevalence and mechanisms of small intestinal obstruction following laparoscopic abdominal surgery. *Arch Surg.* 2000;135:208.
14. Livingston EH. Procedure incidence and in-hospital complication rates of bariatric surgery in the United States. *Am J Surg.* 2004;188:105.
15. Livingston EH, Huerta S, Arthur D, et al. Male gender is a predictor of morbidity and age a predictor of mortality for patients undergoing gastric bypass surgery. *Ann Surg.* 2002;236:576.
16. Shea JA, Healey MJ, Berlin JA, et al. Mortality and complications associated with laparoscopic cholecystectomy: A meta-analysis. *Ann Surg.* 1996;224:609.
17. Feingold DL, Widmann WD, Calhoun SK, et al. Persistent post-laparoscopy pneumoperitoneum. *Surg Endosc.* 2003;17:296.
18. Carucci LR, Levine MS, Rubesin SE, et al. Evaluation of patients with jejunostomy tubes: imaging findings. *Radiology.* 2002;223:241.
19. Crabtree TD, Pelletier SJ, Antevil JL, et al. Cohort study of fever and leukocytosis as diagnostic and prognostic indicators in infected surgical patients. *World J Surg.* 2001;25:739.

25

Urologic Stone Disease

David E. Manthey
Bret A. Nicks

HIGH YIELD FACTS

- Up to 15% of patients with nephrolithiasis will not have microscopic hematuria.
- Stones <5 mm will pass 90% of the time within 4 weeks, while 95% of stones >8 mm will become impacted.
- Stone size on radiographs are magnified; actual size is 80% of measured stone.
- Noncontrast helical computed tomography (CT) is the study of choice for evaluation of patients with suspected renal colic.
- Ultrasound (US) is the study of choice for pregnant patients with suspected renal colic.

EPIDEMIOLOGY

Nephrolithiasis is a common condition with a lifetime incidence of approximately 12%. The recurrence rate is 37% in 1 year and approaches 50% by 5 years with biphasic peaking at 2 and 8 years. The male to female ratio is 3:1. Ethnically, Caucasians develop stones more frequently than African Americans; it is relatively rare in Native American and Asian populations.

Seventy percent of initial nephrolithiasis events occur in patients between 20 and 50 years of age. It is relatively uncommon in patients younger than age 15 accounting for less than 7% of all cases.[1] An initial bout of nephrolithiasis is rare in patients after the age of 60. The highest incidence of stone disease is in Virginia, North Carolina, Georgia, Tennessee, and Kentucky, which forms a "stone belt" but does not include the entire southeast. Peak months of formation are July, August, and September, perhaps due to the peak temperatures during the previous month. Sedentary lifestyles and affluence also increase the incidence of kidney stones. There are also genetic predisposing factors to stone formation with some hereditary diseases (renal tubular acidosis, hyperparathyroidism, cystinuria) augmenting the frequency of nephrolithiasis.

PATHOPHYSIOLOGY

Urologic stone formation occurs when the urine becomes supersaturated with oxalate and calcium. At some point (thermodynamic solubility product), the addition of more solute (calcium, oxalate, urate, etc.) to the solvent (urine) causes crystals to precipitate out of the solution. The thermodynamic solubility product of the solvent (urine) is constantly changing due to changes in dwell time, dilution with other solutes, electrical ion interactions, and presence of inhibitory substances (citrate and urinary proteins). Crystals do not usually aggregate into a stone due to the free flow of urine. However, crystals can coalesce within the renal tubules or adhere to collecting ducts (Randall plaques)[2]; therefore, in the ideal environment, stone formation occurs.

Approximately 85% of renal calculi are composed of calcium combined with either oxalate, phosphate, or a mixture of both. Calcium oxalate stones represent approximately 80% of all stones, and may be associated with chronic dehydration, absorptive hypercalciuria, hypocitraturia, dietary hyperoxaluria, hypernatriuria, or hyperuricosuria. Up to 60% of patients with calcium oxalate stones have elevated urine calcium levels without increased serum calcium levels. Of those patients with hypercalcemia, almost all will have primary hyperparathyroidism with other causes including hyperthyroidism and sarcoidosis. Hyperoxaluria also predisposes one to the formation of calcium oxalate stones.[3]

Struvite stones are the next most common comprising about 2% to 20% of all stones. Known as triple phosphate stones (magnesium, ammonium, and phosphate) they make up the majority of staghorn calculi and are caused by chronic infection with urea-splitting organisms (*Proteus, Klebsiella, Staphylococcus* species, Providencia, and Corynebacterium). The chemical reaction that follows causes the rise in urinary pH, commonly seen with struvite stone formation.

Uric acid stones make up about 6% of all stones. Excessive uric acid secretion is the problem along with excessively acidic urine. Uric acid stones occur about 1% per year after the first gout attack, and approximately 20% of patients with gout suffer from stones. These are the most common radiolucent stone. Cystine stones are rare, account for about 1% of all stones, and occur in patients with cystinuria, an autosomally recessive genetic disorder affecting amino acid transport (COLA: cysteine, ornithine, lysine, arginine). Stones can be made of many other miscellaneous substances, which include indinavir, triamterene, xanthene, and silicate.

The approximate incidence of indinavir urolithiasis in human immunodeficiency virus (HIV) positive patients receiving the drug is 10%. The exact mechanism of lithogenesis is still unknown. Indinavir urolithiasis can be associated with acute unilateral renal colic or severe azotemia. Pure indinavir stones are radiolucent on plain abdominal x-ray or CT scan. Therefore, HIV positive patients with renal colic or renal insufficiency and absence of radio-opaque stone formations should followup with the urologist for consideration of indinavir urolithiasis.[4]

Anatomic considerations and calculus size are important considerations for the resultant disease complications. However, the major cause of progressive renal injury is stone associated infection. As ureteral stones originate in the kidney, gravity and peristalsis contribute to their passage. As they pass, there are five anatomic locations that frequently cause impaction. First, a stone may become wedged in the renal calyx. The narrowing just beyond the distal portion of the renal pelvis is the second impaction location. The third area of impaction occurs at the ureteropelvic junction (UPJ) where the ureter crosses the iliac vessels into the true pelvis. The fourth site, known as the ureterovesicular junction (UVJ), where the ureter enters the intramural bladder is the most common location for impaction as it is the most constricted section of the ureter. The final site that a stone can become impacted is in the vesicular orifice.

With acute ureteral obstruction, there is a triphasic response. In the first 2 hours, both renal blood flow (RBF) and renal pelvic pressure increase (RPP). In the next 4 hours, RBF normalizes and RPP remains elevated. Over longer duration, RBF decreases below baseline while RPP elevation decreases from its peak, but remains elevated above baseline.[5] If the obstruction is unrelieved, irreversible renal damage is sustained within 3 weeks. During acute obstruction, most patients have no rise in serum creatinine or electrolyte abnormalities as the contralateral kidney continues to function. A rise in serum creatinine or electrolyte disturbance suggests the possibility of preexisting renal disease (such that the already impaired contralateral kidney is unable to compensate) or a solitary kidney. Fortunately, most patients have incomplete ureteral obstruction so that the majority can be safely observed over weeks. It is rare for patients to sustain irreversible renal damage from a kidney stone if obstruction has not been present for over one month.[6]

CLINICAL FEATURES

Renal colic is the presenting complaint of most patients. It begins abruptly, causing severe paroxysmal visceral type pain (53%) in the affected flank, radiating anteroinferiorly toward the lateral abdomen and genitals. It is caused by hyperperistalsis of the smooth muscle of the calyces, pelvis, and ureter. Patients are often unable to find a position of comfort, unlike abdominal pathologies associated with peritonitis. Nausea (44%), vomiting (51%), and anorexia (54%) are prominent.[7] Dilation of the ureter and renal pelvis should cause a visceral-type pain without associated peritoneal irritation. However, recent studies have shown that patients with renal colic may have rebound tenderness (29%), guarding (61%), and rigidity (8%) although the numbers vary significantly among studies.[7] Pain may radiate into the testicles in men or the labia in women (15%). As the stone nears the bladder, symptoms of urinary urgency often develop; however, only 3% to 24% of patients with acute renal colic have symptoms referable to micturition.[7] Hematuria is present in 85% to 90% of patients with renal colic while only 30% have gross hematuria. As infection associated with renal colic is concerning, any history of fever and chills should prompt immediate evaluation. Antibiotic choice (i.e., intravenous aminoglycoside or oral fluoroquinolone) should be initially tailored toward *Escherichia coli* as this is the most common pathogen associated with infection.

DIAGNOSIS AND DIFFERENTIAL

The patient with suspected renal colic will require evaluation for life-threatening conditions that mimic its clinical presentation. Beginning with the vital signs, renal colic patients are often tachycardic, hypertensive, and may have mild tachypnea—all typically associated with pain response. The presence of fever is not associated with isolated renal colic and should suggest the possibility of concurrent infection. The presence of hypotension associated with renal colic is exceedingly rare and is associated with the vasovagal response to the pain. If hypotension occurs, a rupturing abdominal aortic aneurysm (AAA) or other vascular or surgical etiology of the pain should be sought immediately (consider bedside US). A clinical diagnostic score revealed three significant predictors of renal colic: acute abdominal pain of short duration (<12 hours), loin (15%) or renal (86%) tenderness, and hematuria (erythrocytes >10).[7]

Renal colic may be associated with tenderness over the site of the impacted stone; however, true peritoneal findings are not a component of this disorder. If peritoneal signs are present, the differential diagnosis should be expanded. In addition, genitourinary examinations are of equal importance during the physical examination. Since the radiating pattern of discomfort often includes the testicles or labia majora, these areas should be evaluated. In males, the testes should be evaluated for torsion or infection. In women, a pelvic examination should be conducted when the diagnosis is unclear to assess for ovarian torsion, cyst, infection or if pregnant, ectopic pregnancy. Differential diagnosis of renal colic is listed in Table 25-1.

Initial evaluation for renal colic should include a urine dipstick for microscopic hematuria, which is present in 85% of patients with renal colic. Urinalysis is recommended to rule out pyuria and bacteriuria. Urine culture is indicated if signs, symptoms, or urinalysis findings suggest infection. Electrolytes with blood urea nitrogen (BUN) and creatinine are helpful for those with profound vomiting or known or possible renal insufficiency (patients who are elderly or who have hypertension, diabetes, or chronic renal insufficiency). Determination of a complete blood count (CBC) is not usually helpful in the evaluation of kidney stones as an elevated white blood cell (WBC) count may be secondary to the stress-pain response. In general, a more extensive metabolic work-up in the emergency department (ED) is inappropriate.

Computed tomography scan without contrast (NCCT) is the study of choice. It is indicated in all patients with the first episode of suspected nephrolithiasis as approximately one third of these patients do not have stones. Computed tomography scanning has a high sensitivity (96%) and a high specificity (92%–100%) overall, with a positive predictive value of 88% and a negative predictive value of 98% in ED patients.[8,9] Computed tomography scanning reveals alternative diagnoses in between 10% and 33% of suspected cases with up to 48% of these diagnoses considered to be significant pathology.[10] The CT findings associated with nephrolithiasis consist of identifying a stone in the ureter or finding secondary changes such as hydronephrosis, fornix rupture, dilation of renal pelvis, or stranding of perirenal and peri-ureteral tissue (Figures 25-1 and 25-2).[11] Noncontrast CT evaluation of stones has been shown to overestimate the

Table 25-1. Differential Diagnosis of Renal Colic

Aneurysm, aortic or iliac
Appendicitis
Biliary colic
Bowel ischemia
Bowel obstruction
Diverticulitis
Drug seeking behavior
Ectopic pregnancy
Endometriosis
Fitz-Hugh-Curtis syndrome
Henoch-Schönlein purpura
Hernia, internal
Malingering
Musculoskeletal pain
Pyelonephritis
Ovarian cyst
Ovarian torsion
Peritonitis
Psoas abscess or hematoma
Renal artery thrombosis or embolism
Renal artery dissection or infarction
Renal papillary necrosis
Retroperitoneal mass or bleed
Rib fracture
Superior mesenteric artery occlusion
Urinary retention

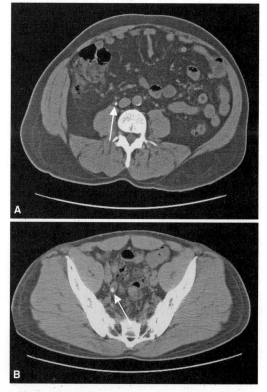

Fig. 25-1. Abdominal CT. The first image A. (top) demonstrates a stone in the ureter without evidence of hydronephrosis (arrow) and the second B (bottom) with hydronephrosis (arrow).

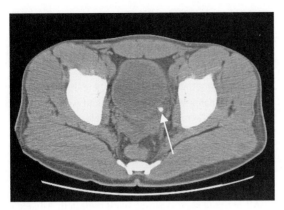

Fig. 25-2. Abdominal CT showing UVJ stone (arrow).

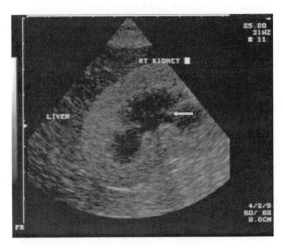

Fig. 25-3. Renal ultrasound. Arrow demonstrates hydronephrosis secondary to downstream ureteral obstruction.

ureteral stone size by 30% to 50%.[12] The NCCT does not evaluate the functional status of the kidney and therefore does not evaluate renal artery or vein occlusion. A negative NCCT may also miss other abnormalities within the abdomen usually evaluated with contrast such as ischemic bowel or appendicitis and does not evaluate for certain causes of back pain such as herniated disc, pelvic inflammatory disease (PID), epidural abscess, and zoster.[13]

Plain radiographs, even when utilized in a retrospective analysis with CT scans have a very limited specificity (60%–77%) and sensitivity (45%–58%). It is currently only utilized after identification of a ureteral stone to follow its passage through the ureter. Intravenous pyelography (IVP) approaches a sensitivity of 90% for detection of nephrolithiasis or obstruction. However, its frequent imaging delays and relative contraindications including dye allergies and renal insufficiency as well as the inability to assess other causes of flank pain limit its usefulness.

Ultrasound, the noncontrasted, noninvasive, nonionizing means of evaluation, has a poor sensitivity (19%)[14] in detecting stones but is approximately 90% sensitive and 94% specific in detecting hydronephrosis (Figure 25-3). The use of resistive index calculation (>0.70), ureteral jet identification, and transvaginal US may improve the diagnostic abilities of US. Resistive indices are based on color Doppler US and may detect subtle renal blood flow changes defined by the formula, resistive index = (peak systolic frequency shift—end diastolic frequency shift)/peak systolic frequency shift. In reevaluation of a known stone, identification of obstruction may be all that is required; however, the accuracy of US studies is operator dependent, with body

habitus limitations, and yields limited information on renal function unless flow studies are added.

Nephrolithiasis in Pregnancy

The consideration of nephrolithiasis in pregnancy highlights two unique issues: the dose of radiation to the fetus and the physiologic dilation of the ureters. The radiation exposure of CT scan in pregnancy is approximately 30 mGy. The National Council on Radiation Protection and Measurements (NCRPM) state that the risk of fetal abnormalities is negligible at 50 mGy or less when compared to other risks of pregnancy.[15] This radiation risk removes CT as the primary study for nephrolithiasis during pregnancy but does not negate its potential use in the appropriate setting.

Ultrasound remains the study of choice for detection of stones during pregnancy. In the normal course of pregnancy, the physiology of the ureter changes with dilation beginning in the first trimester and progressing until delivery, with involvement greatest on the right. Although up to 90% of pregnant patients have dilation of the ureters by the third trimester, the resistive indices are not affected by pregnancy.[16]

Nephrolithiasis in Children

The classic adult presentation of renal colic is uncommon in children. Up to 50% will have some form of abdominal, pelvic, or flank pain. Gross hematuria is found in 33% to 90% of children regardless of age group. In preschool aged children, urinary tract infection is often the presenting complaint. Computed tomography remains the study of choice, but concern for radiation exposure should be considered especially in younger children, in whom US may be more appropriate. All pediatric patients with kidney stones should be worked up for metabolic stone disease as an outpatient.[17, 18]

Complications

Complications include worsening renal function, infection in the face of obstruction, prolonged obstruction greater than 2 weeks, sepsis, hypercalcemia, and obstruction with a single or transplanted kidney. Ureteral stones that remain symptomatic after 4 weeks incur a complication rate of 20% (sepsis, stricture, deterioration of renal function).[6]

EMERGENCY DEPARTMENT CARE AND DISPOSITION

The objectives of therapy for renal colic therapy are to alleviate pain, preserve renal function, and eliminate the obstruction. The basic tenets of ED treatment are hydration, analgesia, and antiemetics, which should be initiated immediately.

Unless the patient has a history of renal or congestive heart failure, or is elderly with concerning comorbidities, normal saline should be infused in volumes sufficient to produce a urine output of at least 100 mL/hr. Overhydration with the desired result of diuresis may increase intraluminal pressures and thereby decrease effective ureteral peristalsis on the obstructed side.[19]

Many drugs can be used to relieve pain: nonsteroidal anti-inflammatory drugs (NSAIDs), opioid analgesics, local or regional anesthesia, and acupuncture.[20] In a recent review, both NSAIDs and opioids lead to clinically significant decrease in patient reported pain scores; however, opioids were noted to have a significant increase in vomiting induced by medication.[21] Nonsteroidal anti-inflammatory drugs, which inhibit renal prostaglandin synthesis, are effective and may be given concurrently with opioids. In patients with preexisting renal disease, administration of NSAIDs can induce renal failure as they interfere with the kidney's auto-regulatory response to obstruction with marked reduction of renal blood flow, and therefore should be used cautiously.[22,23]

A small study of 60 patients showed increased expulsion rate and decreased expulsion time for jux-tavesicular stones when treated with 0.4 mg of tam-sulosin daily for 10 days and 30-mg deflazacort daily

for 10 days.[24] When utilized for stones at the UVJ, there was an increased expulsion rate and decreased expulsion time.

Another small study of 86 patients looked at oral treatment with 30 mg of deflazacort for up to 10 days plus 30-mg nifedipine XL for up to 28 days.[25] This study showed an increased expulsion rate and a reduced need for analgesic therapy with lower ureteral stones. Both studies were small and have specific inclusion and exclusion criteria. An overview of these and other similar recent studies suggests that alpha-blockers may enhance likelihood and speed of stone expulsion from the distal ureter.

All patients should remain well hydrated. Advocate that all urine be strained and any debris or stone collected should be saved for future analysis. Emphasize that patients return for fever, intractable vomiting or pain, foul smelling or cloudy urine, or dysuria. Avoiding rhubarb, beets, spinach, beer, cola, coffee, and citrus fruits is reasonable if the patient has dietary hyperoxaluria and calcium oxalate stones, but not proven for other factors. Moreover, Curhan et al. showed a statistical decrease of stones for moderate beer consumption.[26]

As uric acid stones are managed medically, it is important to determine the type of any previous stones. If the previous stones were urate and the pH of the urine is below 5.5, alkalinize the urine to >6.5 utilizing 20 mmol of potassium citrate 2 to 3 times daily.[27] Discuss treatment with a urologist and have the urine pH reassessed to determine adequacy of treatment.

Admission criteria are listed in Table 25-2. Suggested criteria for consultation with urology by phone or in person are listed in Table 25-3. Patient preference may need to be taken into consideration for disposition, for

Table 25-2. Admission Criteria/Urgent Intervention[6]

Intractable vomiting or pain
Single kidney with high grade obstruction
Transplanted kidney with high-grade obstruction
Anuria
High-grade obstruction, plus UTI and systemic symptoms
Sepsis
Hypercalcemic crisis
Impending renal deterioration (creatinine acutely
    elevated >1.5)

Abbreviation: UTI, urinary tract infection.

Table 25-3. Consult Criteria for Close Follow up

Single kidney **without** high-grade obstruction*
Transplanted kidney **without** high-grade obstruction*
UTI without obstruction
High-grade obstruction with proximal stone*
Urinary extravasation
Stone larger than 6 mm or staghorn
Chronic renal insufficiency (Cr >1.5, but without change)
Input on care in a complicated case

*Based on computed tomography findings.
Abbreviations: UTI, urinary tract infection; Cr, creatinine

example, some patients have occupational requirements that warrant a more aggressive approach, e.g., pilots, or in those cases when the uncertainty of stone passage or pain is unacceptable such as professional athletes, etc.

PITFALLS

- Kidney stones do not cause hypotension. Nephrolithiasis is the most common incorrect diagnosis for an AAA.

- Helical CT stone study does not assess the function of the kidneys.

- A negative CT stone study should prompt further evaluation of etiology of flank pain.

- Infection with obstruction should be considered an emergency.

- Obstruction of a single kidney or transplanted kidney needs prompt treatment to prevent deterioration of renal function.

REFERENCES

1. Drach GW. Urinary lithiasis: Etiology, diagnosis, and medical management. In: Walsh PC, Retik AB, Stamey TA, Vaughn ED, eds. *Campbell's Urology.* 6th ed. Vol 3. Philadelphia: Saunders; 1992.
2. Kim SC, Coe FL, Tinmouth WW, et al. Stone formation is proportional to papillary surface coverage by Randall's plaque. *J Urol.* 2005;173:117.
3. Borghi L, Schianchi T, Meschi T, et al. Comparison of two diets for the prevention of recurrent stones in idiopathic hypercalciuria. *N Engl J Med.* 2002;346:77.
4. Kalaitzis C, Touloupidis S, Patris E, et al. Indinavir urolithiasis in HIV-positive patients: Treatment and prophylaxis *Urologe A.* 2004;43:168.
5. Vaughan ED Jr, Shenasky JH 2nd, Gillenwater JY. Mechanism of acute hemodynamic response to ureteral occlusion. *Invest Urol.* 1971;9:109.
6. Teichman JM. Clinical Practice: Acute renal colic from ureteral calculus. *N Engl J Med.* 2004;350:684.
7. Eskelinen M, Ikonen J, Lipponen P. Usefulness of history-taking, physical examination and diagnostic scoring in acute renal colic. *Eur Urol.* 1998;34:467.
8. Miller OF, Rineer SK, Reichard SR, et al. Prospective comparison of unenhanced spiral computed tomography and intravenous urogram in the evaluation of acute flank pain. *Urology.* 1998;52:982.
9. Nachmann MM, Harkaway RC, Summerton S, et al. Helical CT scanning: the primary imaging modality for acute flank pain. *Am J Emerg Med.* 2001;18:649.
10. Ha M, MacDonald R. Impact of CT scan in patients with first episode of suspected nephrolithiasis. *J Emerg Med.* 2004;27:225.
11. Vaswani KK, El-Dieb A, Vitellas KM, et al. Ureterolithiasis: classical and atypical findings on unenhanced helical computed tomography. *Emerg Radiol.* 2002;9:60.
12. Van Appledorn S, Ball AJ, Patel VR, et al. Limitations of noncontrast CT for measuring ureteral stones. *J Endourol.* 2003;17:851–4; discussion 854.
13. Hamm M, Wawroschek F, Weckermann D, et al. Unenhanced helical computed tomography in the evaluation of acute flank pain. *Eur Urol.* 2001;39:460.
14. Heidenreich A, Desgrandschamps F, Terrier F. Modern approach of diagnosis and management of acute flank pain: Review of all imaging modalities. *Eur Urol.* 2002; 41:351.
15. National Council on Radiation Protection and Measurements. Medical radiation exposure of pregnant and potentially pregnant. NCRP Report No. 54, 1977;6.
16. McAleer SJ, Loughlin KR. Nephrolithiasis and pregnancy. *Curr Opin Urol.* 2004;14:123.
17. Gillespie RS, Stapleton FB. Nephrolithiasis in children. *Pediatr Rev.* 2004;25:131.
18. Bartosh SM. Medical management of pediatric stone disease. *Urol Clin North Am.* 2004;31:575, x-xi.
19. Portis AJ, Sundaram CP. Diagnosis and initial management of kidney stones. *Am Fam Physician.* 2001; 63:1329.
20. Travaglini F, Bartoletti R, Gacci M, et al. Pathophysiology of reno-ureteral colic. *Urol Int.* 2004;72(Suppl 1):20.
21. Holdgate A, Pollock T. Nonsteroidal anti-inflammatory drugs (NSAIDs) versus opioids for acute renal colic. *Cochrane Database Syst Rev.* 2005;2:CD004137.
22. Brater DC. Effects of nonsteroidal anti-inflammatory drugs on renal function: focus on cyclooxygenase 2-selective inhibition. *Am J Med* 1999;107:65S.
23. Perlmutter A, Miller L, Trimble LA, et al. Toradol, an NSAID used for renal colic, decreases renal perfusion and ureteral pressure in a canine model of unilateral ureteral obstruction. *J Urol.* 1993;149:926.

24. Dellabella M, Milanes G, Muzzonigro G. Efficacy of tamsulosin in the medical management of juxtavesical ureteral stones. *J Urol.* 2003;170:2202.

25. Porpiglia F, Destenfannis P, Fiori D, et al. Effectiveness of nifedipine and deflazacort in the management of distal stones. *Urology.* 2000;56:579.

26. Curhan GC, Curhan SG. Dietary factors and kidney stone formation. *Compr Ther.* 1994;20:485.

27. Pak C, Sakhaee K, Fuller C. Successful management of uric acid nephrolithiasis with potassium citrate. *Kidney Int.* 1986;30:422.

26

Urinary Tract Infections

Alan Heins

HIGH YIELD FACTS

- About 5% of febrile infants have urinary tract infections (UTIs) and symptoms may be vague, so urinalysis is indicated in the infant with a fever without a clear source of infection.
- Pyuria and bacteriuria on urine microscopy are sensitive and specific for UTI and should guide empiric therapy in the emergency department (ED).
- Fever, rigors, flank pain, costovertebral angle tenderness, or signs of sepsis syndrome with pyuria and/or bacteriuria should be treated as pyelonephritis.
- Pregnant women with pyelonephritis should be admitted to the hospital for parenteral antibiotics to help prevent premature delivery of low-birth-weight infants.
- All men with UTI should be considered to have a complicated infection and be treated with longer courses of antibiotics.

EPIDEMIOLOGY

Urinary tract infection is a common cause of doctor visits and hospitalization in the United States. In 2000, 9.1 million doctor visits were made for UTI, 1.3 million by men and 7.9 million by women. In 2001, UTI was a diagnosis at hospital discharge for 1.78 million adults—1.29 million women and 0.49 million men.[1] Urinary tract infection is the most common serious bacterial infection in febrile infants, affecting about 5% of infants with fever.[2] In the neonatal period, males are more likely to have UTI than females with a ratio 1.5:1; in adults, women are about 50 times more likely to have UTI than men; and in the elderly, the sex ratio is 1:1.[3] The incidence of UTI is the highest in sexually active women and the elderly.

PATHOPHYSIOLOGY

The urinary tract is usually sterile, but uropathogens can invade the urethra, bladder, and kidneys and cause infection. *Escherichia coli* is by far the most common bacteria causing UTI, isolated in more than 80% of community-acquired infections. Other causes include *Staphylococcus saprophyticus*, *Proteus mirabilis*, *Klebsiella* species, and *Enterobacter* species. In hospitalized patients and those with indwelling bladder catheters, other organisms may cause UTI, including Pseudomonas, Serratia, Citrobacter, and fungi, but *E. coli* remains the most common.[4] In infants, UTI is commonly associated with abnormalities of the genitourinary (GU) tract, with 45% of females and 97% of males demonstrating radiographic abnormalities.[5]

CLINICAL FEATURES

Urinary tract infection is generally separated into lower and upper tract infections, designated cystitis and pyelonephritis, respectively. Localization without expensive imaging is impractical, so clinical signs and symptoms guide diagnosis and therapy.[6] Infections are also considered uncomplicated, usually community acquired in normally healthy adult females, and complicated by GU tract abnormality, comorbidity, or indwelling catheter. Risk factors for UTI include sexual intercourse, delayed postcoital urination, history of recent UTI, indwelling catheter, and abnormality of GU tract, including prostatic hypertrophy.[7,8] The symptoms of cystitis are usually irritative, described as dysuria, urgency, frequency, hematuria, or suprapubic pain. However, the clinical presentation of infants and the elderly with UTI is often nonspecific, and the diagnosis can be missed unless the threshold for ordering urinalysis is low. Pregnant women with UTI and even asymptomatic bacteriuria are at risk for progression to acute pyelonephritis and premature delivery.[9] About 30% of patients with symptoms of cystitis have subclinical kidney involvement, but can be treated as if they have cystitis.[10] Fever, rigors, and flank pain, in association with pyuria and bacteriuria, suggest pyelonephritis.

Physical examination is largely unhelpful in most cases of UTI, except to identify alternative diagnoses that explain the urinary symptoms. Examination should focus on identifying evidence of urosepsis or septic shock, or pyelonephritis. Fever and costovertebral angle tenderness suggest pyelonephritis. Tachycardia, hypotension, and marked leukocytosis are seen in sepsis syndrome and correlate with bacteremia and are predictive of in-hospital death and intensive care unit (ICU) admission.[11]

The clinical course of patients with UTI is usually characterized by rapid recovery once appropriate antibiotic therapy is started. Elderly patients are at increased risk of morbidity and mortality. Almost 5% of elderly patients admitted to the hospital for UTI die during hospitalization.[11] Elderly patients 75 years and older with bacteremia complicating UTI have a 33% in-hospital mortality rate.[12]

DIAGNOSIS AND DIFFERENTIAL

Urinary tract infection is demonstrated by growth of 10^5 colony-forming units (CFU) of a uropathogenic species on urine culture. In symptomatic young women, culture of 100 or more CFU usually indicates infection.[13,14] For a large majority of patients, urine dipstick alone or in combination with microscopy of uncentrifuged specimens is adequate for empiric treatment in the ED. For atypical, recurrent, or complicated infections, culture may help guide therapy in the hospital or at outpatient follow-up visit. Two metaanalyses have investigated the diagnostic accuracy of urine screening tests in diagnosing UTI. Gorelick and Shaw[15] found that the presence of any bacteria on Gram stain of an uncentrifuged urine specimen had the best combination of sensitivity (93%) and specificity (95%). Urine dipstick performed well with sensitivity of 88% for the presence of either leukocyte esterase (LE) or nitrite and specificity of 96% when both LE and nitrite were present. Huicho et al.[16] used the same papers as Gorelick and Shaw and 11 additional papers published later. They found that the best performance, as determined by calculating the area under receiver operating characteristic curves, was the microscopic findings of pyuria $\geq$10 WBC per high power field and any bacteriuria, or bacteriuria $\geq$10 per high power field. Urine dipstick had intermediate performance.

Urine collection methods influence the contamination rates of cultures. Males can provide a clean catch specimen with low contamination rates, so need not be catheterized to obtain urine. Infants, children, and adult women have high contamination rates, even with rigorous cleansing regimens, so suprapubic aspiration or urethral catheterization should be performed to obtain urine for analysis and culture.[17]

Imaging can identify kidney involvement with infection, but is expensive and rarely indicated, except in cases of atypical or recurrent infection where obstruction or an infected stone is suspected. In those complicated cases renal ultrasound (US) or abdominal computed tomography (CT) are most useful to determine hydronephrosis and presence of stones. In the past, routine imaging of infants with a first UTI was recommended to identify GU tract abnormalities, but a recent study found no relation between the presence of vesicoureteral reflux and renal scarring after first UTI in infants.[18]

In severe cases, especially infants and the elderly, the presentation is nonspecific, so other causes of sepsis should be investigated such as pneumonia, occult bacteremia, and meningitis. In adult males <50 years old, the cause of dysuria is almost always urethritis or prostatitis, so sexual history and examination of the penis, urethra, and prostate is indicated. For females, vaginitis caused by *Candida* or *Trichomonas*, cervicitis, and pelvic inflammatory disease may cause similar symptoms as UTI and pyuria.[6] Finally, surgical emergencies such as appendicitis, perforated diverticulitis, and ectopic pregnancy may cause lower abdominal symptoms and pyuria.

EMERGENCY DEPARTMENT CARE AND DISPOSITION

Most patients with uncomplicated cystitis, including children and older women, can be treated successfully with a short course of oral antibiotics as outpatients. Three days of trimethoprim-sulfamethoxazole, cephalosporins, nitrofurantoin, or, for adults, fluoroquinolones, are as effective as longer courses, with lower costs and fewer side effects.[19–21] Local resistance patterns should direct antibiotic choice including consideration for third generation cephalosporins such as cefpodoxime. A multicenter, randomized, controlled trial found that a single dose of gatifloxacin 400 mg was as effective as 3 days of ciprofloxacin twice daily for uncomplicated UTI in women.[22] A Cochrane review found some treatment failures with single-dose therapy compared to short-course therapy (3–6 days) for older women.[19] No specific follow up of these uncomplicated cases is needed, but the patients should be advised to return or seek additional care if symptoms worsen or persist beyond the end of treatment.

Adults with pyelonephritis and patients with complicated UTI, including all men, who do not have signs of severe sepsis or inability to tolerate oral medication, may be treated as outpatients with 7 to 14 days of oral antibiotics.[23] Infants and pregnant women with pyelonephritis and patients with signs of sepsis or persistent vomiting should be admitted to the hospital and have urine and blood cultures obtained. In those patients who are able to tolerate oral antibiotics, there appears to be no significant difference between appropriate oral antibiotic regimens and intravenous antibiotics.[24,25]

PITFALLS

- The clinical presentation of infants and the elderly with UTI is often nonspecific, and the diagnosis can be missed unless the threshold for ordering urinalysis is low.

- In infants, children, and adult women, urine specimens not obtained by suprapubic aspiration or urethral catheterization are frequently contaminated with skin flora.

- *Chlamydia trachomatis* and *Neisseria gonorrhea* are common causes of dysuria in males and females and are not treated by many antibiotic regimens suggested for UTI.

REFERENCES

1. Kidney and Urologic Diseases for the United States. http://kidney.niddk.nih.gov/kudiseases/pubs/kustats/#up, Accessed October 2007.
2. Hoberman A, Chao HP, Keller DM, et al. Prevalence of urinary tract infection in febrile infants. *J Pediatr.* 1993; 123:17.
3. Fang LS, Tolkoff-Rubin NE, Rubin RH. Clinical management of urinary tract infection. *Pharmacotherapy.* 1982; 2:91.
4. Johnson JR, Stamm WE. Diagnosis and treatment of acute urinary tract infections. *Infect Dis Clin North Am.* 1987; 1:773.
5. Ginsburg CM, McCracken GH. Urinary tract infections in young infants. *Pediatrics.* 1982;694:409.
6. Stamm WE, Hooton TM. Current concepts: Management of urinary tract infections in adults. *N Engl J Med.* 1993; 329:1328.
7. Strom BL, Collins M, West SL, et al. Sexual activity, contraceptive use, and other risk factors for symptomatic and asymptomatic bacteriuria: a case control study. *Ann Intern Med.* 1987;107:816.
8. Remis RS, Gurwith MJ, Gurwith D, et al. Risk factors for urinary tract infection. *Am J Epidemiol.* 1987;126:685.
9. Andriole VT, Patterson TF. Epidemiology, natural history, and management of urinary tract infections in pregnancy. *Med Clin North Am.* 1991;75:359.
10. Ronald AR, Boutros P, Mourtada H. Bacteriuria localization and response to single-dose therapy in women. *JAMA.*1976; 235:1854.
11. Ginde AA, Rhee SH, Katz ED. Predictors of outcome in geriatric patients with urinary tract infections. *J Emerg Med.* 2004;27:101.
12. Tal S, Guller V, Levi S, et al. Profile and prognosis of febrile elderly patients with bacteremic urinary tract infection. *J Infect.* 2005;50:296.
13. Stamm WE, Counts GW, Running KR, et al. Diagnosis of coliform infection in acutely dysuric women. *N Engl J Med.* 1982;307:463.
14. Pappas PG. Laboratory in the diagnosis and management of urinary tract infections. *Med Clin North Am.* 1991;75:313.
15. Gorelick MH, Shaw KN. Screening tests for urinary tract infection in children: A meta-analysis. *Pediatrics.* 1999; 104:e54.
16. Huicho L, Campos-Sanchez M, Alamo C. Metaanalysis of urine screening tests for determining the risk of urinary tract infection in children. *Ped Infect Dis J.* 2002;21:1.
17. Lifshitz E, Kramer L. Outpatient urine culture: does collection technique matter? *Arch Int Med.* 2000;160:2537.
18. Moorthy I, Easty M, McHugh K, et al. The presence of vesicoureteric reflux does not identify a population at risk for renal scarring following a first urinary tract infection. *Arch Dis Child.* 2005;90:733.
19. Lutters M, Vogt N. Antibiotic duration for treating uncomplicated, symptomatic lower urinary tract infections in elderly women. *Cochrane Database Syst Rev.* 2002;(3): CD001535.
20. Vogel T, Verreault R, Gourdeau M, et al. Optimal duration of antibiotic therapy for uncomplicated urinary tract infection in older women: A double-blind randomized controlled trial. *CMAJ.* 2004;170:469.
21. Michael M, Hodson EM, Craig JC, et al. Short versus standard duration antibiotic therapy for acute urinary tract infection in children. *Cochrane Database Syst Rev.* 2003;(1): CD003966.
22. Richard GA, Mathew CP, Kirstein JM, et al. Single-dose fluoroquinolone therapy of acute uncomplicated urinary tract infection in women: Results from a randomized, double-blind, multicenter trial comparing single-dose to 3-day fluoroquinolone regimens. *Urology.* 2002;59:334.
23. Gilbert DN, Moellering RC, Eliopoulos GM, et al. *The Sanford Guide to Antimicrobial Therapy.* Hyde Park, VT: Antimicrobial Therapy, Inc., 2005.
24. Bloomfield P, Hodson EM, Craig JC. Antibiotics for acute pyelonephritis in children. *Cochrane Database Syst Rev.* 2003;(3):CD003772.
25. Mombelli G, Pezzoli R, Pinoja-Lutz G, et al. Oral vs intravenous ciprofloxacin in the initial empirical management of severe pyelonephritis or complicated urinary tract infections. *Arch Intern Med.* 1999;159:53.

27

Testicular Torsion

Anjali Bhagra

HIGH YIELD FACTS

> - Testicular torsion is a urologic emergency. It is the commonest surgical emergency in young boys.
> - High index of suspicion is the key for early diagnosis; early diagnosis is essential for testicular salvage. The time window for surgical intervention for testicular salvage is 4 to 8 hours.
> - Delay in correct diagnosis and advanced age are the two main risk factors for orchiectomy after testicular torsion.
> - A patient with a missed diagnosis of torsion, leading to testicular loss, may lead to a successful medical litigation. On the contrary, a clinical suspicion of torsion resulting in an unwarranted scrotal exploration does not lead to medical litigation.

EPIDEMIOLOGY

The incidence of testicular torsion averages to about one case per 4000 men and boys.[1] There is a bimodal pattern of distribution. Pubescent boys are the most frequently affected (65% of all torsions) with another smaller peak during infancy.[2] Although rare, testicular torsion has also been described perinatally and in neonates. It is caused by rotation of the testis with twisting of the spermatic cord, which can subsequently lead to reduced fertility. There are no definite predisposing factors, although it has been postulated that heavy exertion and strenuous exercise may have some association. Interestingly, few cases have been reported during sleep. Over the past several years, there has been an improvement in the testicular salvage rate; however, there still is a large number of patients losing testes.[2]

PATHOPHYSIOLOGY

Testicular torsion can be classified as intravaginal or extravaginal. The anterior surface of the testes is covered by tunica vaginalis, which extends variable distances over the epididymis and the spermatic cord. The covering may extend up to the cord resulting in freely suspended testes in the tunical cavity, also known as the bell clapper variant, which is usually bilateral and has been reported in 12% of testes at postmortem. Bell clapper variant allows the spermatic cord to twist, causing intravaginal testicular torsion (Figure 27-1). It is the leading etiology of torsion in adolescence and childhood, when there is rapid testicular growth. Extravaginal torsion, on the other hand, is more frequent in the neonatal period when the extremely mobile descending or descended testis can twist *en masse*.[2]

CLINICAL FEATURES

The most common presentation is unilateral scrotal pain. Other conditions that can have similar presentation include torsion of the testicular or epididymal appendage. Testicular torsion patients usually present with history of sudden onset pain. Abdominal pain (20%–30%), nausea and vomiting (20%–30%), fever (16%), and urinary frequency (4%) may be the other presenting symptoms. Patients who describe similar previous episodes probably have intermittent testicular torsion with spontaneous detorsion.[3] Patients with previous fixation and presenting with testicular pain can rarely have recurrent torsion.

Physical Examination

Importance of scrotal examination in patients presenting with abdominal complaints cannot be overstated. (It will avoid missing torsion in patients presenting with more "abdominal" symptoms.)[2] A good scrotal examination is extremely important. The examiner should begin the examination on the normal side. Positive physical findings include scrotal swelling and erythema. Lack of resolution of pain upon hemiscrotal elevation differentiates torsion from epididymitis. A horizontal lie and higher position of the testis is suspicious for torsion on the affected side. Cremasteric reflex on the affected side is a sensitive finding. Complete genitourinary, abdominal, and prostate exams should also be carried out.

DIAGNOSIS AND DIFFERENTIAL

Laboratory Studies

One third of the cases may reveal leukocytosis. Urinalysis may be obtained. In patients with torsion, urine is usually clean and may be helpful in differentiating from other

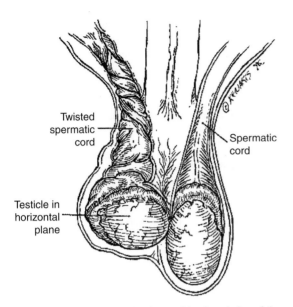

Fig. 27-1. Bell clapper deformity resulting in twisting of the spermatic cord and the testis on the right side. Note that right testis is elevated with a horizontal lie. (Reproduced with permission from *Atlas of Emergency Medicine.* Knoop, Stack and Storrow, 2nd ed., Fig. 8.2. New York, McGraw Hill, 2006.)

conditions such as epididymitis, which may have a similar presentation.

Radiologic Investigations

Physical examination of the testes may be challenging and limiting because of marked pain, tenderness, and swelling. Sonographic evaluation combined with Doppler of the spermatic cord and testes is therefore becoming an essential component of the examination.[4] Color Doppler ultrasonography (CDUS) evaluation of the testes has been shown to have 86% sensitivity, 100% specificity, and 97% accuracy for the diagnosis of testicular torsion and ischemia.[5] Color Doppler ultrasonography may reveal diminished or lack of vascular signal within the affected testis, which may be enlarged, swollen, or hypoechoic with thickened scrotal wall.

Imaging of the spermatic cord with high frequency transducers enables direct visualization of the twist, which remarkably enhances the sensitivity of the examination, thus enabling expeditious surgical intervention. Positive sonographic features include sudden change in the course, echo texture, and increased caliber of the cord

at the level of the "knot" or twist with venous engorgement distal to the site of rotation.[6]

Radionuclide imaging with ^{99m}Tc has reported sensitivity of 90% to 100% and is particularly useful in cases with duration of symptoms greater than 12 hours and prolonged vascular compromise.[7] The findings on scintigraphy include decreased radiotracer uptake on the affected side. Limitations include limited availability, cost, and difficult interpretation in children and patients with comorbidities, such as hydrocele, where localization of the testis is challenging.

Differential

Diagnosis should be promptly made with focused history and comprehensive scrotal examination aided by radiologic tests if needed. Differential diagnoses of testicular torsion include epididymitis, orchitis, torsion of a testicular or epididymal appendage, testicular neoplasm, inguinal hernia, hydrocele, trauma, Fournier gangrene, and peritonitis.

Torsion of the testicular appendage is differentiated by the presence of a paratesticular nodule located at superior pole of the testis. Treatment for this condition is supportive.[8]

Epididymitis is more common in the adolescent age group with most cases being secondary to sexually transmitted diseases. It is important to remember its association with genitourinary abnormalities.[8]

EMERGENCY DEPARTMENT CARE AND DISPOSITION

Time is of the essence in testicular salvage. Testicular torsion warrants early diagnosis and prompt definitive treatment. Once the diagnosis is made, analgesics can be administered for pain relief. Immediate urologic consultation to facilitate surgery for detorsion and orchiopexy should be obtained. In cases where there is anticipated delay in urology referral, manual detorsion should be attempted in the emergency department. Classically, the open book method has been described where the physician stands at the patient's foot end of the bed and attempts to detorse by rotating outward 180 degrees in a medial to lateral direction (Figure 27-2), with pain relief being indicative of the success of the maneuver. Complete detorsion may require two to three attempts at rotation. Reported success rates of this method are 30% to 70%. Definitive treatment is prompt surgery for early detorsion on the affected side and bilateral orchiopexy.

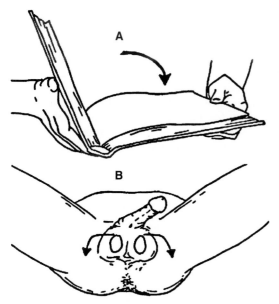

Fig. 27-2. Open book method for detorsion of testis. This procedure is best done standing at the foot of or on the right side of the patient's bed. A. The torsed testis is detorsed in a fashion similar to opening a book. B. The patient's right testis is rotated counterclockwise, and the left testis is rotated clockwise. (Reproduced with permission from Figure 95.7, *Emergency Medicine. A comprehensive study guide.* Tintinalli JE, Kelen GD, stapczynski JS, (eds.) New York, McGraw Hill, 2006.)

PITFALLS

- Hesitancy in seeking medical attention.
- Clinical differentiation between testicular torsion and epididymitis/orchitis is often imprecise and leads to delay in diagnosis.
- Delay in definitive surgical management entails poor prognosis and increased chances of testicular infarction and subsequent infertility.

REFERENCES

1. Blaivas M, Batts M, Lambert M. Ultrasonographic diagnosis of testicular torsion by emergency physicians. *Am J Emerg Med.* 2000;18:198–200.
2. Cuckow PM, Frank JD. Torsion of the testis. *BJU Int.* 2000;86:349–53.
3. Eaton SH, Cendron MA, Estrada CR, et al. Intermittent testicular torsion: diagnostic features and management outcomes. *J Urol.* 2005;174(4 Pt 2):1532–5.
4. Baud C, Veyrac C, Couture A, Ferran JL. Spiral twist of the spermatic cord: A reliable sign of testicular torsion. *Pediatr Radiol.* 1998;28:950–4.
5. Burks DD, Markey BJ, Burkhard TK, et al. Suspected testicular torsion and ischemia: Evaluation with color Doppler sonography. *Radiology.* 1990;175:815–21.
6. Arce JD, Cortes M, Vargas JC. Sonographic diagnosis of acute spermatic cord torsion. Rotation of the cord: A key to the diagnosis. *Pediatr Radiol.* 2002;32:485–91.
7. Lavallee ME, Cash J. Testicular torsion: Evaluation and management. *Curr Sports Med Rep.* 2005;4:102–4.
8. David JE, Yale SH, Goldman IL. Urology: Scrotal pain. *Clin Med Res.* 2003;1:159–60.

28

Acute Urinary Obstruction and Retention

Kristine Thompson

ACUTE URINARY OBSTRUCTION

High Yield Facts

- Urinary tract obstruction is a reversible cause of acute renal failure and should be considered in every patient with unexplained azotemia, anuria, or flank pain.
- Unenhanced helical computed tomography has a 97% sensitivity and 99% specificity to detect the need for intervention in acute flank pain.
- The most common causes of acute urinary obstruction vary by age; congenital anomalies in children, calculi in young adults, and benign prostatic hypertrophy (BPH) in elderly men.

Epidemiology

Urinary tract obstruction (UTO) is a reversible cause of acute renal failure that must be diagnosed quickly to preserve renal function. However, renal failure is unusual unless the level of obstruction is at or below the bladder neck, the ureteral obstruction occurs in a patient with a single kidney, or in the rare event that the ureteral obstruction is bilateral. The causes of acute UTO vary by age. Anatomic anomalies cause the majority of pediatric obstructions, calculi are most common in young adults, and BPH or neoplasms tend to affect the elderly.

Routine use of prenatal ultrasound (US) has dramatically improved antenatal detection of urinary tract anomalies. Most abnormalities can be detected as early as 12 weeks' fetal gestation by skilled ultrasonographers. Ureteropelvic junction (UPJ) obstruction is the most common cause of hydronephrosis in the neonate and child. The male to female ratio is 2:1, and 60% occur on the left.[1]

Acute urinary retention secondary to outlet obstruction is a common complication of BPH in elderly male patients. Advanced age and larger prostate size have been associated with a higher risk of developing acute urinary obstruction. The relative risk of urinary retention was estimated to be 0.9 in the fifth decade of life, increasing to 4.8 in the eighth decade.[2]

Pathophysiology

There are multiple congenital anomalies that can restrict urinary flow through intrinsic or extrinsic compression. The most common finding on antenatal US is hydronephrosis; however, this finding is not pathognomonic for obstruction. The pathophysiology behind the development of acute obstruction depends on the location and extent of the lesion and the age at which it is discovered. The final common pathway is dilation of the renal pelvis indicated by hydronephrosis with increasing intranephric pressures, which can ultimately lead to renal failure. Young adults with acute UTO most often have kidney stones (see Chapter 25). In older patients, external compression is the most frequent etiology behind acute UTO. For elderly males, this most commonly occurs in the setting of BPH. Symptoms are attributed to a gradually enlarging or thickening prostate gland, which eventually blocks flow through the prostatic urethra leading to outlet obstruction. Less common causes of extrinsic compression include vascular impingement, fibrotic lesions, and neoplasms.

Clinical Features

The clinical presentation depends on the location and extent of obstruction. This can be partial or complete, can be unilateral or bilateral, and can occur at any point along the urinary tract. Acute, complete obstruction tends to cause severe pain, vomiting, and diaphoresis. Upper tract lesions often present with flank pain, whereas lower tract lesions tend to cause pain that radiates to the ipsilateral testicle or labia. A complete bilateral or urethral obstruction will often present with anuria; however, normal urine output is possible with a partial or unilateral obstruction. Most cases of congenital anomalies leading to pediatric obstructions are detected through prenatal US. However, they can present acutely in the emergency department (ED) with sepsis, azotemia, failure to thrive, urinary infection, or voiding difficulties. Infection and sepsis may be the first indication of UTO in infants with potential for significant morbidity and mortality. Benign prostatic hypertrophy is clinically distinguished by progressive symptoms of lower urinary tract dysfunction. These symptoms are variable but frequently include nocturia, urinary hesitancy, dribbling, or progressive decrease in the force of the urinary stream. If infection is present, a history of dysuria, frequency, urgency, or fever may be elicited. Constitutional symptoms such as bone pain or weight loss are concerning for neoplasm, and previous urethral instrumentation or radiation therapy in the setting of acute urinary output obstruction suggests the presence of a urethral stricture.

The physical exam begins with the overall appearance of the patient. Those with acute, complete UTO appear very uncomfortable. They are often unable to maintain one position and are often diaphoretic and nauseated or vomiting. Abnormal vital signs including fever should be noted. Hypertension may be seen in acute unilateral renal or urethral obstruction secondary to the activation of the renin-angiotensin system. The back exam includes palpation and percussion of the costovertebral angles as hydronephrosis or pyelonephritis often produces tenderness in these areas. The abdominal exam includes palpation of the suprapubic area. A bladder containing more than 250 mL of urine is easily palpated or percussed. In men, the penis should be examined for phimosis or paraphimosis and a rectal exam performed to elicit the size and consistency of the prostate. The length of the urethra must be palpated for evidence of foreign body or abscess. In either sex, the meatus should be examined for signs of stenosis.

Diagnosis and Differential

Adult male UTO is statistically most common with BPH, which is characterized by progressive obstruction, usually in the sixth decade or later. Other causes include neoplasms, retroperitoneal fibrosis (fibrous histiocytoma), bladder or urethral clots, or ureteral or urethral calculi. Urethral obstruction due to phimosis or stricture must also be considered. Urinary tract obstruction in women is very uncommon but causes may include calculi, ureteroceles, urethral polyps and strictures, neoplasms, or clots. In children, the etiology of acute obstruction is most often due to anatomic abnormalities such as UPJ obstruction, posterior urethral valves in boys, and hydrocolpos in girls. The diagnosis is suggested by the detection of a distended bladder, costovertebral angle tenderness, oliguria or anuria, worsening renal function, urinary tract infection (UTI), or sepsis. The differential diagnosis of acute urinary obstruction or retention also includes nonmechanical causes. These include inflammatory or infectious disorders, neurogenic dysfunction, and medication induced retention (see Urinary Retention section). The differential of flank pain in adults must also include abdominal aortic aneurysm and retroperitoneal hematoma. In addition, patients of all ages, but especially children, may introduce foreign bodies into the urethra leading to bladder outlet obstruction.

Laboratory studies should be obtained to assess renal function and look for infection in those at risk. Hematuria suggests the presence of infection, tumor, or calculi. Renal insufficiency can occur with acute complete or partial bilateral obstructions, which are otherwise asymptomatic. For this reason, obstruction should be considered in any patient with unexplained renal insufficiency. Conversely, renal function tests should be performed whenever obstruction is complete, prolonged, or the patient is at risk for renal insufficiency (such as in the elderly). Serum prostate specific antigen (PSA) may be helpful to the urologist, but is rarely available in the time frame required to be of assistance to the emergency medicine physician.

Radiographic studies are generally used to look for obstruction of the ureters. These procedures attempt to identify the dilatation of the collecting system proximal to the obstruction. Renal ultrasonography (US) has traditionally been considered the test of choice to exclude hydronephrosis since it is noninvasive and does not require contrast. However, the sensitivity of US to detect hydronephrosis may be as low as 85%.[3] Computed tomography scanning should be performed if the kidneys are not well visualized or if the US results are equivocal. Unenhanced helical CT has a 97% sensitivity and 99% specificity to detect the need for intervention in acute flank pain.[4] Intravenous pyelogram (IVP) has the advantage of being able to identify the site of obstruction. However, it is cumbersome to perform and requires a contrast agent and should be reserved for those cases in which CT cannot identify the level of obstruction or when multiple renal cysts are present limiting the ability to detect hydronephrosis. Plain films of the abdomen offer minimal information and should be reserved for suspected urethral foreign bodies.

Emergency Department Care and Disposition

Regardless of the cause, treatment of an acute UTO ultimately focuses on elimination of the obstruction. However, if acute renal failure is present, care should be initially directed at correcting the potentially lethal complications such as hyperkalemia or volume overload. An attempt at placement of a standard urinary catheter should be made. If successful, the catheter should be left in place. Antibiotic therapy is initiated when a urine sample displays evidence of infection. In the case of bladder outlet obstruction, no further emergency treatment is needed and the patient may be instructed in catheter care and sent home with urologic follow-up arranged. Conversely, complete ureteral obstruction or an inability to easily pass a urethral catheter will require emergent urologic specialty consultation as percutaneous drainage may be urgently required. Patients with pyelonephritis, decreased renal function, bilateral complete obstruction (or complete obstruction of a solitary kidney), or evidence of volume overload should be considered for admission to the hospital.

Pitfalls

- Urethral foreign bodies are an uncommon, but important cause of obstruction.
- Multiple attempts at passage of a urinary catheter or forceful catheter insertion may lead to iatrogenic urethral trauma.
- Uncomplicated UTI is a common diagnosis in the emergency department, which is amenable to outpatient treatment. However, UTO with infection is an emergency requiring urologic consultation and admission for intravenous (IV) antibiotics.

URINARY RETENTION

High Yield Facts

- Rapid decompression of the obstructed urinary bladder is safe and effective. Hematuria, hypotension, and postobstructive diuresis are rarely clinically significant. The exception is cases of high pressure chronic retention, seen most commonly with BPH.
- Commonly prescribed medications and over-the-counter "cold" remedies are a frequent cause of urinary retention in young, healthy individuals.

Epidemiology

While the etiology of urinary retention is often obstructive such as in the case of BPH, there are several other causes that must be considered. These include inflammatory or infectious processes, neurogenic disorders, and pharmacologic complications and postsurgical states.

Pathophysiology

The process of voiding involves a coordinated series of muscular activities. The bladder wall is innervated by beta-adrenergic receptors, which relax the detrusor muscle, allowing filling. The vesical outlet and proximal urethra are predominantly alpha-adrenergic and stimulation maintains contraction and outlet resistance. The external urethral sphincter is primarily skeletal muscle, which is contracted to maintain continence. The process of voiding involves reversal of all three functions. This series of functions can be disrupted by pharmacologic agents, neurologic disorders, and inflammatory or infectious etiologies resulting in acute urinary retention.

There are many pharmaceutical agents that can lead to retention. The most common are anticholinergics, which inhibit contraction of the detrusor muscle. Alpha-adrenergic agents such as ephedrine compounds, amphetamines, and certain "cold" remedies cause bladder neck smooth muscle contraction leading to retention if abused or taken by susceptible individuals. Retention may also occur with the use of some antispasmotics, antipsychotics, and narcotics. In postsurgical patients urinary retention is common even in the absence of significant medication.

Inflammatory or infectious processes can produce enough swelling or sediment to obstruct the flow of urine from the bladder causing a mechanical obstruction. Additionally, the dysuria associated with certain infections may lead to functional obstruction. The most common cause of urinary retention related to infection is acute prostatitis. Other infectious etiologies include urethral herpes, abscesses, and tuberculous cystitis.[5]

Neurogenic causes can include upper motor neuron lesions, lower motor neuron lesions, or peripheral nerve lesions. Upper motor neuron etiologies of urinary retention include cerebrovascular accidents, multiple sclerosis, Parkinson disease, and neoplasm. Lower motor neurons may be affected by spinal cord injury or compression secondary to neoplasm. Peripheral lesions include diabetic neuropathy, intervertebral disk herniation, and iatrogenic disruption of the pelvic plexus.

Clinical Features

Patients experiencing acute urinary retention appear uncomfortable. Younger patients more typically do not present to the ED until they are no longer able to tolerate the pain associated with a markedly distended bladder. Another frequently encountered scenario is the noncommunicative elderly patient who is sent from a care facility with change in mental status or abdominal pain.

The history should include inquiries into voiding difficulties, recent surgeries or procedures, and constitutional symptoms. In addition, a detailed medication history, including over-the-counter medications and supplements and illicit drug use is imperative as many cases of acute retention are the result of a pharmacologic agent. The presence of prostatitis, urethritis, or cystitis may produce symptoms such as dysuria, frequency, and urgency prior to retention. Vaginal or urethral discharge, skin lesions, or fever may be reported in patients with gonococcal or herpetic disease. Recent trauma, back pain, and lower extremity weakness suggest a spinal cord lesion or compression.

Most patients with acute urinary retention are in distress. An appropriate physical examination includes inspection of the meatus for signs of stenosis, palpation of the urethral length for masses, palpation of the abdomen, back, costovertebral angles, and a rectal exam to evaluate the size and consistency of the prostate as well as sacral sensation and sphincter tone. A bladder containing >250 mL of urine should be easily palpable and percussible. The perineum is examined for skin lesions, vaginal or urethral discharge, and any evidence of trauma.

It is clear that prolonged urinary retention or obstruction may lead to tubular atrophy and irreversible renal injury. The prognosis for recovery of function depends on the extent and duration of the obstruction or retention. Most functional recovery will be seen within the first 7 to 10 days, but patients can regain partial function after several weeks of dialysis as well.

Diagnosis and Differential

Laboratory evaluation is focused on looking for signs of infection or renal insufficiency. A urinalysis and serum electrolytes should be collected on all patients with acute urinary retention. If perineal lesions are present, consider sending samples for viral and bacterial culture. Any urethral or vaginal discharge also must be sent for culture.

Radiologic studies in acute urinary retention are most helpful in the case of neurogenic etiologies; however, they are rarely needed to manage the acute episode. Radiographs of the spine may indicate lytic neoplasms, acute fractures, or suggest intervertebral disc herniation, which can be further defined on CT or magnetic resonance imaging (MRI). Brain CT is indicated to rule out acute stroke when clinically suggested. In all cases of urinary retention, bedside ultrasonography can be helpful to establish the quantity of postvoid residual urine in the bladder and examine the kidneys for signs of hydronephrosis.

The differential diagnosis for acute urinary retention includes obstructive etiologies including calculi, BPH, neoplasms, congenital anomalies, urethral strictures, blood clots, and foreign bodies. Psychogenic urinary retention is also a possibility, but it is a diagnosis of exclusion.

Emergency Department Care and Disposition

Acute urinary retention can result from a variety of illness, injuries, or ingestions. As such, treatment must be individualized according to the cause. However, in all cases, decompression of the bladder will provide initial relief. An attempt at placement of a standard urinary catheter should be made. Lidocaine jelly should be inserted into the urethra both to anesthetize and lubricate it. If this fails, the next step is to try a Coude catheter. If this will not pass, efforts at further instrumentation should be stopped as the creation of false tracts and hemorrhage are possible complications. If a specialist is not available, or immediate bladder decompression is needed, a percutaneous bladder aspiration may be required.

It is widely taught that once the catheter is in place, the rate of bladder emptying needs to be carefully controlled. In fact, this is largely myth. There are two complications that can be induced by rapid bladder decompression: gross hematuria and reflex hypotension. The risk of gross hematuria resulting from sudden release of pressure on compressed veins of the bladder wall is 2% to 16%.[6] However, the bladder pressure is very sensitive to the release of small amounts of urine. The pressure is reduced by 50% after the removal of 100 mL.[7] Clamping the catheter at 500 mL or 1000 mL is unlikely to prevent hematuria and if it does occur, it is most often self limited and of little consequence. An extensive review by Nyman recommends rapid, complete emptying of the obstructed urinary bladder in all cases.[6]

Another common belief is that postobstructive diuresis requires quantitative replacement. While some patients with chronic obstruction sustaining high bladder pressures may experience excessive diuresis, the urine output after an acute episode of retention most often represents an appropriate attempt to remove excess fluid and does not require replacement.[8] The patients who appear to be most at risk are those with chronic obstruction, signs of volume overload, or a history of renal insufficiency. A 4- to 6-hour observation period for signs of hypovolemia or hypotension is recommended for this group; if significant diuresis continues, the patient should be admitted to the hospital.

Acute urinary retention is a symptom of an underlying disorder that will require further investigation. If placement of a urinary catheter provides relief, the patient is reliable, and there are no signs of renal failure, spinal cord compression, or systemic illness (i.e., sepsis), the patient may be sent home with the catheter in place and outpatient urologic consultation arranged. If this follow-up cannot be assured, the patient has an acute neurologic lesion, renal failure, or sepsis, or develops hypotension with diuresis, emergent urologic consultation and admission to the hospital will likely be required.

Pitfalls

- Failure to consider acute urinary retention as a cause for acute abdominal pain or altered mental status in the elderly population may lead to prolonged retention and permanent loss of renal function.

- A history that does not include specific questions regarding the use of supplements or illicit drugs may miss the etiology of a case of acute urinary retention.

REFERENCES

1. Behrman RE, Kleigman R, Jenson HB, (Eds): *Nelson Textbook of Pediatrics.* 17th ed. Elsevire Science, St. Louis MO, 2004: 1798.
2. Wei JT, Calhoun E, Jacobsen SJ. Urologic diseases in America project: benign prostatic hyperplasia. *J Urol.* 2005; 173:1256.
3. Henderson SO, Hoffner RJ, Aragona JL, et al. Bedside emergency department ultrasonography plus radiography of the kidneys, ureters, and bladder versus intravenous pyelography in the evaluation of suspected renal colic. *Acad Emerg Med.* 1998;5:666.
4. Dalrymple NC, Verga M, Anderson KR, et al. The value of unenhanced helical computerized tomography in the management of acute flank pain. *J Urol.* 1998;159:735.
5. Fontanarosa PB, Roush WR. Acute urinary retention. *Emerg Med Clin North Am.* 1988;6:419.
6. Nyman MA, Schwenk NM, Silverstein MD. Management of urinary retention: Rapid versus gradual decompression and risk of complications. *Mayo Clin Proc.* 1997;72:951.
7. Christensen J, Ostri P, Frimodt-Moller C, Juul C. Intravesical pressure changes during bladder drainage in patients with acute urinary retention. *Urol Int.* 1987;42:181.
8. Howards SS. Post-obstructive diuresis: A misunderstood phenomenon. *J Urol.* 1973;110:537.

29

Complications of Urologic Devices

Simon A. Mahler

Lekshmi Vaidyanathan

COMPLICATIONS OF URETERAL STENTS

High Yield Facts

- Sixty percent to 80% of patients experience irritative voiding symptoms.
- Plain films are sensitive for diagnosis of stent migration, encrustation, malposition, or fracture.
- Urinary tract infection (UTI) in patients with ureteral stents can typically be treated with ciprofloxacin without stent removal.

Epidemiology

Ureteral stents are used to treat or prevent ureteral obstruction from stones, malignancy, or periprocedural edema. They are frequently associated with complications and up to 80% of patients report a reduced quality of life.[1] Irritative voiding symptoms are the most common complication occurring in 60% to 80% of patients with ureteral stents.[1–4] Other common complications include flank pain in 16% to 43% of patients, infection in 15% to 38%, gross hematuria in 13% to 18%, incontinence in up to 20%, and stent migration in approximately 1% to 8% of patients.[4–7] Encrustation, malposition, malfunction (obstruction), fracture, fistula formation, vesicorenal reflux, and forgotten stent are other complications (Table 29-1).[8–10]

Ureteral stents that remain in place for longer than 3 months are at increased risk for complications such as infection, encrustation, and fracture.[9–12] Diabetes mellitus, chronic renal insufficiency, female gender, and emergent placement also increase the risk of stent associated UTI.[11,12]

Pathophysiology

Ureteral stents are hollow tubes typically made of silicone or polyurethane. They are designed with curves at each end, pigtails or Js, which help prevent stent migration. Urine presents a harsh environment, which can lead to stent obstruction or fracture due to mineral deposition and bacterial colonization.

Clinical Features

The most common complaints voiced by patients with ureteral stents are irritative voiding symptoms such as dysuria, urgency, frequency, and nocturia. Flank pain, hematuria, and fever are frequent presentations. Many patients report persistent discomfort with an indwelling stent. Although persistent discomfort is common, a sudden change in symptoms such as fever, new onset hematuria, or pain that has changed in character, intensity, or location may indicate a serious complication.

Diagnosis and Differential

The differential diagnosis for patients with irritative voiding symptoms, flank pain, fever, or hematuria includes the complications of ureteral stents summarized in Table 29-1. However, it is important to retain a broad differential to avoid missing conditions unrelated to the indwelling stent.

Urinalysis should be obtained. Patients with fever or a urinalysis suggestive of infection should have urine culture and sensitivities. The presence of bacteriuria is not specific for infection, as it is seen in stent colonization, although infection is more likely if there is significant pyuria (white blood cell [WBC] >30 per high power field).[12]

Microscopic hematuria is often seen in patients with normal, functional stents but gross hematuria requires evaluation for infection, stent migration, ureteral erosion, or vascular fistula formation. Erosions and fistulas communicating with the abdominal arterial vasculature are rare, but potentially life threatening. Patients with suspected vascular fistulas should undergo angiography.[8]

Patients with ureteral stents and new symptoms should have an abdominal x-ray to evaluate stent position. Ureteral stents are typically radio-opaque or have distal markers facilitating identification on anteroposterior (AP) abdominal plain film. The proximal loop of an appropriately placed stent is located in the renal pelvis and the distal loop is located above the base of the bladder. A malpositioned stent refers to a stent placed incorrectly initially. Stent migration refers to stent movement following initial placement due to peristalsis of the ureter and may occur proximally or distally. Stent migration is recognized on plain film by inappropriate positioning, straightening of the J or pigtail, or coiling of

Table 29-1. Complications of Ureteral Stents[8]

Irritative voiding symptoms	Obstruction
Flank pain	Encrustation
Suprapubic pain	Ureteral erosion
Hematuria	Fistulization
Pyuria	Vesicorenal reflux
Urinary tract infection	Incontinence
Stent malposition	Stent fracture
Stent migration	Forgotten stent

the stent (Figure 29-1). Plain films can also identify moderate to severe stent encrustation, forgotten stents, and stent fracture.[8]

Stent malfunction from occlusion may occur secondary to hematuria, mineral deposition, or stone debris. Computed tomography (CT) and ultrasound (US) can be used to detect stent malfunction demonstrated by hydronephrosis. Doppler US can detect stent flow by measuring stent jets in the bladder. Blood urea nitrogen (BUN)

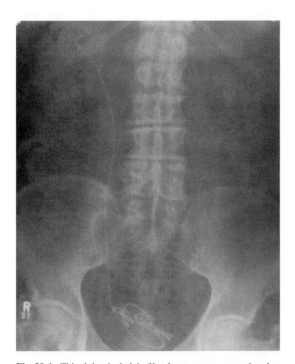

Fig. 29-1. This abdominal plain film demonstrates stent migration with the distal portion of the stent coiled with in the bladder.

and creatinine have poor sensitivity and specificity for unilateral ureter obstruction in patients with two functioning kidneys.[5,8]

Emergency Care and Disposition

The majority of patients with irritative voiding, flank pain, infection, and hematuria can be treated on an outpatient basis with urologic follow up. Exceptions that require admission and emergent consultation include gross hematuria from a vascular-ureter fistula, stent malfunction or obstruction in patients with a single kidney, and patients with severe or systemic infections.

Patients with irritative voiding symptoms or flank pain without complications such as infection, obstruction, and stent migration can be treated with opiate analgesics and anticholinergics on an outpatient basis. Recent evidence suggests that alpha$_1$ blockers such as alfuzosin or tamsolusin may also decrease pain and irritative voiding symptoms.[3]

Patients with simple UTIs can be treated as outpatients with antibiotics such as ciprofloxacin (consider local resistance patterns) and do not require stent removal or exchange. Admission and intravenous (IV) antibiotics are required for patients with evidence of pyelonephritis, toxic appearance, or comorbid illness. Treatment and disposition decisions regarding stent related infections should be discussed with the patient's urologist. Prophylactic antibiotics are not recommended for patients with ureteral stents.[15,16]

Patients with stent migration, fracture, encrustation, and forgotten stent require stent removal or repositioning. Urology should be consulted as these problems require timely treatment.[8–10] Stent malfunction requires emergent intervention in patients with a single kidney, underlying renal disease, or any signs of acute renal insufficiency. However, any patient with evidence of persistent or worsening hydronephrosis with a stent in place should receive urologic consultation. Patients with gross hematuria should also be evaluated by urology for ureteral erosions or vascular fistula formation.[8]

Pitfalls

- Failure to collaborate with urology in the diagnosis and treatment of stent complications.
- Failure to obtain an abdominal plain film on a patient with new, irritative voiding symptoms, flank pain, or hematuria.
- Relying on elevation of BUN and creatinine to diagnose stent obstruction.

COMPLICATIONS OF PERCUTANEOUS NEPHROSTOMY TUBES

High Yield Facts

- Up to 30% of patients experience kinking or tube dislodgment.
- Inadvertent puncture of bowel or adjacent organs may not be recognized in the immediate postoperative period.
- Severe bleeding several days after nephrostomy tube insertion or removal requires angiography to evaluate for vascular fistula, pseudoaneurysm, or vessel laceration.

Epidemiology

By creating urinary diversion, percutaneous nephrostomy tubes treat or prevent urinary tract obstruction from stones, malignancy, or periprocedural edema. Nephrostomy tubes are also used to facilitate endo-urologic procedures. The reported complication rate for nephrostomy tubes is approximately 10% with a reported range of 4% to 34%.[17–20] Tube kinking and dislodgment are common and occur in 11 % to 30% of patients. [19,21,22] Hematuria is nearly universal, but severe bleeding requiring transfusion or intervention occurs in less than 4% of cases.[17,23] Fever commonly follows nephrostomy tube insertion, with septic shock occurring in 1% to 3% of patients.[17,21,23] The risk for sepsis is increased in patients requiring emergent stent placement for UTI with concomitant urinary obstruction.[17,20,23] Less common complications include encrustation, obstruction, urine leakage, urinoma formation, injury to adjacent organs including bowel perforation, pneumothorax, hydrothorax, vascular injury, or fistula formation.[17,18,24,25]

Pathophysiology

Percutaneous nephrostomy refers to a tube that is passed through the skin, body wall, and renal parenchyma entering the urinary collecting system. These devices are placed by urologists or interventional radiologists under fluoroscopic, US, or CT guidance.[24] The typical approach is below the 12th rib, because supracostal access is associated with a higher complication rate including pneumothorax.[26,27] Manipulation of nephrostomy tubes in patients with UTIs is thought to precipitate bacteremia and possibly septic shock.[24]

Clinical Features

Patients with dislodgment, tube kinking, or obstruction may complain of urine leakage or lack of urine output. Although hematuria is nearly universal, the development or worsening of hematuria several days after tube insertion or removal is ominous and may indicate a vascular injury or fistula.[28,29] Patients with pyelonephritis following nephrostomy tube insertion may present with fever, nausea, vomiting, flank pain, and change in urine appearance or smell. Patients who develop urosepsis may have mental status changes, hypotension, or appear toxic.[24,25]

Diagnosis and Differential

Urinalysis and urine culture should be obtained in any patient with flank pain, fever, or hematuria. Patients with fever or a urinalysis suggestive of infection should have urine culture and sensitivities obtained. The presence of bacteriuria and pyuria are consistent with infection, but culture remains the standard. Patients who appear toxic, are hypotensive, or have altered mental status should be evaluated for urosepsis.

Coagulation studies, platelet count, hemoglobin, hematocrit, and type and screen or cross should be considered in patients with suspected vascular complications. Angiography should be performed to evaluate for vascular fistula, pseudoaneurysm, or vessel laceration.

Puncture of adjacent organs such as bowel, spleen, liver, or pleural space is rare and is usually apparent in the immediate postoperative period. However, some bowel injuries may take days to manifest. These patients may present to the emergency department with fever, abdominal pain, or other nonspecific complaints such as nausea and vomiting. Computed tomography can be used to evaluate intraabdominal injury while patients with clinically significant pneumothorax can usually be diagnosed with a chest x-ray. Patients with tube dislodgment, kinking, or obstruction can typically be diagnosed clinically.[24,25]

Emergency Care and Disposition

Most cases of minor hematuria can be managed with irrigation and tube clamping by the urologist with outpatient follow up. Patients with severe or late onset bleeding require angiography and possibly embolization if a vascular fistula or injury is identified. These patients should also have an emergent urology consultation because surgery may be necessary to control bleeding if interventional techniques fail.[24,25,28]

Patients with irritative symptoms and bacteriuria should be treated with antibiotics in consultation with urology. Patients with pyelonephritis or urosepsis require broad spectrum IV antibiotics and inpatient care. Patients with peritoneal signs or CT evidence of intraabdominal organ injury require IV antibiotics and immediate surgical consultation.

Nephrostomy tube kinking, obstruction, and dislodgment require management by urology. Dislodgment within the first week of placement usually requires the creation of a new tract. After the first week, nephrostomy tubes can be replaced under fluoroscopic guidance through the old tract. Kinked and obstructed catheters may be corrected under fluoroscopy.[25]

Pitfalls

- Failure to collaborate with urology in the diagnosis and treatment of nephrostomy tube complications.

- Failure to consider vascular fistula or vascular injury in patients with delayed or severe hematuria.

- Failure to consider intraabdominal injury in patients with abdominal pain and fever several days after nephrostomy tube insertion.

- Failure to recognize urosepsis as a cause of altered mental status or fever.

COMPLICATIONS OF URETHRAL CATHETERS

High Yield Facts

- The most common complication of urethral catheters is infection.
- Treatment of infection should include antibiotics and catheter replacement.
- Patients with hematuria that fails to clear with irrigation should have a urology consultation.

Epidemiology

Between 15% and 25% of hospitalized patients have a urethral (Foley) catheter placed.[30] Chronic indwelling Foley catheters are often placed in debilitated patients with neurogenic bladders, spinal cord injuries, or neurologic disorders such as multiple sclerosis.

Table 29-2. Complications of Urethral Catheters[36]

Infectious	Traumatic
Asymptomatic: Asymptomatic bacteriuria	Traumatic hematuria Urethral injury
Symptomatic:	Bladder rupture
Cystitis	False passage
Periurethral abscess	Balloon inflation in
Prostatic abscess	urethra or prostate
Prostatitis	Removal with inflated
Pyelonephritis	balloon
Urosepsis	

Inflammatory	Functional
Urethral necrosis	Nondeflating balloon
Urethral stricture	Knot formation
Erosion of the glans penis	Obstruction:
Polypoid cystitis	Blood clots
Squamous cell carcinoma	Encrustation
of the bladder	Prostate chips
Fistulization	Lubricating jelly
Bladder stones	

Patients with chronic indwelling Foley catheters are at substantially increased risk of complications, particularly infection, compared to patients with shorter catheter duration.[31–34] Urinary tract infection is the most common nosocomial infection in the United States with the majority of cases associated with urinary catheters.[35,36] Obstruction, encrustation, urethral or bladder trauma, and nondeflating balloons are less frequent complications of urethral catheterization (Table 29-2).[36]

Pathophysiology

Urethral catheters are hollow tubes typically made of latex with a retention balloon near the tip. Silicone catheters are available for patients with latex allergy. Urethral catheters, like other urinary devices, are subjected to bacterial biofilm formation and mineral deposition. Bacterial colonization and infection occur primarily from enteric gram negative bacteria ascending from the urethral meatus along the external surface of the Foley catheter. Infectious complications include asymptomatic bacteriuria, cystitis, prostatitis, pyelonephritis, periurethral abscess, and urosepsis. Encrustation or blood clots from trauma, recent urologic surgery, or irritation to the urethra, prostate, or bladder, can lead to catheter obstruction.[30,33,37] Balloon nondeflation is caused by an obstruction of the balloon inflation channel by debris or a faulty valve. Inappropriate balloon inflation with saline or tap water instead of sterile water can cause obstruction secondary to mineral deposits.[38–40]

Clinical Features

Patients with urethral catheter associated infection may present to the emergency department with any combination of the following: fever, suprapubic pain, flank pain, hematuria, nausea, vomiting, altered mental status, or change in urine smell or appearance. Emergency physicians should have a high index of suspicion for infection associated with a catheter and urosepsis in patients with chronic indwelling Foley catheters, particularly in patients presenting with altered mental status or fever.[32,41–43]

Patients with urethral catheter obstruction may present with leakage around the catheter, or oliguria and suprapubic pain from bladder distension. Patients with catheter trauma or irritation may present with gross hematuria and pain. Hematuria may cause obstructive symptoms due to blockage of the catheter lumen from large clots.[36]

Diagnosis and Differential

Urinalysis and culture should be obtained in any catheterized patient with fever, suprapubic pain, flank pain, hematuria, nausea, vomiting, change in mental status, or change in urine smell or appearance. Patients with fever or a urinalysis suggestive of infection should have urine culture and sensitivities obtained. Infection is more likely if there is significant pyuria (WBC >30 per HPF) but culture is recommended; positive criteria is 10^5 colony forming units/mL.[30,35]

Leakage of urine around the catheter may indicate catheter obstruction, bladder spasm, or infection. Attempts to flush the catheter may differentiate the cause of leakage. For example, the catheter should flush easily if leakage is secondary to bladder spasm or infection. Difficulty flushing the catheter indicates obstruction; however, blood clots can create a ball-valve effect allowing flush to enter the bladder but not impeding return of the irrigant.[36]

Gross hematuria requires evaluation for infection, urethral or bladder trauma, or erosion. Coagulation studies, platelet count, hemoglobin, hematocrit, and type and screen or cross should be considered in patients on anticoagulants and those with significant hemorrhage. Flushing the bladder provides information about the degree of hemorrhage and often stops the bleeding. Traumatic Foley catheter insertion or removal can result in urethral or bladder injury. Most cases are minor, but urethral disruption, creation of a false passage, and bladder perforation have been described.[36] Bladder perforation should be suspected in patients with hematuria, peritoneal signs, and diminished urine output. If there is concern for urethral disruption or bladder rupture, a retrograde cystourethrogram should be preformed.

Emergency Care and Disposition

Oral fluoroquinolones (ciprofloxacin or levofloxacin) for 7 to 14 days (consider local resistance patterns) for mild UTI.[43] Patients with pyelonephritis or urosepsis require admission and broad-spectrum IV antibiotic coverage with antipseudomonal penicillins, such as piperacillin-tazobactam, a combination of ampicillin and gentamicin, and/or flouroquinolones.[43] Admission should also be considered in patients with mild to moderate UTI and chronic indwelling catheters and significant comorbidities. Catheter replacement is also recommended because antibiotics may fail to eradicate urinary pathogens sequestered within a catheter's biofilm.[30,35]

Patients with asymptomatic bacteriuria do not require antimicrobial therapy. Exceptions include patients at high risk of serious complications such as those with transplants or neutropenia.[30] Prophylactic antibiotics are not indicated in the prevention of catheter associated infections.[30,33]

Most patients with Foley catheter trauma from insertion or removal do not require intervention. However, Foley replacement may be harmful in patients with significant urethral injury. Discussion with the urologist or a retrograde urethrogram should precede replacement of the catheter. Urethral disruption or bladder perforation requires emergent urology consultation.

Nontraumatic gross hematuria requires catheter replacement and copious bladder irrigation. Triple lumen Foley catheters are often used for bladder irrigation.[44] However, some urologists advocate the use of a large, single lumen catheter to facilitate passage of large blood clots or debris. Once the bladder irrigant has cleared, patients can usually be managed as outpatients with close urology follow up. If there is evidence of active bleeding following irrigation, urology should be consulted for possible cystoscopy.[36]

Patients with urethral catheter obstruction require catheter replacement. Obstruction secondary to blood clots requires bladder irrigation. Patients with urine leakage who do not have a catheter obstruction or infection can be treated for bladder spasms with anticholinergics such as oxybutinin.

Emergency physicians should be familiar with techniques for retrieving a catheter with a nondeflating balloon. Since nondeflation is often caused by a faulty valve, the first step is to cut the balloon inflation channel distal to the valve. If the balloon remains inflated, a lubricated guide wire can be inserted to dislodge the obstruction. If these standard techniques fail, further interventions should be performed by the urologist. Urology may deflate the balloon by overinflation or needle deflation. Emergency physicians should avoid balloon overinflation because it often causes balloon fragmentation requiring cystoscopic removal. Ultrasound guided needle deflation, with a 22-gauge spinal needle in a suprapubic approach, is preferable because it is less likely to cause balloon fragmentation.[38–40]

Pitfalls

- Failure to recognize urosepsis as a cause of altered mental status or fever in patients with chronic indwelling urethral catheters.

- Treating patients with asymptomatic bacteriuria is not indicated and may encourage antimicrobial resistance.

- Failure to consider urethral disruption and bladder rupture in patients with traumatic Foley catheter placement or removal.

MISCELLANEOUS UROLOGIC DEVICES

High Yield Facts

- Urethral catheters should be avoided in patients with artificial urinary sphincters.

- Infection of artificial urinary sphincters or implantable penile prostheses requires treatment with anti-staphylococcal antibiotics and device removal.

- Genital piercing may be associated with significant infectious and traumatic complications.

Epidemiology

Continence is achieved in approximately 73% of patients with artificial urinary sphincters, but revision is required in 32% of patients due to mechanical failure, urethral erosion, or infection.[45] Penile prosthetics have an 80% to 90% satisfaction rate, but between 5% and 20% will require revision for infection or mechanical failure.[46] Genital piercing is associated with infectious and traumatic complications.[47]

Pathophysiology

An artificial urinary sphincter consists of three parts: an inflatable cuff that fits around the urethra, a pump that inflates the cuff, and a pressure regulating balloon that acts as a reservoir. The pump is placed in the scrotum for men and in the labia for women. The system is filled with a liquid, typically contrast medium, which is pumped into the cuff to maintain continence. Squeezing the pump moves fluid from the cuff to the balloon allowing the sphincter to relax so that micturation can occur. The cuff slowly reinflates spontaneously over about 2 minutes.[48] The most common complication of this device is mechanical failure, often due to fluid leakage from the cuff. Erosion through the urethra can be caused by infection or pressure necrosis from cuff inflation.[48] It is important to note that placement of urethral catheters in patients with artificial sphincters increases the risk of urethral erosion and infection.[49]

Penile prosthetics used for erectile dysfunction are of two basic types: semi-rigid or inflatable. Inflatable prostheses are used most commonly and are similar in design to artificial urinary sphincters. They consist of two inflatable columns that are inserted into the penis, a reservoir filled with radiopaque fluid, and a pump in the scrotum. The more complicated inflatable devices are more susceptible to mechanical failure, usually from fluid leakage. Erosion of the device through the skin and penile deformities are other common complications.[46]

Infection is the most feared complication of both penile prosthesis and artificial urinary sphincters. Infection occurs in 1% to 10% of penile prosthetics and approximately 5% of artificial urinary sphincters.[45] Infection is usually from skin flora contamination at the time of surgery, but hematogenous seeding can occur.[50,51] The most common organisms are *Staphylococcus epidermitis*, *Staphylococcus aureus*, gram-negative bacteria (*Pseudomonas*), and anaerobes.[52–54] Necrotizing infections, such as Fournier gangrene, have been reported.[55]

Infections from genital piercing typically involve skin flora. They range in severity from minor local infections to necrotizing infections such as Fournier gangrene. The erythema and skin changes from infection should be differentiated from the commonly occurring contact dermatitis due to nickel allergy.

Accidental pulling on genital jewelry may cause significant genital lacerations and bleeding. Jewelry that is inserted through the glans penis can disrupt urine flow and cause a paraphimosis in uncircumcised men. Penile rings causing engorgement and vascular compromise can lead to gangrene of the penis. Clitoral jewelry may interfere with barrier contraception and sexually transmitted disease prevention by tearing condoms. [47]

Clinical Features

Patients with artificial urinary sphincters may present with recurrent incontinence, indicating mechanical failure of the device. Patients with a penile prosthesis who have a mechanical failure may complain of impotence or penile deformity. Infection of urinary sphincters or erectile prosthetic devices may cause pain, swelling, induration, erythema, purulent drainage, or fever. Persistent pain for more than 6 weeks postoperatively may be the sole indication of an indolent infection. [52]

Local infectious complications of genital piercing may present with pain, induration, erythema, and warmth. Systemic symptoms such as fever, nausea, and vomiting indicate a more severe infection. Patients with penile rings may present with a priapism. Genital trauma from piercing causes pain and bleeding. [47]

Diagnosis and Differential

Patients with artificial urinary sphincters who present with recurrent or new onset incontinence should be evaluated with plain films of the device. Since most devices are contrast filled, an open and closed cuff plain film can evaluate the function and continuity of the device. If plain films fail to identify the malfunction, urology should be consulted for possible cystoscopy or urodynamic studies. [56]

Penile prosthetic devices should also be evaluated with plain films. Unfortunately, newer prosthetics may not be filled with radiopaque fluid. In these cases, magnetic resonance imaging, CT, or US may be required to evaluate prosthetic deformity and malfunction. [57] Urine cultures and urinalysis should be obtained in patients with artificial urinary sphincters or penile prosthetic devices who present with pain or infectious symptoms.

Patients with genital piercing typically have minor local infections. In diabetics, immunocompromised, or those with systemic symptoms, more serious infections including Fournier gangrene should be considered. Patients with traumatic removal of transurethral jewelry may require a retrograde urethrogram. [47]

Emergency Care and Disposition

Mechanical failure of artificial urinary sphincters or penile prostheses often requires revision by the urologist. [49,55,56] Infection of these devices requires removal as well as antibiotic administration. Anti-staphylococcal antibiotics such as vancomycin and rifampin are indicated with gentamicin or ciprofloxacin added for gram negative coverage. [52,55] Cutaneous or urethral erosions from the artificial sphincter cuff or penile prostheses require device removal. [48,49]

Patients with minor infections or dermatitis from a genital piercing can often be managed with jewelry removal. Antibiotics to cover skin flora can be administered. Patients with evidence of more severe infections such as Fournier gangrene require immediate surgical consultation and IV antibiotics. Traumatic removal or genital tears associated with genital piercing may require surgical repair. Priapism from a penile ring requires immediate ring removal and urology consultation. [47]

Pitfalls

- Failure to collaborate with urology in the diagnosis and treatment of artificial urinary sphincter, penile prostheses, and genital piercing complications.

- Placement of a urethral catheter in a patient with an artificial urinary sphincter.

- Failure to consider necrotizing infections in patients with genital piercing, penile prosthesis, or artificial urinary sphincters.

REFERENCES

1. Joshi HB, Sianthorpe A, MacDonagh RP, et al. Indwelling ureteral stents: Evaluation of symptoms, quality of life and utility. *J Urol.* 2003;169:1065.
2. Joshi HB, Okeke A, Newns F, et al. Characterization of urinary symptoms in patients with ureteral stents. *Urology.* 2003;59:511.
3. Deliveliotis C, Chrisofos M, Evagelso G, et al. Is there a role for alpha$_1$ blockers in treating double-J stent-related symptoms. *Urology.* 2006;67:35.
4. El-Nahas AR, El-Assmy AM, Shoma AM, et al. Self-retaining ureteral stents: Analysis of factors responsible for patients' discomfort. *J Endourol.* 2006;20:33.
5. Richter S, Ringel M, Shaley M, et al. The indwelling ureteric stent: a friendly procedure with unfriendly high morbidity. *BJU Int.* 2000;85:408.
6. Damiano R, Oliva A, Esposito C, et al. Early and late complications of double pigtail ureteral stent. *Urol Int.* 2002; 69:136.

7. El-Faqih SR, Shamsuddin AB, Chakrabarti A, et al. Polyurethane internal stents in treatment of stone patients: Morbidity related to indwelling times. *J Urol.* 1991; 146:1487.

8. Dyer RB, Chen MY, Zagoria RJ, et al. Complications of ureteral stent placement. *Radiographics.* 2002;22:1005.

9. Bultitude, MF, Tiptaft RC, Glass JM, et al. Management of encrusted ureteral stents impacted in upper tract. *Urology.* 2003;62:622.

10. Singh I, Gupta NP, Hemal AK, et al. Severely encrusted polyurethane ureteral stents: management and analysis of potential risk factors. *Urology.*2001;58:526.

11. Kehinde EO, Rotimi VO, Al-Awadi KA, et al. Factors predisposing to urinary tract infection after J uretetal stent insertion. *J Urol.* 2002;167:1334.

12. Paick SH, Park HK, Oh SJ, et al. Characteristics of bacterial colonization and urinary tract infection after indwelling of double-J ureteral stent. *Urology.* 2003;62:214.

13. Paz A, Amiel GE, Pick N, et al. Febrile complications following insertion of 100 double-J ureteral stents. *J Endourol.* 2005;19:147.

14. Auge BK, Preminger GM. Ureteral stents and their use in endourology. *Curr Op Urol.* 2002;12:217.

15. Riedl CR, Plas E, Hubner WA, et al. Bacterial colonization of ureteral stents. *Eur Urol.* 1999;36:53.

16. Reid G, Habash M, Vachon D, et al. Oral flurroquinolone therapy results in drug absorption on ureteral stents and prevention of biofilm formation. *Int J Antimicrob Agents.* 2001;17:317.

17. Ramchandani P, Cardella JF, Grassi CJ, et al. Quality improvement guidelines for percutaneous nephrostomy. *J Vasc Interv Radiol.* 2003;14:S227.

18. Lee WJ, Smith AD, Cubelli V, et al. Complications of percutaneous nephrolithotomy. *AJR Am J Roentgenol.* 1987; 148:177.

19. Ekici S, Sahin A, Ozen H. Percutaneous nephrostomy in the management of malignant ureteral obstruction secondary to bladder cancer. *J Endourol.* 2001;15:827.

20. Lee WJ, Patel U, Patel S, et al. Emergency percutaneous nephrostomy: results and complications. *J Vasc Interv Radiol.* 1994;5:135.

21. Mahaffey KG, Bolton DM, Stoller ML. Urologist directed percutaneous nephrostomy tube placement *J Urol.* 1994; 152:1982.

22. Farrell TA, Wallace M, Hicks ME. Long-term result of transrenal ureteral occlusion with use of Gianturco coils and gelatin sponge pledgets. *J Vasc Interv Radiol.* 1997; 8:449.

23. Lewis S, Patel U. Major complications after percutaneous nephrostomy-lessons from a department audit. *Clin Radiol.* 2004;59:171.

24. Dyer RB, Regan JD, Kavanagh PV, et al. Percutaneous nephrostomy with extensions of the technique: Step by step. *Radiographics.* 2002;22:503.

25. Millward SF. Percutaneous nephrostomy: A practical approach. *J Interv Radiol.* 2000;11:955.

26. Munver R, Delvecchio FC, Newman GE, et al. Critical analysis of supracostal access for percutaneous renal surgery. *J Urol.* 2001;166:1242.

27. Kekre NS, Gopalakrishnan GG, Gupta GG, et al. Supracostal approach in percutaneous nephrolithotomy: Experience with 102 cases. *J Endourol.* 2001;15:789.

28. Martin X, Murat FJ, Feitosa LC, et al. Severe bleeding after nephrolithotomy: results of hyperselective embolization. *Eur Urol.* 2000;37:136.

29. Martinez-Valls GPL, Villaplana HG, Lopez MB, et al. Lower massive hematuria deferred by arteriovenous fistula following percutaneous nephrostomy. *Arch Esp Urol.* 2003; 56:1158.

30. Warren JW. Catheter-associated urinary tract infections. *Int J Antimicrob Agents.* 2001;17:299–303.

31. Platt R, Polk BF, Murdock B, et al. Risk factors for nosocomial urinary tract infection. *Am J Epidemiol.* 1986; 124:977.

32. Larsen LD, Chamberlin DA, Khonsari F, et al. Retrospective analysis of urologic complications in male patients with spinal cord injury managed with and without indwelling urinary catheters. *Urology.* 1997;50:418.

33. Thomsen TW, Setnik GS. Male urethral catheterization. *N Engl J Med.* 2006;354:e22.

34. Warren JW, Platt R, Thomas RJ, et al. Antibiotic irrigation and catheter-associated urinary-tract infections *N Engl J Med.* 1978;299:570.

35. Wagenlehner FME, Naber KG. Hospital-acquired urinary tract infections. *J Hosp Infect.* 2000;46:171.

36. Cancio LC. Managing the Foley catheter. *Am Fam Physician.* 1993;48:829.

37. Stine RJ, Avila JA, Lemons MF, et al. Diagnostic and therapeutic urologic procedures. *Emerg Med Clin North Am.* 1988;6:547.

38. Hessl JM. Removal of the Foley catheter when balloon does not deflate. *Urology.* 1983;22:219.

39. Kleeman, FJ. Technique for removal of Foley catheter when balloon does not deflate. *Urology.* 1983;22:416.

40. Siamak D, Youssefzadeh D, Skinner EC. Review of techniques to remove a Foley catheter when the balloon does not deflate. *Urology.* 2002;59:127.

41. Warren JW. Catheter associated bacterriuria in long-term care facilities. *Infect Control Hosp Epidemiol.* 1994; 15:557.

42. Warren JW, Muncie HL, Hebel E, et al. Long-term urethral catheterization increases risk of pyelonephritis and renal inflammation. *J Am Geriatr Soc.* 1994;42:1286.

43. Gilbert DN, Moellering RC, Eliopoulos GM, et al. *The Sanford Guide To Antimicrobial Therapy.* 36th ed. Antimicrobial Therapy Inc, Sperryville, VA 2006.

44. Braasch M, Antolak C, Henlin K, et al. Irrigation and drainage properties of three-way urethral catheters. *Urology.* 2006; 67:40.

45. Hajivassiliou CA. A review of the complications and results of implantation of the AMS artificial urinary sphincter. *Eur Urol.* 1999;35:36.

46. Minervini A, Ralph DJ, Pryor JP. Outcome of penile prosthesis implantation for treating erectile dysfunction: experience with 504 procedures. *BJU Int* 2005;97:129.

47. Meltzer DI. Complications of body piercing. *Am Fam Physician.* 2005;72:2029.

48. Hussain M, Greenwell TJ, Venn SN, et al. The current role of the artificial urinary sphincter for the treatment of urinary incontinence. *J Urol.* 2005;174:418.

49. Ratan HL, Summerton DJ, Wilson SK, et al. Development and current status of the AMS 800 artifical urinary sphincter. *Eur Assoc Urol Update Series.* 2006;4:117.

50. Carson CC. Efficacy of antibiotic impregnation of inflatable penile prosthesis in decreasing infection in original implants. *J Urol.* 2004;171:1611.

51. Carson CC, Robertson CN. Late hematogenous infection in penile prosthesis. *J Urol.* 1988;139:50.

52. Carson CC. Management of prosthesis infections in urologic surgery. *Urol Clin North Am.* 1999;26:829.

53. Nickel JC, Heaton J, Morales A, et al. Bacterial biofilm in persistent penile prosthesis-associated infection. *J Urol.* 1986;135:586.

54. Licht MR, Montague DK, Angermeier KW, et al. Cultures from genitourinary prostheses at reoperation: questioning the role of *Staphylococcus epidermidis* in periprosthetic infection. *J Urol.* 1995;154:387.

55. Walther PJ, Adriani RT, Maggio MI, et al. Fournier's gangrene: A complication of penile prosthetic implantation in a renal transplant patient. *J Urol.* 1987;137:299.

56. Montague DK, Angermeier KW. Artificial urinary sphincter troubleshooting. *Urology.* 2001;58:779.

57. Moncada I, Jara J, Cabello JI, et al. Radiological assessment of penile prosthesis: The role of magnetic resonance imaging. *World J Urol.* 2004;22:371.

30

Pelvic Pain in the Nonpregnant Patient

Howard K. Mell

HIGH YIELD FACTS

- Ectopic pregnancy must be considered in any patient who presents with complaints of lower abdominal or pelvic pain or abnormal uterine bleeding.
- A thorough history and careful, complete physical exam is needed to distinguish gynecologic pain from pain arising from orthopedic, gastrointestinal, urologic, neurologic, or psychosomatic origin.
- The most common gynecologic causes of acute pelvic pain include ruptured ectopic pregnancy, salpingitis/pelvic inflammatory disease (PID), hemorrhagic ovarian cyst, torsion of adnexa, degenerating leiomyoma, or endometriosis/adenomyosis.
- Nongynecologic causes of pelvic pain include appendicitis (most common), colitis, ileitis, gastroenteritis, diverticulitis, gastric or duodenal ulcers, pancreatitis, cholecystitis, urinary tract infection, inflammatory bowel disease, or irritable bowel syndrome.
- The potentially life-threatening etiologies of pelvic pain include appendicitis, ruptured ectopic pregnancy, salpingitis/PID, tuboovarian abscess, adnexal torsion, or ruptured ovarian cyst.

EPIDEMIOLOGY

Pelvic pain is a common complaint. One study estimated the prevalence of pelvic pain in female patients of two obstetric and gynecologic clinics and three family medicine practice clinics at 39%.[1] Pelvic pain was most common among women aged 26 to 30. African American race was also identified as a risk factor. Otherwise parity, marital status, income, or education was not identified as a risk factor.[1] Another study found the reported prevalence of chronic pelvic pain (defined as "recurrent or constant pelvic pain of ≥6 months' duration unrelated to periods, intercourse, or pregnancy") to be 21% among a random sample of women aged 18 through 49 years selected from the Oxfordshire (UK) Health Authority Register.[2]

Ultrasound (US) is playing an increasing role in the diagnosis of pelvic pain[3–5] but laparoscopy remains the gold standard. However, studies[6,7] suggest that a majority of patients suffering from pelvic pain are not helped by diagnostic and operative laparoscopy. Given the complexity of definitive diagnosis, the emergency physician should be mindful that many causes of pelvic pain do not require emergent treatment or diagnosis. Therefore, clinical efforts should be focused on excluding sources of pelvic pain with the potential for significant sequelae. These include appendicitis, ruptured ectopic pregnancy, salpingitis/PID, tuboovarian abscess, adnexal torsion, or ruptured ovarian cyst.

Most patients with pelvic pain who present in shock will require surgical intervention. Resuscitation should focus on fluid replacement and hemodynamic stability. Computerized tomography (CT) can be used to guide diagnosis prior to surgery if the patient's condition allows. Otherwise, bedside US in the emergency department (ED) may prove useful in guiding surgical efforts.[8]

PATHOPHYSIOLOGY

The pathology of acute pelvic pain varies by etiology. There are five general sources of acute pelvic pain: gynecologic, obstetric, gastrointestinal, orthopedic, and psychosomatic. The pelvis contains the vagina, uterus, fallopian tubes, and ovaries. Therefore, gynecologic or obstetric pathologies often present with pelvic pain. The pelvis also contains the urinary bladder, ureters, sigmoid colon, and rectum. The pelvic organs share visceral pain afferent nerves with the appendix, ureters, and colon. This can make localization of visceral pain (resulting from inflammation, stretching, or distension of an organ) very difficult. Appendicitis and other gastrointestinal problems can present as "pelvic pain." Pelvic pain can also be parietal in nature. This occurs in case of inflammation to the parietal peritoneum adjacent to an organ, such as in peritonitis.

Orthopedic pelvic pain is most often the result of direct trauma causing disruption of the bony pelvic ring; however, insufficiency fractures at the sacroiliac joint can also result in pelvic pain.[9]

Psychosomatic pelvic pain is a challenge to the clinician. Studies suggest that women who have been physically and/or sexually abused, either as children or adults, suffer an increased incidence of psychosomatic pelvic

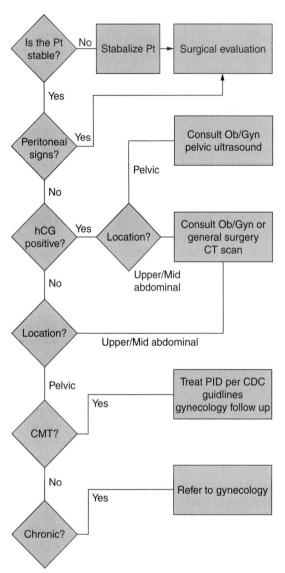

Fig. 30-1. Algorithm for evaluation of pelvic pain. (Courtesy of Dr. Mark Amols.)

pain.[10,11] However, their incidence of structural pathophysiology is unchanged. Separating the physical causes of pelvic pain from the psychosomatic ones requires a consistent diagnostic approach.

The pathology of chronic pelvic pain is more poorly understood. It has been suggested that chronic pelvic pain be considered as a chronic visceral pain syndrome.[12] Several possible etiologies for chronic pelvic pain have been suggested. These include 1. subclinical or undiagnosed

irritable bowel syndrome, 2. alteration of nervous system processing, and 3. dilatation of pelvic veins resulting in reduced blood flow to pelvic organs ("pelvic congestion syndrome"). Given that the pathophysiology of chronic pelvic pain is not well understood, its treatment is often limited to symptom relief and is often ineffective. The main approaches to management include counseling or psychotherapy, attempting to provide reassurance using laparoscopy to exclude serious pathology, hormone therapy, and surgery to interrupt nerve pathways. None has been demonstrated to be clearly superior to the others.[13]

CLINICAL FEATURES

The specific cause of pelvic pain may not always be determined in the ED. Instead, specific focus should be placed on the exclusion or diagnosis of those causes associated with significant morbidity or mortality. A systematic approach to the patient with pelvic pain should be taken (see Figure 30-1).

1. Is the patient hemodynamically stable?
   - If not, immediate fluid resuscitation should be started and a stat OB/GYN consult obtained. If shock persists despite fluid resuscitation, emergent laparoscopy is indicated.
   - If the patient can be stabilized, consider computed tomography (CT) imaging or pelvic US to guide further treatment.

2. Is the patient pregnant?
   - This should be confirmed by urine or serum beta hCG testing in all patients of child bearing age regardless of lack of menarche or onset of menopause as these conditions can mask a pregnancy.

3. What is the pain like, specifically what is the location, duration, and characterization?
   - Provoking and palliative factors can often provide valuable clues.

4. Are there any associated symptoms?
   - Specific inquires as to the presence of fever, nausea and vomiting, urinary symptoms, gastrointestinal symptoms, vaginal bleeding or discharge, and/or syncope should be made.
   - If vaginal bleeding is present, the quantity and duration should be assessed.

5. A complete past medical history should be taken.
   - A sexual history is absolutely essential with emphasis on screening for intimate partner violence,

recent sexual contact, and previous history of sexually transmitted disease.
- Any history of recent significant trauma should be ascertained.

DIAGNOSIS AND DIFFERENTIAL

If the diagnosis of pelvic pain is to be made in the ED, it will be on the basis of history, physical exam, and ancillary studies.

Determining the nature and duration of the pain is a key component of history taking in pelvic pain. Mild, ill-defined (visceral) pain is associated with mild or early PID, ovarian cysts, menstrual disorders (e.g., endometriosis or uterine fibroids) or menstrual cramping, unruptured ectopic pregnancy, appendicitis, gastroenteritis, or cystitis. More severe visceral pain (accompanied by vomiting, diaphoresis, restlessness, fever, and/or hypotension) is associated with ovarian torsion, ectopic pregnancy, PID, incarcerated hernia, ischemic bowel, bowel obstruction, or renal colic.

The sudden onset of pain suggests a more acute process such as the rupture of a hollow viscous (e.g., ruptured ectopic pregnancy), acute intraperitoneal hemorrhage (e.g., ruptured hemorrhagic ovarian cyst), or sudden, peritoneal contamination (e.g., rupture of a tuboovarian abscess). Retroperitoneal injuries or insults, such as acute pancreatitis, leaking abdominal aortic aneurysm, and renal trauma, can allow blood or other fluids to collect in the retroperitoneum from the diaphragm to the pelvic floor.[14] Such patients might present with the sudden onset of peritoneal pelvic pain.

Provoking factors can also provide clues. Dyspareunia is associated with PID, endometriosis, and psychosomatic pelvic pain[15]; it can also be associated with interstitial cystitis.[16] Sitting upright or standing may exacerbate orthopedic pelvic pain. Painful defecation is associated with endometriosis.[17]

The physical exam may reveal hypotension (associated with perforated/ruptured viscous, sepsis, or secondary to heavy menstrual bleeding); fever (associated with infection from PID, UTI, appendicitis, or ovarian torsion); peritonitis (associated with ovarian torsion, appendicitis, PID, or intraabdominal/retroperitoneal hemorrhage); cervical motion tenderness (associated with PID, ovarian cyst, ovarian torsion, or endometriosis); purulent discharge from the cervical os (associated with PID); or adnexal mass (associated with ovarian pathology, such as cyst, torsion, tumor, or abscess). Findings associated with pelvic pain are described in Table 30-1.

Table 30-1. Findings in Acute Pelvic Pain

Finding	Associated Diagnosis
Positive urine pregnancy test	Ectopic pregnancy
Unilateral pain	Ovarian cyst
	Acute appendicitis
	Pelvic inflammatory disease
Tense, tender adnexal mass	Ovarian torsion
Cyst fluid in cul-de-sac	Ruptured ovarian cyst
Right-sided pain, GI symptoms, and low-grade fever	Acute appendicitis
Positive cervical gram stain	Pelvic inflammatory disease
Chronic pelvic pain	Endometriosis
	Uterine leiomyoma
	Pelvic Neoplasia
Positive urine gram stain	Infectious cystitis
Hematuria	Urolithiasis

Abbreviation: GI, gastrointestinal.

Table 30-2. Differential Diagnosis of Acute Pelvic Pain

Gynecologic	Nongynecologic
Ectopic pregnancy	Appendicitis
Pelvic inflammatory disease	Urinary tract infection
	Pyelonephritis
Ovarian cyst	Interstitial cystitis
Menstrual cramps	Gastroenteritis
Uterine fibroids	Diverticulitis
Endometriosis	Hemorrhoids
Ovarian torsion	Incarcerated hernia
Hydrosalpinx rupture	Ischemic bowel
Pyosalpinx rupture	Bowel obstruction
Mittelschmerz	Renal colic
	Ruptured spleen
	Ruptured abdominal aneurysm
	Perforated viscous
	Inflammatory bowel disease
	Psychosomatic

EMERGENCY DEPARTMENT CARE AND DISPOSITION

Patients with pelvic pain who present in clinical shock require immediate fluid resuscitation and surgical consult. Laparoscopy is indicated. If the patient can be stabilized, CT may prove useful to differentiate the etiology in atypical presentations.[8] The stable patient of childbearing age requires urine beta-HCG testing and urinalysis. If the urine pregnancy test is positive, obtain a pelvic US and consult OB. If the urinalysis is suggestive of a UTI, provide antibiotic therapy and analgesia. If the urinalysis is suggestive of urolithiasis, obtain a noncontrast CT. Nonpyogenic stones may be treated with fluids and analgesia, whereas pyogenic urolithiasis requires a urology consult. If the urine tests are negative, assess for peritonitis. If present, consider an US or CT (unless the presentation is classic for specific pathology) and obtain a general surgical (or gynecology, if indicated) consult. If no peritonitis is present, proceed with the physical examination. If a significantly tender adnexal mass is appreciated, obtain an US and consult gynecologist. If localized right lower quadrant tenderness is appreciated, obtain a CT and consult general surgery if indicated.[8] If no tender adnexal mass is present, and no right lower quadrant pain is appreciated, assess for cervical motion tenderness (CMT). If CMT is present and there is fever, purulent discharge from the cervical os, or an elevated white blood cell count, a presumptive diagnosis of PID should be made. The patient should be provided with appropriate antibiotic therapy and a gynecology follow up. If the infection is clinically severe or the patient has an inability to take and absorb oral antibiotics because of nausea, vomiting, or other causes, then hospitalization is indicated. If no CMT is present, or if CMT is present without fever, purulent discharge from the cervical os, or elevated white blood cell, then the patient should follow up with gynecology for an outpatient workup.

PITFALLS

- Ectopic pregnancy must be considered in all female patients of childbearing age who present complaining of lower abdominal or pelvic pain.

- Patients complaining of pelvic pain who have been previously diagnosed with psychosomatic pelvic pain still require a full pelvic pain work up with emphasis on excluding etiologies associated with high morbidity or mortality.

- Clinical shock in the setting of pelvic pain is an indication for laparoscopy.

- The definitive diagnosis of pelvic pain etiology might not be made in the ED, instead efforts should be made to exclude pathology associated with significant morbidity and mortality.

REFERENCES

1. Jamieson DJ, Steege JF. The prevalence of dysmenorrhea, dyspareunia, pelvic pain, and irritable bowel syndrome in primary care practices. *Obstet Gynecol.* 1996;87:55.
2. Zondervan KT, Yudkin PL, Vessey MP, et al. Chronic pelvic pain in the community—symptoms, investigations, and diagnoses. *Am J Obstet Gynecol.* 2001;184:1149.
3. Lambert MJ, Villa M. Gynecologic ultrasound in emergency medicine. *Emerg Med Clin North Am.* 2004;22:683.
4. Nezhat C, Santolaya J, Nezhat FR. Comparison of transvaginal sonography and bimanual pelvic examination in patients with laparoscopically confirmed endometriosis. *J Am Assoc Gynecol Laparosc.* 1994;1:127.
5. Harris RD, Holtzman SR, Poppe AM. Clinical outcome in female patients with pelvic pain and normal pelvic US findings. *Radiology.* 2000;216:440.
6. Kontoravdis A, Chryssikopoulos A, Hassiakos D, et al. The diagnostic value of laparoscopy in 2365 patients with acute and chronic pelvic pain. *Int J Gynaecol Obstet.* 1996; 52:243–8.
7. Howard FM. The role of laparoscopy in chronic pelvic pain: promise and pitfalls. *Obstet Gynecol Surv.* 1993; 48:357.
8. Terasawa T, Blackmore CC, Bent S, Kohlwes RJ. Systematic review: Computed tomography and ultrasonography to detect acute appendicitis in adults and adolescents. *Ann Intern Med.* 2004;141:537.
9. Soubrier M, Dubost JJ, Boisgard S, et al. Insufficiency fracture. A survey of 60 cases and review of the literature. *Joint Bone Spine.* 2003;70:209.
10. Hilden M, Schei B, Swahnberg K, et al. A history of sexual abuse and health: a Nordic multicentre study. *BJOG.* 2004; 111:1121.
11. Bodden-Heidrich R, Kuppers V, Beckmann MW, et al. Psychosomatic aspects of vulvodynia. Comparison with the chronic pelvic pain syndrome. *J Reprod Med.* 1999; 44:411.
12. Wesselmann U, Czakanski PP. Pelvic pain: A chronic visceral pain syndrome. *Curr Pain Headache Rep.* 2001; 5:13.
13. Stones RW, Mountfield J. Interventions for treating chronic pelvic pain in women. *Cochrane Database Syst Rev.* 2000;(4): CD000387.
14. Scialpi M, Scaglione M, Angelelli G, et al. Emergencies in the retroperitoneum: assessment of spread of disease by helical CT. *Eur J Radiol.* 2004;50:74.

15. Ferrero S, Esposito F, Abbamonte LH, et al. Quality of sex life in women with endometriosis and deep dyspareunia. *Fertil Steril.* 2005;83:573.

16. Parsons CL, Tatsis V. Prevalence of interstitial cystitis in young women. *Urology.* 2004;64:866.

17. Thomassin I, Bazot M, Detchev R, et al. Darai E. Symptoms before and after surgical removal of colorectal endometriosis that are assessed by magnetic resonance imaging and rectal endoscopic sonography. *Am J Obstet Gynecol.* 2004; 190:1264.

31

Pelvic Inflammatory Disease

Scott M. Silvers

HIGH YIELD FACTS

- Risk factors for the development of PID include young age, multiple sexual partners, prior history of PID, sexually transmitted infection, and failure to use a barrier form of contraceptive.
- Pelvic inflammatory disease may present with minimal symptoms and signs.
- No single symptom or sign reliably rules in or rules out the diagnosis of PID.
- An elevated serum white blood cell count (WBC) is neither sensitive nor specific for the diagnosis of PID.
- Women with a history of PID have a tenfold greater incidence of both infertility and ectopic pregnancy compared to those who have never had the disease, and this incidence nearly doubles following recurrent disease.
- Patients should be reminded that, in the setting of a sexually transmitted disease, their sexual partners should be informed and medical evaluation recommended.

EPIDEMIOLOGY

It is estimated that in the United States approximately 800,000 women are diagnosed with acute pelvic inflammatory disease (PID) annually.[1] However, this incidence may be an underestimate given that PID is not a reportable disease, and many cases maybe subclinical or even asymptomatic.[2]

Approximately two thirds of proven cases of PID are caused by *Neisseria gonorrhea* and *Chlamydia trachomatis* followed by other bacteria typically associated with bacterial vaginosis (Table 31-1).[3] Accepted risk factors for the development of PID include young age, multiple sexual partners, prior history of PID, sexually

transmitted infection (gonorrhea, *Chlamydia*), and failure to use a barrier form of contraceptive. Other, more controversial risk factors include low socioeconomic status, use of an intrauterine device (IUD), and douching.[4] Nonuse of contraception imparts a higher risk for the development of PID, while conversely, the use of barrier contraceptive methods reduces the risk of acquiring sexually transmitted diseases and subsequent development of PID.[5-9] While use of oral contraceptives have also been linked to a lower risk for developing PID, the exact mechanism in unclear. Oral contraceptive use may be associated with "less risky" sexual behavior, or it may exert its effects by altering the receptivity of the uterus to pathogens by thickening the cervical mucous and lessening the amount and duration of menstrual flow.[4]

PATHOPHYSIOLOGY

Pelvic inflammatory disease specifically refers to a polymicrobial, inflammatory condition resulting from the atraumatic migration of microorganisms (e.g., bacteria) from the vagina or cervix into the upper structures of the female reproductive tract (i.e., uterus, fallopian tubes) and potentially into the peritoneal cavity.[4] Pelvic inflammatory disease includes such conditions as endometritis, salpingitis, tuboovarian abscess, and pelvic peritonitis.[10]

CLINICAL FEATURES

Diagnosing PID can be challenging due to the variability in presentation of the disease (which may include asymptomatic disease), other diseases that may mimic PID such as ovarian cysts and endometriosis, and the imperfect performance of diagnostic testing. Corroborating this difficulty in diagnosis, the CDC in 2002 reported the positive predictive value of a clinical diagnosis of PID to range from 65% to 90% compared to laparoscopy.[10] This means that approximately one quarter of patients clinically diagnosed with PID are diagnosed incorrectly.

No single symptom or sign reliably rules in or rules out the diagnosis of PID. Classically, patients with PID may complain of dull abdominal pain, fevers, vaginal discharge, onset of symptoms after menstruation, and abnormal vaginal bleeding.[4] The magnitude and character of the symptoms vary greatly. Symptoms of PID may be confused with other diagnoses such as appendicitis. Right lower quadrant pain of shorter duration (approximately 21 hours) appears to be more specific to the diagnosis of appendicitis while patients with PID more commonly present with more diffuse pain of at least 48 hours in duration.[11] One study revealed that abdominal

Table 31-1. Common Etiologic Agents of Pelvic Inflammatory Disease

Common Etiologic Agents of PID	
Aerobic bacteria	*Neisseria gonorrhoeae*
	Chlamydia trachomatis
	Gardnerella vaginalis
	Escherichia coli
	Streptococcus spp.
	Haemophilus influenzae
Anaerobic bacteria	*Bacteroides* spp.
	Peptostreptococcus spp.
	Peptococcus spp.
	Prevotella spp.
	Porphyromonas spp.
Mycoplasmas	*Mycoplasma hominis*
	Mycoplasma genitalium

Used with permission from Cohen J, and Powderly WG, (eds). *Infectious Diseases.* 2nd ed. New York: Mosby; 2004;694.

pain is absent in 5% of women with PID.[12] Some data also support the presence of subclinical or asymptomatic disease. In 1995, the World Health Organization reported that among women found to have tubal occlusion and serologic evidence of prior exposure to gonococcus or chlamydia, nearly two thirds denied having symptoms consistent with PID.[13]

Findings on physical examination typically include cervical motion tenderness, adnexal tenderness, and vaginal discharge. However, these findings individually are similar to historical data in that alone they do not reliably predict the presence or absence of PID. When compared to the pelvic examination findings of patients with appendicitis, adnexal tenderness is more commonly bilateral in PID and right-sided in appendicitis.[11] Although an elevated temperature greater than 38°C (100.4°F) is only present in approximately one-third of patients with PID, the presence of this finding among patients suspected of having PID makes the diagnosis significantly more likely (Table 31-2).[14]

Laboratory blood analysis is of limited value in diagnosing PID. An elevated serum WBC is neither sensitive nor specific for the diagnosis of PID. In fact, only about one half of patients with PID have an elevated WBC.[15] An erythrocyte sedimentation rate (ESR) and C-reactive protein (CRP) both have moderate sensitivity for the diagnosis of PID and are positive in approximately 80% to 85% of patients.[13] However, if this test were relied upon alone as a screen, it would miss 15% to 20% of patients with the disease.

The presence of polymorphonuclear leukocytes (PMNs) on microscopy of a vaginal wet smear, although imperfect, is one of the best screening tests for PID. The presence of 3 or more PMNs per high power field (HPF) has a sensitivity of approximately 90%.[16] Therefore, among patients with a low or intermediate pretest probability for PID, fewer than 3 PMNs per HPF on vaginal wet smear makes the diagnosis of PID very unlikely.

There are serious, life-altering complications associated with PID. Acutely, patients may develop a tuboovarian abscess from progression of the infection in the pelvis, or perihepatitis (Fitz-Hugh-Curtis syndrome) from spilling of the infection into the peritoneum and up to the liver.[4] Long-term complications include infertility, ectopic pregnancy, and chronic pelvic pain. Women with

Table 31-2. Sensitivity and Specificity for the Diagnosis of Pelvic Inflammatory Disease of Selected Objective Findings

Finding	Sensitivity (% range)	Specificity (% range)
Physical examination		
Vaginal discharge	26–81	42–83
Temperature (>38°C)	24–40	79–91
Palpable mass present	24–49	74–79
Laboratory		
Elevated C-reactive protein	74–92	50–90
Elevated erythrocyte sedimentation rate (ESR >15)	75–81	25–57

Data from Kahn JG, Walker CK, Washington, AE, et al. Diagnosing pelvic inflammatory disease: a comprehensive analysis and considerations for developing a new model. *JAMA.* 1991;266:2594.

a history of PID have a ten-fold greater incidence of both infertility and ectopic pregnancy compared to those who have never had the disease, and this incidence nearly doubles following recurrent disease.[9,17] Chronic pelvic pain develops in approximately 20% of women following an episode of PID.[18]

DIAGNOSIS

The 2002 Centers for Disease Control and Prevention (CDC) Guidelines for diagnosing PID state that PID should be presumed present and treatment initiated among "sexually active young women and other women at risk for STDs if the following minimum criteria are present and no other cause for the illness can be identified: uterine/adnexal tenderness, or cervical motion tenderness."[10] The presence of additional criteria such as fever, mucopurulent cervicitis, elevated ESR or CRP, and proven cervical infection with *Chlamydia trachomatis* or *Neisseria gonorrhea* make the diagnosis of PID more likely.[10]

Imaging investigations have evaluated the role of transvaginal ultrasound in the diagnosis of PID. Ultrasound findings may include large, dilated fallopian tubes, fluid collections in the pelvis, and the presence of a tuboovarian abscess. Transvaginal ultrasound is a poor study for screening for PID as it has a sensitivity of only 32% for this disease.[19] However, its high specificity of 97% makes it useful for ruling in disease when positive findings are present.[19]

Endometrial biopsy has a moderate sensitivity and specificity of approximately 80%.[20] However, endometrial biopsies are typically performed by specialists in the field, and the turn around time prior to reporting is usually 2 or more days making this test less desirable in the acute setting.

Laparoscopy has generally been considered the "gold standard" for diagnosing PID. Laparoscopic findings of PID may include edema, erythema, and purulence of the fallopian tubes as well as peritubal adhesions.[21] However, several more recent biopsy-based studies have called into question the accuracy of laparoscopy stating that visualization alone by laparoscopy may miss 17% to 50% of cases of PID.[22–24] Although diagnostic laparoscopy has a higher associated cost and risk of surgery, it is typically warranted in cases of possible PID when the patient is ill appearing and the diagnosis is uncertain. Diagnostic laparoscopy also has the added advantage of providing the ability to culture and drain inflammatory masses should they be present.

DIFFERENTIAL DIAGNOSIS

The differential diagnosis of PID includes urinary tract infection, bacterial vaginosis, endometriosis, fibroids, ectopic pregnancy, hemorrhagic corpus luteal cyst, ovarian torsion, ovarian tumors, appendicitis, and diverticulitis.

EMERGENCY DEPARTMENT CARE AND DISPOSITION

Treatment for PID should be guided by local bacterial prevalences and susceptibilities. Initial therapy typically includes polymicrobial coverage until a definitive organism and susceptibilities are identified (Table 31-3, note: fluoroquinolones no longer recommended). Clinical cure rates with antibiotic therapy are approximately 95%.[4]

Patients with tuboovarian abscess often require surgical intervention depending on the size of the mass. Approximately, 70% of women with a tuboovarian abscess greater than 10 cm in diameter require surgical drainage.[25]

The CDC recommends hospital admission and parenteral antibiotics for patients with PID in the setting of the following conditions:[10]

1. Pregnancy.
2. Inability to exclude a surgical emergency (e.g., appendicitis).
3. Failure to respond to oral therapy.
4. Inability to tolerate oral therapy.
5. Severe Illness (e.g., high fever, peritonitis).
6. Presence of tuboovarian abscess.

Patients may also be considered for inpatient therapy if there is a significant concern for poor compliance with therapy as an outpatient. Patients should also be reminded that, in the setting of a sexually transmitted disease, their sexual partners should be informed and offered treatment as well if necessary.

PITFALLS

- Not considering PID in the differential diagnosis of undifferentiated lower abdominal pain in a female patient.
- Failure to recognize that PID may present with minimal symptoms and signs.
- Overreliance on any one symptom, sign, or test for ruling in or ruling out the diagnosis of PID.

Table 31-3. 2007 Centers for Disease Control and Prevention Recommended Treatment Regimens for Pelvic Inflammatory Disease

Parenteral

Recommended

A. Cefotetan 2 g IV q12h OR Cefoxitin 2 g IV q6h + Doxycycline 100 mg po/IV q12h[a]

B. Clindamycin 900 mg IV q8h + Gentamicin IV/IM (2 mg/kg load, then 1.5 mg/kg q8h)[*a]

Alternative

C. Ampicillin/Sulbactam 3 g IV q6h + Doxycycline 100 mg po/IV q12h[a]

Oral

A. Ceftriaxone 250 mg IM × 1 dose OR Cefoxitin 2 g IM × 1 dose and Probenicid 1 g po × 1 dose OR other third generation cephalosporin IM + Doxycycline 100 mg po bid × 14 days with or without Metronidazole 500 mg po bid × 14 days

[a]After clinical improvement, therapy is continued with oral doxycycline 100 mg bid (regimen A & C) or either oral doxycycline or oral clindamycin 450 mg qid (regimen B) to complete a 14-day treatment course.

[*]Single daily dosing can be substituted.

Adapted from CDC's Sexually Transmitted Diseases Treatment Guidelines, 2006; Fuoroquinolones. No Longer Recommended for Treatment of Ganococcal Infections. *MMWR Mortal Wkly Rep.* 2007;56:332.

- Failure to inform the patient about the importance of informing and treating all sexual partners as necessary.

REFERENCES

1. Rein DB, Kassler WJ, Irwin KL, et al. Direct medical cost of pelvic inflammatory disease and its sequelae: Decreasing but still substantial. *Obstet Gynecol.* 2000;95:397.

2. Wiesenfeld HC, Hillier SL, Krohn MA, et al. Lower genital tract infection and endometritis: insight into subclinical pelvic inflammatory disease. *Obstet Gynecol.* 2002;100:456.

3. Cohen J. and Powderly WG, (Eds). *Infectious Diseases.* 2nd ed. New York: Mosby;2004:694.

4. Beigi RH, Wiesenfeld HC. Pelvic inflammatory disease: new diagnostic criteria and treatment. *Obstet Gynecol Clin N Am.* 2003;30:777.

5. Kelaghan J, Rubin GL, Ory HW, et al. Barrier-method contraceptives and pelvic inflammatory disease. *JAMA.* 1982; 248:184.

6. Cramer DW, Goldman MB, Schiff I, et al. The relationship of tubal infertility to barrier method and oral contraceptive use. *JAMA.* 1987;257:2446.

7. Darrow WW. Condom use and use-effectiveness in high-risk populations. *Sex Transm Dis.* 1989;16:157.

8. Wolner-Hanssen P, Eschenbach DA, Paavonen J, et al. Decreased risk of symptomatic chlamydial pelvic inflammatory disease associated with oral contraceptive use. *JAMA.* 1990;263:54.

9. Westrom L. Incidence, prevalence, and trends of acute pelvic inflammatory disease and its consequences in industrialized countries. *Am J Obstet Gynecol.* 1980;138:880–892.

10. CDC's Sexually Transmitted Diseases Treatment Guidelines, 2006; Fuoroquinolones. No Longer Recommended for Treatment of Ganococcal Infections. *MMWR Mortal Wkly Rep.* 2007;56:332.

11. Bongard F, Landers DV, Lewis F. Differential diagnosis of appendicitis and pelvic inflammatory disease. *Am J Surg.* 1985;150:90.

12. Bowie WR, Jones H. Acute pelvic inflammatory disease in outpatients: Association with *Chlamydia trachomatis* and *Neisseria gonorrhoeae. Ann Intern Med.* 1981;95:685.

13. World Health Organization Task Force on the Prevention and Management of Infertility. Tubal infertility: serologic relationship to post chlamydial and gonococcal infection. *Sex Trans Dis.* 1995;22:71.

14. Kahn JG, Walker CK, Washington AE, et al. Diagnosing pelvic inflammatory disease: A comprehensive analysis and considerations for developing a new model. *JAMA.* 1991; 226:2594.

15. Eschenbach DA. Epidemiology and diagnosis of acute pelvic inflammatory disease. *Obstet Gynecol.* 1980;55: 142S.

16. Yudin MH, Hillier SL, Wiesenfeld HC, et al. Vaginal polymorphonuclear leukocytes and bacterial vaginosis as markers for histologic endometritis among women without symptoms of pelvic inflammatory diease. *Am J Obstet Gynecol.* 2003;188:318.

17. Westrom L, Joesoef R, Reynolds G, et al. Pelvic inflammatory disease and fertility: A cohort study of 1844 women with laparoscopically verified disease and 657 control women with normal laparoscopic results. *Sex Transm Dis.* 1992;19:185.

18. Westrom L. Sexually transmitted diseases and infertility. *Sex Transm Dis.* 1994;21:S32.

19. Boardman LA, Peipert JF, Brody JM, et al. Endovaginal sonography for the diagnosis of upper genital tract infection. *Obstet Gynecol.* 1997;90:54.

20. Paavonen J, Teisala K, Heinonen PK, et al. Microbiological and histopathological findings in acute pelvic inflammatory disease. *Br J Obstet Gynecol.* 1987;94:454.

21. Jacobson L, Westrom L. Objectivized diagnosis of acute pelvic inflammatory disease. *Amer J Obstet Gynecol.* 1969;105:1088.

22. Sellors JW, Mahony J, Goldsmith C, et al. The diagnosis of pelvic inflammatory disease: the accuracy of clinical and laparoscopic findings. *Am J Obstet Gynecol.* 1991; 164:113.

23. Kenney A, Greenhalf JO. Limitation of laparoscopy in the diagnosis of gonococcal salpingitis. *BMJ.* 1974;4:519.

24. Eckert LO, Hawes SE, Wolmer-Hanssen PK, et al. Endometritis: The clinical-pathologic syndrome. *Am J Obstet Gynecol.* 2002;186:690.

25. Reed SD, Landers DV, Sweet RL. Antibiotic treatment of tuboovarian abscess: Comparison of broad-spectrum β-lactam agents versus clindamycin-containing regimens. *Am J Obstet Gynecol.* 1991;164:1556.

32

Ectopic Pregnancy and Abdominal Pain in the Pregnant Patient

Stacie Zelman

HIGH YIELD FACTS

- Ectopic pregnancy is one of the leading causes of first trimester morbidity and mortality, as well as one of the leading malpractice risks for emergency physicians.[1]

- Diagnosis of ectopic pregnancy can be safely ruled out in a stable patient with a viable intrauterine pregnancy (IUP) by ultrasound (US), and a B-hCG above discriminatory zone.

- In hemodynamically unstable patients with a positive pregnancy test, immediate gynecologic consultation for laparoscopy is indicated, even if quantitative B-hCG and US have not yet been obtained.

- Stable patients with a B-hCG below the discriminatory zone, and a nondiagnostic US, can be discharged for serial quantitative B-hCGs, with OB/GYN evaluation and follow up within 2 days.

EPIDEMIOLOGY

Ectopic pregnancy is one of the leading causes of maternal morbidity and mortality in the first trimester. Rates of ectopic pregnancy have been increasing in the United States over the last several decades, increasing from 0.5% of pregnancies in 1970 to 1.97% in 1992.[1-3] Increases in ectopic pregnancy rates are thought to stem from increasing incidence of risk factors such as pelvic inflammatory disease, but earlier diagnosis and early recognition, stemming from improvement in diagnostic techniques, is also reflected in these increasing rates.[1] With earlier diagnosis, overall mortality rates from ectopic pregnancy have decreased almost 90% from 1970 to 1989.[2] However, ectopic pregnancy still accounts for up to 13% of all pregnancy related deaths, and 80% of deaths in the first

trimester. Missed ectopic pregnancy remains one of the leading causes of emergency medicine malpractice risk.[2,4]

PATHOPHYSIOLOGY

The pathophysiology of ectopic pregnancy is multifaceted and complex. The etiology of ectopic pregnancy is thought to be a combination of hormonal and anatomic factors. An ectopic pregnancy occurs when a fertilized ovum implants outside the uterus. The most common site of extrauterine implantation is the fallopian tube (97%), with the ampullary region being the most common. Other sites of implantation such as the ovaries, cervix, abdomen, and interstitium, account for less than 3% of ectopic pregnancies.[1]

During the initial phases of an ectopic pregnancy, the patient may be asymptomatic, and the B-hCG may rise appropriately. However, as trophoblastic tissue continues to invade tubal submucosa, hematoma formation and tubal swelling begin to cause unilateral pelvic pain. The growth of the trophoblast eventually begins to outgrow the blood supply within the fallopian tube. As the trophoblastic tissue is responsible for the production of B-hCG, B-hCG levels will begin to level off or start falling.[1] Uterine and vaginal bleeding may begin shortly after, with falling progesterone levels and decidual sloughing.[1,5] Tubal rupture finally occurs when continued growth of the trophoblast and continued hemorrhage burst the already compromised tubal serosa.[1] Actual rupture of the fallopian tube is estimated to occur in up to 5% of cases.[6]

CLINICAL FEATURES

Ectopic pregnancy is a significant cause of maternal mortality accounting for approximately 6% of maternal deaths, yet the presentation of ectopic pregnancy can vary widely, owing to an up to 40% rate of error or delay in diagnosis.[7] The traditional symptom triad for ectopic pregnancy is vaginal bleeding, amenorrhea, and abdominal or pelvic pain. However, this complete triad is actually only manifested in 50% of ectopic pregnancies, the majority of these ruptured.[8] Of individual presenting symptoms, the most common is abdominal pain. A study in 1990 by Stovall et al. reported a 100% incidence of abdominal pain in patients with ruptured ectopics, but only 30% of patients had abdominal pain in unruptured ectopic pregnancies.[9] Clinically, absence of pain in a patient with a suspected ectopic is useful as a negative predictor for rupture.[1,10] The second most common presenting symptom is amenorrhea or irregular vaginal bleeding. Amenorrhea may be present in up to 85% of presenting patients, while 70% may have irregular bleeding.[7] Other less common, but significant presenting symptoms include nausea/vomiting, dizziness, and syncope.[7]

Intrinsic in the clinical evaluation of a patient with a suspected ectopic pregnancy is the evaluation of inherent risk factors for ectopic. Risk factors include any condition that is thought to prevent the passage of the fertilized ovum to the uterus. This includes conditions such as pelvic inflammatory disease, previous ectopic pregnancy, or pelvic surgery (including tubal ligation) all of which may result in scarring of the fallopian tubes.[11] However, up to 50% of ectopic pregnancies occur in patients without defined risk factors.[1]

Physical exam findings in ectopic pregnancy can vary widely from patient to patient. The clinician must assess the patient's vital signs, and conduct a problem-focused exam of the abdomen and pelvis. Initial presentation of clinical shock, manifested by severe hypotension and tachycardia, is becoming less common because of improved diagnostic techniques and earlier patient presentation. It is now reported in less than 5% of ectopic pregnancies.[1] The most common physical exam finding is abdominal tenderness, found in 90% of patients, with adnexal tenderness accounting for 50% to 80% of pain.[1,7] However, the presence of adnexal tenderness alone is unreliable in determining ectopic pregnancy from other sources of pelvic pathology.[1] Cervical motion tenderness is another important physical exam finding, found in 50% of ectopic pregnancies,[1] and vaginal bleeding is found in up to 60%.[7] It is important to note that the pelvic exam can be normal in 10% of ectopic pregnancies.[5] Other pertinent physical exam findings include normal uterine size (71%),[12] and inaudible fetal heart tones with appropriate dating (exceptions include advanced/live ectopics).[1,13] Overall, Stovall et al. found that clinical diagnosis is only 55.3% sensitive in predicting ectopic pregnancy on the initial visit, while Weckstein found clinical diagnosis to have a predictive value of only 49%, indicating that clinical diagnosis alone is inadequate for the diagnosis of ectopic pregnancy.[9,14]

Once a pregnancy has been established, it is the duty of the emergency department (ED) physician to determine whether the patient is safe to be discharged or whether immediate intervention is indicated. An algorithm noted in the article "An Update on the Medical Treatment of Ectopic Pregnancy," by Barnhart et al.[11] has been validated as a useful tool to make this determination. In summary, for quantitative B-hCGs above the discriminatory zone of 1500 mIU/mL, a transvaginal ultrasound is performed (many institutions use 1000 mIU/mL as their cut off). If a viable intrauterine pregnancy is established, the patient may be discharged with follow up. If no IUP, or

findings suggestive of an abnormal or ectopic pregnancy are discovered, OB/GYN is consulted for either laparoscopy or dilation and curettage. In the stable patient with a B-hCG below the discriminatory zone, the patient is discharged for outpatient serial B-hCG measurements.[11,15] A falling, plateauing, or abnormal rise in B-hCG over the next couple of days indicates an abnormal pregnancy (but not necessarily an ectopic).[16] However, a small number of normal IUPs can have an initial abnormal rise in B-hCG.[17] A clinically ill-appearing patient with a quantitative B-hCG below the discriminatory zone should have an US for evaluation of abdominal free fluid, adnexal masses, or other nonspecific indicators of ectopic pregnancy, and immediate gynecologic consultation should be established.

DIAGNOSIS AND DIFFERENTIAL

One of the first principles in the diagnosis of ectopic pregnancy is developing an index of suspicion for the diagnosis in any reproductive age female who presents with abdominal pain and/or vaginal bleeding.[16] Early suspicion may result in timely diagnosis, and thus, intervention. An index of suspicion may be peaked when taking into account patient's history, symptomatology, and risk factors for ectopic pregnancy.

Lab Evaluation

The initial step in the diagnosis of ectopic pregnancy is obtaining a qualitative B-hCG (typically a urine sample). Once the determination of pregnancy has been established, obtaining a quantitative B-hCG is the next step. The quantitative B-hCG has several uses. First, it is used to determine the "discriminatory zone," i.e., the level of hormone at which all IUPs should be visualized by US.[16] For abdominal US, this B-hCG level approaches 6500 mIU/mL, while for transvaginal US the discriminatory zone is reduced to 1000 to 1500 mIU/mL.[16] If the quantitative B-hCG has not yet reached the discriminatory zone, monitoring the rising trend can be utilized. In a normal pregnancy, B-hCG should double on average every 2 days, until a B-hCG value of 10,000 mIU/mL, where doubling is less reliable.[17] A falling or inadequately rising B-hCG indicates an abnormal (but not necessarily an ectopic pregnancy) in the majority of cases.[16]

Imaging

By and large, the preferred imaging modality in evaluation of ectopic pregnancy is transvaginal US. It has largely replaced culdocentesis and exploratory laparoscopy as the diagnostic screening modality of choice. In one study in the United Kingdom, transvaginal US had a sensitivity and specificity of 89.9% and 99.8%, respectively, for ectopic pregnancy, with corresponding positive and negative predictive values of 92.5% and 99.8%.[4,18] An ectopic pregnancy can be either visualized directly by transvaginal US (Figure 32-1), or the images may suggest ectopic when combined with B-hCG markers. When combined with a B-hCG less than 1800 mIU, US has been shown to have a sensitivity of only up to 40% in diagnosing ectopic pregnancy, intrauterine pregnancy, or miscarriage.[19] The positive predictive value of US in diagnosing an ectopic pregnancy and IUP below the B-hCG discriminatory zone of 1800 mIU is 60% and 80%, respectively.[19] In one study, a B-hCG of 1000 IU/L with an ultrasonographically visualized adnexal mass had a diagnostic sensitivity and specificity of 97% and 99%, respectively, for ectopic pregnancy, with positive and negative predictive values of 98%.[3,20] Rapid advances in US technology have helped to determine findings suggestive of ectopic pregnancy, such as small amounts of free fluid, adnexal masses, and the like, long before the B-hCG discriminatory zone for IUP has been reached. However, below the discriminatory zone, US is only useful as an adjunct to laboratory evaluation and clinical exam and should not be the sole diagnostic tool.

Differential

The differential diagnosis of acute abdominal pain in early pregnancy is broad, encompassing both pregnancy and nonpregnancy related etiologies. In the care of the pregnant patient with acute abdominal pain, life-threatening etiologies must be uncovered quickly. As this chapter discusses, ectopic pregnancy should be high on the differential because of its potentially high mortality. Some of the more common pregnancy-related causes that should be considered include spontaneous or missed abortion, occurring in up to 15% of pregnancies, 80% of these in

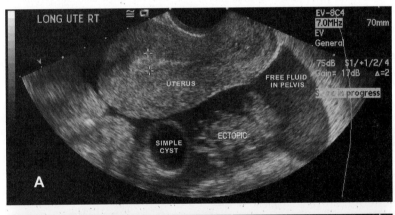

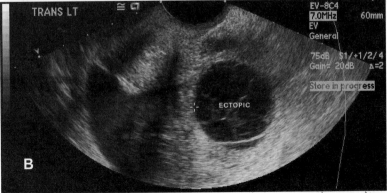

Fig. 32-1 Transvaginal ultrasound of an ectopic pregnancy. A. Longitudinal view. B. Transverse view.

the first trimester.[21] Adnexal torsion, which is relatively common in pregnancy, occurs in 1 in 1800 pregnancies.[22] This is thought to be due to increasing laxity of ovarian ligaments in pregnancy.[6,23] In addition, pelvic inflammatory disease and ruptured ovarian cysts should be considered in the differential.

Some of the more common nonpregnancy related causes of pelvic pain include appendicitis, which is considered one of the leading causes of nonobstetrical surgery in the obstetric patient. Appendicitis has an incidence ranging between 0.38 and 1.69 per 1000 pregnancies (similar incidence to ovarian torsion of pregnancy).[24] Pyelonephritis stemming from an existing cystitis or bacturia can occur in 1% to 2% of pregnancies.[6] The constellation inflammatory/irritable bowel diseases can also be a source of pelvic pain, but the diagnosis usually pre-exists the pregnancy.

EMERGENCY DEPARTMENT CARE AND DISPOSITION

Any patient presenting to the ED with a clinical history suspicious for an ectopic pregnancy warrants an immediate qualitative pregnancy test. Patients must then be stratified into stable versus unstable based on hemodynamic status and overall clinical condition. If the patient shows any measure of hemodynamic instability, such as hypotension or tachycardia, with or without severe abdominal pain, or excessive bleeding, immediate resuscitative measures should be instituted.[2] Along with immediate gynecologic consultation, the patient should be placed on a monitor, have two large bore IVs placed with aggressive fluid resuscitation, and blood sent for compete blood count (CBC) and type and cross-match (T&C) Type specific or O–blood products should be considered in the persistently hypotensive patient. If the patient is Rh–, RhoGAM should be administered.[2]

In the stable patient, the initial work-up should consist of a quantitative B-hCG, with diagnostic US. Using only quantitative B-hCG measurements to determine whether an US is warranted is a risky practice. Several studies have shown a high incidence of ectopic pregnancy even when B-hCG is below the discriminatory zone. Studies by Mol and Dart both show confirmed ectopic pregnancy rates of 39% and 38%, respectively, with quantitative B-hCGs less than 1000 mUI/mL.[2,25,26]

In the stable patient with a US determinate for ectopic pregnancy, blood should be sent for T&C and CBC, and gynecologic consultation obtained for laparoscopy or methotrexate therapy.[2] Methotrexate therapy should only be instituted in consultation with an OB/GYN, as close

follow-up is needed. If US is indeterminate, but suggestive of ectopic, gynecologic consultation is also warranted. Patients may be discharged from the ED if they exhibit one of the following: (1) Definite viable IUP on US, (2) Early ectopic without signs of rupture, with methotrexate therapy in consultation with OB/GYN, (3) Nonviable IUP with expectant management, (4) B-hCG below the discriminatory zone, hemodynamically stable, no definititive US findings, and close OB/GYN follow up.

PITFALLS

- Clinical history and physical exam *alone* are highly unreliable in the diagnosis of ectopic pregnancy. Ten percent of patients with ectopic pregnancy present with normal pelvic exams.[5] A combination of quantitative B-hCG and transvaginal US are necessary to confirm diagnosis.

- Risk factors for ectopic pregnancy, while important to determine, are only present in 50% of patients with the diagnosis.[8] Any patient with a history suspicious for ectopic pregnancy, regardless of risk factors, should be evaluated as such.

- Not all sources of abdominal pain in the pregnant patient are pregnancy related. Don't forget alternative diagnoses!

REFERENCES

1. Brennan DF. Ectopic pregnancy—Part I: Clinical and laboratory diagnosis. *Acad Emerg Med.* 1995;2:1081.
2. Della-Giustina D, Denny M. Ectopic pregnancy. *Emerg Med Clin North Am.* 2003;21:565.
3. Pisarska MD, Carson SA, Buster JE. Ectopic pregnancy. *Lancet.* 1998;351:1115.
4. Sowter MC, Farquhar CM. Ectopic pregnancy: an update. *Curr Opin Obstet Gynecol.* 2004;16:289.
5. Cartwright PS. Diagnosis of ectopic pregnancy. *Obstet Gynecol Clin North Am.* 1991;18:19.
6. Cappell MS, Friedel D. Abdominal pain during pregnancy. *Gastroenterol Clin North Am.* 2003;32:1.
7. Mayer IE. Abdominal Pain During Pregnancy. *Gastroenterology Clinics of North America.* 1998;27:1.
8. Emerson DS, McCord ML. Clinician's approach to ectopic pregnancy. *Clin Obstet Gynecol.* 1996;39:199.
9. Stovall TG, Kellerman AL, Ling FW, Buster JE. Emergency department diagnosis of ectopic pregnancy. *Ann Emerg Med.* 1990;19:1098.
10. Hirata AJ, Soper DE, Bump RC, Hurt WG. Ectopic pregnancy in an urban teaching hospital: can tubal rupture be predicted? *South Med J.* 1991;84:1467.

11. Barnhart K, Esposito M, Coutifaris C. An update on the medical treatment of ectopic pregnancy. *Obstet Gynecol Clin North Am.* 2000;27:653. viii.

12. Weckstein LN. Current perspective on ectopic pregnancy. *Obstet Gynecol Surv.* 1985;40:259.

13. Sanfilippo J, Woodworth, SH. *Ectopic Pregnancy.* 4th ed. Philadelphia: J.B. Lippincott; 1992.

14. Weckstein LN, Boucher AR, Tucker H, et al. Accurate diagnosis of early ectopic pregnancy. *Obstet Gynecol.* 1985; 65:393.

15. Barnhart K, Mennuti MT, Benjamin I, et al. Prompt diagnosis of ectopic pregnancy in an emergency department setting. *Obstet Gynecol.* 1994; 84:1010.

16. Fylstra DL. Tubal pregnancy: a review of current diagnosis and treatment. *Obstet Gynecol Surv.* 1998;53:320.

17. Kadar N, Caldwell BV, Romero R. A method of screening for ectopic pregnancy and its indications. *Obstet Gynecol.* 1981;58:162.

18. Zane SB, Kieke BA, Jr., Kendrick JS, Bruce C. Surveillance in a time of changing health care practices: estimating ectopic pregnancy incidence in the United States. *Matern Child Health J.* 2002;6:227.

19. Barnhart KT, Simhan H, Kamelle SA. Diagnostic accuracy of ultrasound above and below the beta-hCG discriminatory zone. *Obstet Gynecol.* 1999;94:583.

20. Cacciatore B, Stenman UH, Ylostalo P. Diagnosis of ectopic pregnancy by vaginal ultrasonography in combination with a discriminatory serum hCG level of 1000 IU/l (IRP). *Br J Obstet Gynaecol.* 1990;97:904.

21. Coppola PT, Coppola M. Vaginal bleeding in the first 20 weeks of pregnancy. *Emerg Med Clin North Am.* 2003; 21:667.

22. Johnson TR, Jr., Woodruff JD. Surgical emergencies of the uterine adnexae during pregnancy. *Int J Gynaecol Obstet.* 1986;24:331.

23. Mancuso A, Broccio G, Angio LG, Pirri V. Adnexal torsion in pregnancy. *Acta Obstet Gynecol Scand.* 1997;76:83.

24. Kennedy A. Assessment of acute abdominal pain in the pregnant patient. *Semin Ultrasound CT MR.* 2000;21:64.

25. Mol BW, Hajenius PJ, Engelsbel S, Ankum WM, Van der Veen F, Hemrika DJ, Bossuyt PM. Serum human chorionic gonadotropin measurement in the diagnosis of ectopic pregnancy when transvaginal sonography is inconclusive. *Fertil Steril.* 1998;70:972.

26. Dart RG, Kaplan B, Cox C. Transvaginal ultrasound in patients with low beta-human chorionic gonadotropin values: How often is the study diagnostic? *Ann Emerg Med.* 1997;30:135.

33

Ovarian Torsion

Heather L. Farley

HIGH YIELD FACTS

- The two most common presenting features in ovarian torsion are lower abdominal pain and an adnexal mass.[1]
- Ultrasound (US) is the imaging modality of choice in evaluating suspected ovarian torsion; however, a negative US does not rule out the diagnosis.
- Operative evaluation and management are the definitive treatment for ovarian torsion.

EPIDEMIOLOGY

Ovarian torsion is the fifth most common gynecologic emergency, with a prevalence of approximately 2.7%.[1] Although it can affect women of all ages, those of reproductive age have the highest incidence.

Women with ovarian cysts or neoplasms account for over 94% of cases of ovarian torsion.[2] The likelihood of malignancy in any such identified neoplasm is greater in postmenopausal women, but the majority of the neoplasms found during surgery for suspected adnexal torsion are benign in nature.[1]

Certain patient populations may be at particular risk for developing ovarian torsion, including those women who are pregnant or have undergone fertility treatments. The incidence of ovarian torsion during pregnancy has been reported to be 1:10,000 to 5:10,000 pregnancies,[3] occurring most commonly between 6 and 14 weeks gestation and in the immediate puerperium.[4] After gonadotropin stimulation, however, the incidence rises dramatically to 6%, and in patients with hyperstimulation, to 16%.[3] Suspicion of ovarian torsion should therefore be increased in patients undergoing such infertility treatments. Women who have undergone tubal ligation may also be at increased risk.[1]

While rare, concurrent bilateral ovarian torsion has been reported.[1] In addition, approximately 10% of women who have experienced ovarian torsion will go on to have a recurrent episode involving the contralateral adnexum.[5]

PATHOPHYSIOLOGY

The ovary lies suspended in the abdomen by three main structures: (a) the ligament of the ovary, which attaches the ovary to the uterus, (b) the suspensory ligament of the ovary, which attaches the ovary to the abdominal wall and contains the ovarian vessels, and (c) the mesovarium, which attaches the ovary to a portion of the broad ligament and thereby to the fallopian tube.[6]

In adnexal torsion, the ovary twists upon its vascular pedicle, resulting in obstruction of venous and lymphatic drainage. Over time, the arterial supply of the ovary becomes compromised, leading to infarction. Torsion of the ovary may occur separately from the fallopian tube, but the two structures usually torse as a unit. In addition, the adnexa may twist either partially or completely, and may intermittently twist and untwist. Interestingly, some reports suggest that the right ovary may be more likely to torse than the left.[5] It has been proposed that the sigmoid colon may decrease available space on the left, affording relative protection from torsion to the left ovary.

Torsion is a known complication of ovarian cysts, and typically occurs with the production of a corpus luteum in the second half of the menstrual cycle.[7] The development of ovarian cysts is not limited to reproductive age women and may occur even in utero. The pathogenesis of neonatal ovarian cysts is not well understood, but may involve the stimulation of fetal ovaries by maternal estrogens and fetal pituitary and placental gonadotropins.[8] While the majority of these cysts resolve without complication over the first year of life, neonatal cysts >4 cm in size are particularly prone to torsion. The likelihood of torsion in young children is greatest in months 2 to 12 of life.[9] A second peak period of ovarian torsion in the pediatric population occurs around the time of menarche. It has been proposed that the increased hormonal stimulation surrounding the initiation of menstruation leads to the development of a greater number of functional ovarian cysts. In fact, up to 20% of girls may have multicystic and enlarged ovaries during menarche, thus increasing the risk of torsion in this population.[10]

Torsion may also occur in the absence of ovarian pathology. Proposed mechanisms whereby a normal ovary may undergo torsion include tortuosity and elongation of the fallopian tube or mesosalpingeal vessels, congenitally long supportive ligaments, tubal spasm, or abrupt changes in intraabdominal pressure such as with vomiting or coughing.[10]

CLINICAL FEATURES

While the clinical presentation of ovarian torsion can be quite nonspecific, the "classic" history includes the abrupt onset of pain in either lower quadrant with radiation to the flank or groin.[11] Indeed, the most commonly reported symptom is the sudden onset of lower abdominal pain, often associated with waves of nausea and vomiting. However, these symptoms are not universally present in patients with ovarian torsion.[1] In one series, the frequency of symptoms was as follows:

- Seventy percent of patients experienced nausea and vomiting.
- Seventy percent described the pain as stabbing or sharp in nature.
- Fifty-nine percent related that the onset of pain was sudden.
- Fifty-one percent complained of pain radiating to the back, flank, or groin.
- Less than 2% of patients reported fevers.[11]

Of special mention, parents of neonates experiencing torsion may relate a history of feeding intolerance, vomiting, abdominal distension, or irritability.

Physical examination findings in patients with ovarian torsion may include unilateral adnexal tenderness and/or an ovarian mass. In one study, the presence of a palpable ovarian mass was reported in 72% of patients with torsion.[1] Despite these findings on pelvic exam, the abdominal exam is often nondiagnostic, with peritoneal signs present in only 3% of patients.[11]

DIAGNOSIS AND DIFFERENTIAL

The diagnosis of ovarian torsion in the emergency department is primarily a clinical one. While certain aspects of the history, physical exam, and imaging studies may suggest the presence or absence of torsion, definitive diagnosis is made by surgical exploration. To maximize the chances of ovarian salvage, the possibility of torsion must be considered early in the patient's presentation and should be suspected in any woman who presents with lower abdominal pain and/or an adnexal mass. Despite the importance of early detection, ovarian torsion was suspected in less than half of confirmed cases in one study.[11]

Laboratory testing is rarely helpful in establishing the diagnosis. However, a drop in hemoglobin may result if significant hemorrhage has occurred and leukocytosis may be observed following ovarian necrosis. Elevated serum interleukin-6 (IL-6) levels were significantly associated with the occurrence of ovarian torsion in one study.[12] Further investigation is necessary to determine the role of IL-6 as a potential diagnostic tool.

Ultrasound is considered the imaging modality of choice in the diagnosis of ovarian torsion. As US poses no risk of ionizing radiation exposure and it is an ideal diagnostic tool for the evaluation of both children and gravid patients presenting with lower abdominal pain. Pelvic US may also be performed at the time of the pelvic examination by qualified practitioners. Sonographic findings in ovarian torsion are variable, depending on the duration and degree of vascular compromise and whether an adnexal mass is present. The most common sonographic finding is ovarian enlargement.[7] A cystic or solid adnexal mass may be identified in over 70% of patients with ovarian torsion, and free fluid in the cul-de-sac is common.[13] Another common finding, the presence of large, peripherally located follicles, may result from the transudation of fluid into the follicles following vascular compromise (Figure 33-1a).[7] Additional gray-scale US findings suggestive of ovarian torsion include a heterogeneous central ovarian stroma, cystic necrosis of the ovary, and a twisted vascular pedicle. One small study detected the presence of a positive "whirlpool" sign in the twisted vascular pedicle in 20 out of 20 patients studied with ovarian torsion.[14] The "whirlpool" sign is described as the appearance of hypoechoic vessels wrapping around a central axis when the probe is moved along the axis of the pedicle (Figure 33-1b).[7]

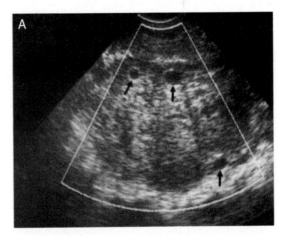

Fig. 33-1a. Doppler ultrasound of ovarian torsion. The ovary is enlarged with several small, peripherally located cysts (arrows). The central ovarian stroma is heterogeneous, with echogenic areas representing hemorrhage and hypoechoic areas representing edema. No flow is detected.[4]

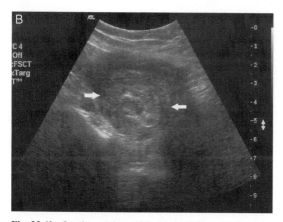

Fig. 33-1b. Ovarian torsion whirlpool sign. The twisted pedicle appears as a large echogenic mass (arrows). Used with permission from Dr. S. Boopathy Vijayaraghavan, Sonographic Whirlpool Sign in Ovarian Torsion. *J Ultrasound Med.* 2004; 23:1643–1649.

The utilization of Doppler has made it possible to identify the presence of blood flow in the adnexa. While abnormal Doppler flow is highly predictive of torsion, a normal flow Doppler scan does not exclude the diagnosis. Numerous studies and reports have documented the presence of blood flow in surgically proven cases of ovarian torsion.[5,7,11] Part of the challenge with Doppler examination of ovarian vasculature results from the natural progression of ovarian torsion, in which venous outflow is compromised prior to arterial inflow. Thus, the detection of arterial flow does not exclude the possibility of ovarian torsion early in the disease process.[7] Spectral Doppler, however, enables the sonologist to differentiate venous from arterial flow. One study found that the positive predictive value of the absence of venous flow on spectral Doppler was 94%. This same study reported a misdiagnosis rate of only 2% if normal venous flow was noted on spectral Doppler.[15] Finally, three-dimensional power Doppler provides a quantitative assessment of vessel density and perfusion. By enabling the operator to evaluate overall tissue vascularization, this technology may prove a useful adjunct in the diagnosis of ovarian torsion.[16] Despite all of these advances, it is important to note that the presence of spectral, or power Doppler flow within ovarian tissue cannot definitively rule out ovarian torsion. If torsion is suspected clinically in the face of a normal US,

laparoscopic exploration is emerging as the recommended diagnostic and therapeutic tool.[17]

A computed tomography (CT) scan of the abdomen and pelvis, ordered to evaluate the patient for alternate diagnoses such as appendicitis or diverticulitis, may reveal certain findings which, when present, are suggestive of ovarian torsion. Clinical suspicion of ovarian torsion should be increased when either a central, round lesion surrounded by a thickened "shell"[18] or a markedly enlarged ovary with small peripheral cystic structures is observed on CT scan.[19]

Magnetic resonance imaging (MRI) findings in ovarian torsion include a thick, edematous vascular pedicle and a lack of enhancement of the affected ovary.[20] Non-contrast-enhanced MRI has been proposed as an adjunct to ultrasonography in the diagnosis of ovarian torsion in pregnant women, since it poses no risk of ionizing radiation to the fetus.[21]

The differential diagnosis of ovarian torsion includes ectopic pregnancy, hemorrhagic/ruptured ovarian cyst, ovarian neoplasm, mittelschmerz, appendicitis, pelvic inflammatory disease, degenerating leiomyoma, tubo-ovarian abscess, diverticulitis, renal colic, and endometriosis. Later in pregnancy, the differential diagnosis must also include labor, uterine rupture, placental abruption, and hemolysis, elevated liver enzymes, and low platelet count (HELLP) syndrome.

EMERGENCY DEPARTMENT CARE AND DISPOSITION

The most important factor for preserving ovarian function and minimizing complications in ovarian torsion is expeditious diagnosis and treatment. As the mainstay of treatment is operative evaluation and management, the earlier in the course of the disease the patient is taken to the operating room, the greater the chances of ovarian salvage. In one series, among those patients operated on within 8 hours of initial examination, the salvage rate was 40%; among those operated on within 24 hours of initial examination, the salvage rate was 33%; and among those with operative intervention more than 24 hours after initial examination, none had ovaries salvaged.[22] The duration of symptoms prior to examination, however, does not serve as a reliable guide for determining tissue viability, as torsion may be partial, complete, and/or intermittent in nature.[1] In fact, recuperation of the ovary has been reported for up to 72 hours after torsion has occurred.[17] Therefore, while it is essential to identify ovarian torsion as quickly as possible, it should not be assumed that the ovary is nonviable based on an extended duration of symptoms.

After identifying a probable ovarian torsion, the main responsibility of the emergency physician lies in obtaining prompt surgical consultation, adequately resuscitating the patient, and preparing the patient for the operating room. Intravenous access should be obtained, and crystalloid infused as needed to correct volume losses. Hemodynamically unstable patients should be closely monitored until definitive treatment can be rendered. Routine laboratory studies including a complete blood count, electrolyte panel, urinalysis, and urine pregnancy test should be considered, and any significant anemia or coagulopathy corrected. Finally, antiemetics and analgesia should be administered as needed.

Once in the operating room, the affected adnexum is most commonly evaluated laparoscopically. If torsion is identified, the involved adnexum is usually excised in the postmenopausal woman.[1] In the premenopausal woman, however, the surgical paradigm has shifted over time from one of ovarian removal to one of ovarian detorsion, possible cystectomy or aspiration, and stabilization of the ovary whenever possible.[5] Several studies have demonstrated the return of ovarian function in the majority of women who undergo laparoscopic detorsion, even in the presence of necrotic-appearing adnexa.[23] Intravenous fluorescein has been used by some investigators as an adjunctive method of evaluating viability of the torsed ovary.[24] Following detorsion, many surgeons advocate oophoropexy, whereby the ovary is secured in order to prevent recurrent torsion. Oophoropexy of the contralateral ovary may also be performed, either at the time of the original surgery or on an elective basis. This may be particularly important in children and reproductive-age women who undergo oophorectomy in order to secure future fertility of the remaining ovary.[25]

PITFALLS

- Failure to consider ovarian torsion in the differential diagnosis, particularly in infants or those patients with intermittent symptoms.

- Reliance on a negative US to rule out the diagnosis of ovarian torsion.

- Delay in obtaining definitive surgical management.

REFERENCES

1. Bayer AI, Wiskind AK. Adnexal torsion:can the adnexa be saved? *Am J Obstet Gynecol.* 1994;171:1506.
2. Varras M, Tsikini A, Polyzos D, et al. Uterine adnexal torsion:pathologic and gray-scale ultrasonographic findings. *Clin Exp Obstet Gynecol.* 2004;31:34.
3. Djavadian D, Braendle W, Jaenicke F. Laparoscopic oophoropexy for the treatment of recurrent torsion of the adnexa in pregnancy: case report and review. *Fertil Steril.* 2003;82:933.
4. Webb EM, Green GE, Scoutt LM. Adnexal mass with pelvic pain. *Radiol Clin North Am.* 2004;42:336.
5. Stenchever MA, Droegemueller W, Herbst AL, et al. Benign gynecologic lesions. In: Stenchever MA (ed.). *Comprehensive Gynecology.* 4th ed. St. Louis. Missouri: Mosby Inc.; 2001:519.
6. Agur AMR, Lee MJ. The perineum and pelvis. In: Gardner RJM, (ed.). *Grant's Atlas of Anatomy.* 9th ed. Baltimore. Maryland; Williams & Wilkins:1991:176.
7. Lambert MJ, Villa M. Gynecologic ultrasound in emergency medicine. *Emerg Med Clin North Am.* 2004;22:63.
8. Hamrick HJ. Ovarian cyst and torsion in a young infant. *Arch Pediatr Adolesc Med.* 1998;152:1245.
9. Alrabeeah A, Galliani CA, Giacomantonio M, et al. Neonatal ovarian torsion: report of three cases and review of the literature. *Pediatr Pathol.* 1988;8:143.
10. Kokoska ER, Keller MS, Weber TR. Acute ovarian torsion in children. *Am J Surg.* 2000;180:462.
11. Houry D, Abbott JT. Ovarian torsion: a fifteen-year review. *Ann Emerg Med.* 2001;38:156.
12. Cohen SB, Wattiez A, Stockheim D, et al. The accuracy of serum interleukin-6 and tumour necrosis factor as markers for ovarian torsion. *Hum Reprod.* 2001;16:219.
13. Varras M, Tsikini A, Polyzos D, et al. Uterine adnexal torsion: Pathologic and gray-scale ultrasonographic findings. *Clin Exp Obstet Gynecol.* 2004;31:37.
14. Vijayaraghavan SB. Sonographic whirlpool sign in ovarian torsion. *J Ultrasound Med.* 2004;23:1643.
15. Ben-Ami M, Perlitz Y, Haddad S. The effectiveness of spectral and color Doppler in predicting ovarian torsion. *Eur J of Obstet Gynecol Reprod Biol.* 2002;104:64.
16. Yaman C, Ebner T, Jesacher K. Three-dimensional power Doppler in the diagnosis of ovarian torsion. *Ultrasound Obstet Gynecol.* 2002;20:513.
17. Aziz D, Davis V, Allen L, et al. Ovarian torsion in children: Is oophorectomy necessary? *J Pediatr Surg.* 2004;39:752.
18. Schlaff WD, Lund KJ, McAlesse KA, et al. Diagnosing ovarian torsion with computed tomography. *J Reprod Med.* 1998;43:827.
19. Gittleman AM, Price AP, Goffner L, et al. Ovarian torsion: CT findings in a child. *J Pediatr Surg.* 2004;39:1270.
20. Born C, Wirth S, Stabler A, et al. Diagnosis of adnexal torsion in the third trimester of pregnancy: a case report. *Abdom Imaging.* 2003;29:123.

21. Birchard KR, Brown MA, Hyslop WB, et al. MRI of acute abdominal and pelvic pain in pregnant patients. *AJR Am J Roentgenol.* 2005;184:452.

22. Anders JF, Powell EC. Urgency of evaluation and outcome of acute ovarian torsion in pediatric patients. *Arch Pediatr Adolesc Med.* 2005;159:532.

23. Shalev E, Bustan M, Yarom I, et al. Recovery of ovarian function after laparoscopic detorsion. *Hum Reprod.* 1995; 10:2965.

24. McHutchison LL, Koonings PP, Ballard CA, et al. Preservation of ovarian tissue in adnexal torsion with fluorescein. *Am J Obstet Gynecol.* 1993;168:1386.

25. Crouch NS, Gyampoh B, Cutner AS, et al. Ovarian torsion: To pex or not to pex? Case report and review of the literature. *J Pediatr Adolesc Gynecol.* 2003;16:381.

34

Intussusception

Melissa W. Costello
W. Scott McNair

HIGH YIELD FACTS

- The classic triad is abdominal pain, vomiting, and bloody stools ("currant jelly") but less than one-third of patients have all three elements. Seventy-five percent of patients are hemoccult positive.
- It is the most common cause of intestinal obstruction in children under the age of 2.[1]
- Computed tomography (CT) scan of the abdomen is the test of choice in adult intussusception.
- Contrast enema is the principal diagnostic/therapeutic test of choice in children.
- Clinical signs of perforation, peritonitis, or hypovolemic shock/sepsis are clear contraindications to enemas.[2]

EPIDEMIOLOGY

Intussusception is the predominate cause of obstruction in children aged 3 months to 6 years. It occurs most commonly between 5 and 12 months[3] with two thirds of cases prior to the first birthday and 80% prior to age 2.[4] It is the second most common cause of gastrointestinal (GI) bleeding in infants and the overall incidence is 1 to 4 cases per 1000 live births.[4] In pediatric cases there is a statistically significant gender difference. The male to female ratio is 2:1 in infancy but this disparity increases with age. By the age of 4 the male-to-female ratio is up to 8:1. Despite the marked difference in later childhood, recent studies have shown that this gender discrepancy disappears in the adult population.[5]

PATHOPHYSIOLOGY

Intussusception is the telescoping of a segment of intestine (intussusceptum) into the lumen of the adjoining segment of intestine (intussuscipiens).[6] Idiopathic intussusception most commonly occurs at the terminal ileum with the segment telescoping into the large bowel. This type is referred to as ileocolic or ileocecal and accounts for nearly 90% of all cases. Enteroenteral intussusception involving jejunum, ileum, or both (jejunojejunal, jejunoileal, or ileoileal) is much less common and occurs almost exclusively in adult patients.

Generally the intestine will begin to invaginate into the distal segment and draw the mesentery along with it. Once this mesentery is compressed into the intussuscipiens, lymphatic drainage is impaired resulting in swelling. This swelling will progress to the point where first the venous, then ultimately the arterial flow, is impaired producing ischemia and bowel obstruction.[2,3] The mucosal lining of the bowel is extremely sensitive to ischemia and will begin to slough off causing heme-positive stool followed closely by the classic "currant jelly" appearance of mixed stool, mucous, blood, and sloughed mucosa.[4] If the intussusception remains untreated, bowel infarction leading to gangrene, perforation, peritonitis, and sepsis will follow.

Multiple sources discuss the possible etiology of idiopathic intussusception. A combination of factors is postulated to play a role in the development of this condition. There is also good correlation with recent viral illness, leading to the theory that lymphatic hypertrophy of the Peyer patches in the distal ileum may be involved.[3] These lymphatic patches are present throughout the bowel, but have the highest concentration in the ileum, the most common starting point for the intussusceptum. Nonetheless, it is difficult to determine conclusively whether the enlarged Peyer patches seen in resected segments of bowel are the primary cause of the intussusception or the secondary effect of the lymphatic obstruction. Also, there is evidence that an imbalance in the peristaltic contractions along the wall of the small bowel contributes to the development of a lead point.[6] This would explain the cases of intussusception that develop in the setting of an early postoperative ileus.

In older children and adults, intussusception typically occurs in the presence of a pathologic lead point. There is some debate in the pediatric literature regarding the appropriate cut-off for increased suspicion about a pathologic lesion. The consensus seems to be that under the age of 3 approximately 90% of intussusception cases will be idiopathic. After the age of 5, a pathologic lesion such as polyps, lymphoma, Meckel diverticulum, Henoch-Schönlein purpura or carcinoma, can be identified in more than 75% of cases.[2,5]

CLINICAL FEATURES

The typical presentation is of a healthy male child, age 6 to 12 months with sudden onset of paroxysmal colicky abdominal pain lasting 2 to 10 minutes and recurring after 15- to 30-minute pain free intervals.[1,2,7] All three components of the classic clinical triad: colicky abdominal pain, vomiting, and "currant jelly" stool, are present in only about 20% of patients at the time of presentation. Up to 60% of patients may have two of the three components.[2] The classic "currant jelly" appearing stool can develop rather late in the clinical course of the disease although Hemoccult positive stool may be present as early as 2 hours after the onset of symptoms.[3] In some instances lethargy or convulsion is the predominant sign or symptom.[8] Therefore, it is critical to keep in mind the possibility of intussusception and to perform a stool guaiac in any child presenting to the emergency department (ED) with altered mental status.[9]

In older children and adults the presentation may be more indolent and is attributable to the intermittent partial bowel obstruction that results from the intussusception. Seventy-five to 80% of patients will report crampy abdominal pain, and slightly fewer will report nausea and vomiting.[10] An acute presentation (symptom duration of hours to days) of intussusception in an adult patient is rare. In one study more than 50% of patients reported symptoms that had lasted from 3 weeks up to 1 year before presentation.[6]

Physical exam may reveal a sausage-like mass in the right upper quadrant with the absence of bowel contents in the right lower quadrant (Dance sign) representing the movement of the cecum out of its normal position.[1] This clinical finding is pathognomonic for intussusception, but is present in less than 10% to 15% of cases and is often not able to be felt, even when present, in a crying infant.[7,11] The patient may or may not have grossly bloody ("currant jelly") stool at presentation, but Hemoccult testing will reveal positive occult blood in up to 75% of cases where stool is not grossly positive.[12]

Complications of intussusception include bowel obstruction progressing to perforation, peritonitis, and sepsis as discussed in the pathophysiology section above. With recognition and appropriate treatment most patients will recover in approximately 24 hours and overall mortality of treated patients is approximately 1% to 3%. Without treatment, the progressive dehydration and strangulating intestinal obstruction of intussusception is usually fatal within 5 days.[13]

DIAGNOSIS AND DIFFERENTIAL

The diagnosis of intussusception is made by a suggestive history and physical exam in combination with radiologic imaging. There are no laboratory tests specific to this disease. Complete blood count (CBC) with differential and electrolytes with blood urea nitrogen (BUN) may be normal, though leukocytosis becomes more common as obstruction progresses. The finding of a heme-positive stool may also aid in the diagnosis. A high index of suspicion is required.

Plain abdominal films are routinely obtained and may show evidence of a soft tissue mass or paucity of gas in the right lower quadrant. The findings of intestinal obstruction are present in up to 54%.[14] In 30% to 50% of cases, plain radiographs may be normal though intussusception is present.[14,15] Ultrasound (US) is the least invasive and most commonly used modality for visualizing intussusceptions in children. Its use avoids radiation exposure to the child. Ultrasound has a sensitivity of 98% to 100% with specificity 88% to 100% for intussusception even in inexperienced hands.[15,16] Sonography will usually show a mass 3 to 5 cm in diameter, with a target appearance on transverse images (Figure 34-1) or the "pseudokidney" sign when seen longitudinally (Figure 34-2).[8,15] Contrast enema with fluoroscopic guidance is routinely used for diagnosis and therapeutic reduction of an intussusception. Water-soluble contrast has replaced barium as the material of choice for this procedure. The common radiographic finding is that of a coiled spring (Figure 34-3), produced by contrast filling the narrow intraluminal space between the intussusceptum and the intussuscipiens (Figure 34-4). Pneumatic reduction under fluoroscopic guidance and hydrostatic (saline) reduction with US guidance have also been used with excellent results.

The diagnosis of intussusception in adults remains a diagnostic challenge due to its relative rarity and the vague clinical presentation. Although CT scanning of the abdomen is the diagnostic test of choice in adults, the diagnosis will often be made on routine scanning of the abdomen when intussusception is not suspected. A target lesion (Figure 34-5), "pseudokidney" or sausage-shaped mass defines the intussusception. Proximal bowel dilatation is commonly noted. Computed tomography is rarely able to define the underlying pathology.[6]

The differential diagnosis of intussusception in children includes constipation, acute appendicitis, gastroenteritis, malrotation/midgut volvulus, strangulated hernia, mesenteric adenitis, bleeding or perforated Meckel

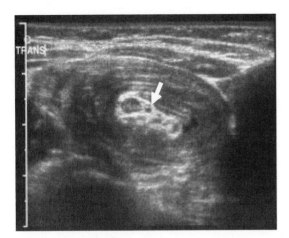

Fig. 34-1. Target appearance of intussusception by ultrasound. Transverse sonographic view demonstrates the intussusception. The hypoechoic outer layer represents the intussuscipiens and the central echogenic layer represents the intussusceptum (arrow). Reprinted with permission from: Vasavada P: Ultrasound evaluation of acute abdominal emergencies in infants and children. *Radiol Clin N Am.* 2004;42:445.

diverticulum, Henoch-Schönlein purpura, inflamatory bowel disease (IBD), Hirsch-sprung enterocolitis, protein-sensitive enterocolitis, and pancreatitis. In adults, any obstructive bowel process will have findings similar to intussusception.

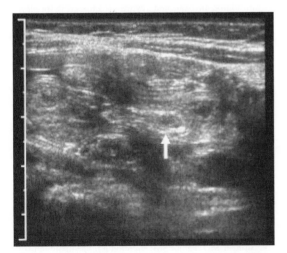

Fig. 34-2. "Pseudokidney" appearance of intussusception by ultrasound. Long-axis sonographic view shows an elongated appearance resulting in a pseudokidney appearance (arrow). Reprinted with permission from Vasavada P: Ultrasound evaluation of acute abdominal emergencies in infants and children. *Radiol Clin N Am.* 2004;42:445.

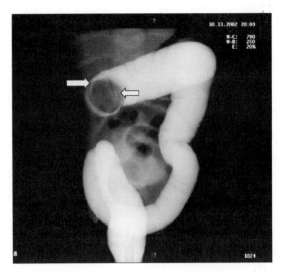

Fig. 34-3. Fluoroscopic findings during water-soluble contrast enema in an infant. Note the "coiled spring" (arrows) appearance of the contrast material in this cross-sectional view of a reduction attempt. Proximal bowel dilatation is also present.

EMERGENCY DEPARTMENT CARE AND DISPOSITION

The initial treatment of intussusception involves the evaluation of airway, breathing, and circulation (ABCs) in any unstable patient. Fluid resuscitation to maintain blood pressure and adequate urine output is required prior

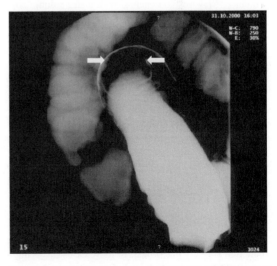

Fig. 34-4. Fluoroscopic findings during water-soluble contrast enema in an infant. Contrast material between the intussuceptum and the intussuscipiens is responsible for this appearance.

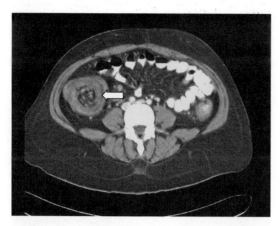

Fig. 34-5. CT findings of intussusception in an adult. This contrasted abdominal CT reveals the classic target or bowel-within-bowel sign of intussusception (arrow).

to any attempts at reduction. Normal saline is used in 20 cc/kg boluses in children. In cases of persistent hypotension despite adequate fluid resuscitation, dopamine at 2 to 20 mcg/kg/min may be initiated. Oral intake should be withheld and a nasogastric tube inserted for decompression. Ampicillin, metronidazole, and an anti-pseudomonal aminoglycoside should be the antibiotics of choice if evidence of peritonitis or shock exists.[17]

The treatment of choice for intussusception in pediatric patients is air contrast enema with fluoroscopic guidance.[15] Hydrostatic enemas with water-soluble contrast under fluoroscopic or ultrasound guidance are also routinely used. Both of these procedures mitigate the risk of peritoneal contamination if perforation is present or results. Ultrasound use also avoids radiation exposure. Successful reduction rates of 70% to 90% have been reported with both pneumatic and hydrostatic procedures.[18] Many institutions mandate surgical consultation prior to attempts at image guided reduction. Surgical intervention should supercede reduction attempts if signs of peritonitis, evidence of shock, multiple recurrences, or evidence of a lead point are present. Children should be observed for 24 to 48 hours after a successful reduction due to a significant recurrence risk of 5% to 10%.

Definitive surgical resection is the recommended treatment in adult intussusception.[19] Due to the high likelihood of a pathologic lead point, attempt at nonoperative reduction is rarely performed. In those cases involving a large portion of small bowel, intraoperative manual reduction may help limit the extent of resection and help prevent short-gut syndrome.[10] In the colon, resection

without manipulation or reduction is advocated due to the high association with malignant pathology and the potential for intraluminal or intraperitoneal seeding of tumor cells.[10,20]

PITFALLS

- A "normal" plain film series of the abdomen does not rule out intussusception.

- Failure to consider intussusception in an infant presenting with altered mental status may lead to delayed or missed diagnosis.

- Failure to admit and observe patients for recurrence following successful enema reduction.

REFERENCES

1. Marx JA. Hockberger RS, Walls RM et al. *Rosen's Emergency Medicine: Concepts and Clinical Practice.* 5th ed. St. Louis, MO: Mosby, Inc.; 2002.
2. McCollough M. Abdominal surgical emergencies in infants and young children. *Emerg Med Clin N Am.* 2003; 21:909.
3. Neblett WW, Pietsch JB, Holcomb GW. Acute abdominal condition in children and adolescents. *Surg Clin North Am.* 1988;68:415.
4. Behrman RE. *Nelson Textbook of Pediatrics.* 17th ed., Philadelphia: Elsevier; 2004.
5. Eisen LK, Cunningham JD, Aufses AH. Intussusception in adults: Institutional review. *J Am Coll Surg.* 1999; 188:390.
6. Huang B, Warshauer D. Adult intussusception: diagnosis and clinical relevance. *Radiol Clin N Am.* 2003;41:1137.
7. D'Agostino J. Common abdominal emergencies in children. *Emerg Med Clin N Am.* 2002;20:139.
8. Vasavada P. Ultrasound evaluation of acute abdominal emergencies in infants and children. *Radiol Clin N Am.* 2004;42:445.
9. Heldrich FJ. Lethargy as a presenting symptom in patients with intussusception. *Clin Pediatr.* 1986;25:363.
10. Weilbacher D, Bolin JA, Hearn D, et al. Intussusception in adults: Review of 160 cases. *Am J Surg.* 1971;121:531.
11. Luks FI, Yazbeck S, Perreault G, et al. Changes in the presentation of intussusception. *Am J Emerg Med.* 1992; 10:574.
12. Losek JD. Intussusception and the diagnostic value of testing stool for occult blood. *Am J Emerg Med.* 1991;9:1.
13. Stringer MD, Pablot SM, Brereton RJ. Paediatric intussusception. *Br J Surg.* 1992;79:867.
14. Hernandez JA. Validity of plain films in intussusception. *Emerg Radiol.* 2004;10:323.
15. Grainger R, Allison D, Andreas A, et al (eds.). *Grainger and Allison's Diagnostic Radiology: A Textbook of Medical Imaging, 4th edn.* Churchill Livingstone Orlando, FL; 2001.

16. Koumanidou C, Vakaki M, Pitsoulakis G, et al. Sonographic detection of lymph nodes in the intussusception of infants and children: Clinical evaluation and hydrostatic reduction. *AJR Am J Roentgenol.* 2002;178:455.

17. Ferzoco L, Raptopoulous V, Silen W. Acute diverticulitis. *N Engl J Med.* 1998;338:1521.

18. Hadidi AT. Childhood intussusception: A comparative study of nonsurgical management. *J Pediatr Surg.* 1999;34:304.

19. Nagorney MD, Sarr M, McIlrath DC. Surgical management of intussusception in the adult. *Ann Surg.* 1981;1903:230.

20. Haas E, Etter E, Ellis S, et al. Adult intussusception. *Am J Surg.* 2003;186:75.

35

Malrotation and Volvulus in Infants

David Magilner

HIGH YIELD FACTS

- Bilious emesis in the first year of life should always be considered a surgical emergency until proven otherwise because it may be the only sign of volvulus.
- Eighty percent of patients who have malrotation present in the first month of life.
- Plain films of the abdomen are usually normal in patients with malrotation. An upper gastrointestinal (UGI) study is the preferred method to diagnose malrotation.

"Malrotation" refers to any congenital defect in the rotation or fixation of the intestines anywhere from the stomach to the descending colon. Malrotation may be asymptomatic. "Volvulus" may be the result of malrotation; it refers to an abnormal twisting of a hollow viscus that leads to obstruction.

EPIDEMIOLOGY

Because it may be asymptomatic throughout a lifetime, the exact incidence of malrotation is not known. It is thought that malrotation occurs in 1 in 500 live births.[1] Although malrotation can become symptomatic at any age, 80% of cases of malrotation present in the first month of life, and 50% present in the first week of life.[1] Males and females are equally affected. Of those children in whom diagnosis is delayed beyond the first month of life, diagnosis is delayed an average of 1.7 years.[2] At surgery, 25% to 50% of symptomatic pediatric patients with malrotation are found to have volvulus.[3,4]

PATHOPHYSIOLOGY

Malrotation results from the failure of normal progression of the embryonic development of the intestinal tract, a brief discussion of which is given here. Although there is a continuous progression of growth and rotation

that results in formation of the c-loop of the duodenum, development is traditionally broken down into three distinct stages. In the first stage (5 to 10 weeks), the intestines (then called the "midgut") herniate through the umbilicus in order to facilitate their growth. As they grow longer, there is a 90-degree counterclockwise rotation around the superior mesenteric artery (SMA) followed by a 90-degree bend posteriorly and inferiorly.

In the second stage, from 10 to 12 weeks, the gut regresses back into the abdominal cavity, proximal portion first, and there is a final 90-degree rotation at the duodenal-jejunal junction, which results in the duodenum crossing posterior to the SMA and coursing back toward the left upper quadrant. This is followed by regression of the distal portion of the gut, which rotates 180 degrees upward and results in the typical configuration of the large intestine.

The third stage of embryonic development is characterized by further growth of the intestine, and, more importantly, by fixation of various portions of the GI tract. The duodenum is fixed to the retroperitoneum. The ligament of Treitz, a fibrous band extending from the crux of the right hemidiaphragm, fixes the duodenal-jejunal junction. The ascending, descending, and sigmoid portions of the colon are fixed to the retroperitoneum, and the transverse colon is attached to the greater omentum. The transverse and sigmoid colon also have mesenteries to keep them fixed. The remainder of the small bowel is attached by a broad mesentery that extends from the duodenal-jejunal junction to the cecum.

Malrotation refers to the failure of any of the above steps in the normal embryonic development of the intestinal tract. This can result in a wide array of abnormalities and configurations of the intestines, all of which have in common a variable decrease in the mesenteric attachment of the small bowel. Without this attachment, the cecum usually "floats" toward the right upper quadrant. More importantly, the midgut is also poorly fixed, and this may lead to characteristic twisting of volvulus. A drawing of malrotation immediately prior to surgical correction is seen in Figure 35-1. Volvulus then leads to intestinal obstruction and disruption of the blood supply, which may lead rapidly to intestinal necrosis, shock, and death. Malrotation may also be complicated by the presence of fibrous bands, known as Ladd bands, which extend from the cecum or ascending colon to the retroperitoneum in the right upper quadrant. These bands may cause a partial or complete obstruction of the duodenum as they pass across it. Ladd bands are present in approximately 60% of patients with malrotation.[5] Malrotation is most often idiopathic, but may occur in with eating, failure to thrive (thought to be due to venous compression and subsequent malabsorption), chronic diarrhea, and intermittent vomiting.[2,4]

Radiologic evaluation is indicated in all patients with suspected malrotation with or without volvulus. Evaluation usually starts with plain radiographic images of the abdomen (Figure 35-2). It is important to remember that plain films are usually normal in cases of malrotation[7]; these are done to rule out other causes of the patient's symptoms. Although a contrast enema may be considered, this study will be normal in 25% of patients with malrotation.[4] Therefore, a UGI series with barium or water-soluble contrast is the study of choice to make the diagnosis (Figure 35-3). This test is 95% sensitive in making the diagnosis but may occasionally give a false positive result.[5] If the UGI series is inconclusive, computed tomography (CT) may be helpful. Ultrasound (US) has also been reported to be sensitive for making the diagnosis of malrotation. On US, a "whirlpool" appearance of the duodenum around the SMA has been described.[8] At this point, there is insufficient evidence to recommend

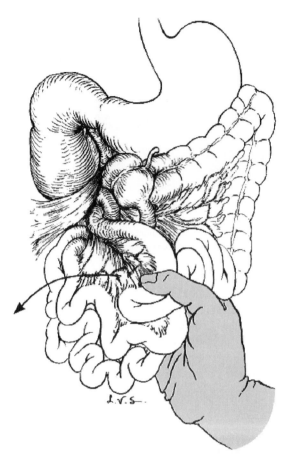

Fig. 35-1. Malrotation. This drawing illustrates malrotation immediately prior to surgical derotation and fixation. Used with permission from Albaese CT, Sylvester KG, Pediatric surgery, in *current surgery,* Doherty GM, Way LW, (eds.), Fig. 45-11. New York, Mcgraw-Hill, 2006,

association with other congenital abnormalities, including congenital diaphragmatic hernia and asplenia syndromes.

CLINICAL FEATURES

Intestinal malrotation may be asymptomatic, or it can present with a variety of signs and symptoms. In all ages, bilious emesis is the cardinal symptom. This symptom occurs in approximately 95% of patients.[3,6] In neonates, other common symptoms include constipation (89% of patients) or blood in the stool. If volvulus has occurred, additional symptoms may include abdominal distension, fussiness, lethargy, fever, and shock. In children past the neonatal period, symptoms may be less obvious and may include intermittent abdominal pain, pain associated

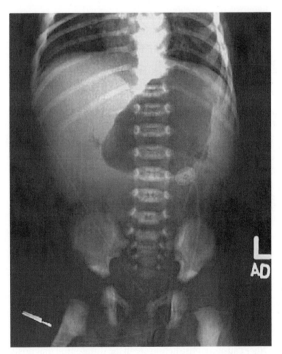

Fig. 35-2. Malrotation; Abdominal plain film. Abdominal x-ray of a 10-day-old infant with bilious emesis. Note the dilated proximal bowel and the paucity of distal bowel gas, characteristic of a volvulus. Schwartz's Principles of surgery, 8th ed., Brunicardi FC, Anderson DK, Pollack RE, et al. (eds.). Fig. 38-16. New York, Mcgraw-Hill, 2005.

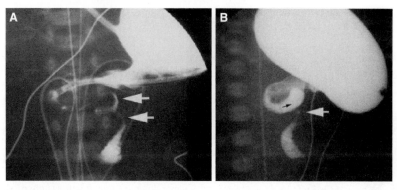

Fig. 35-3. Malrotation; Upper GI Malrotation with volvulus: 1-day-old with bilious vomiting and abdominal distension. **A.** A UGI, anteroposterior projection. Barium opacifies a downward, narrow, "corkscrew" course of the distal duodenum and proximal jejunum (arrows). **B.** Upper GI, lateral projection. The "corkscrew" pattern is again seen (white arrow). Note the anterior course of the distal duodenum (black arrow).

ultrasound over a UGI series; however, when performing US to rule out other diseases (i.e., pyloric stenosis) the diagnosis of malrotation may be suspected.

DIAGNOSIS AND DIFFERENTIAL

The diagnosis of malrotation should be suspected in all neonates with bilious vomiting or in patients with more subtle clinical presentations discussed above. The diagnosis is confirmed by the appropriate radiologic studies. In any ill-appearing patient in whom the diagnosis of volvulus is suspected, laboratory tests such as a complete white count, electrolytes, and an arterial blood gas may help assess the severity of illness.

In the neonatal period, the differential diagnosis of malrotation includes all causes of vomiting and obstruction. The most common alternate diagnoses to be considered include pyloric stenosis and gastroesophageal reflux disease (GERD). Classically, these latter diagnoses present with nonbilious emesis, but both can present with bilious emesis as well. Pyloric stenosis tends to present after one month of age, whereas the majority of patients with malrotation present before that time. Upper GI studies can distinguish among these diagnoses; ultrasonography can confirm the diagnosis of pyloric stenosis. Other causes or obstruction are in the differential diagnosis as well; if Ladd bands are present and cause duodenal obstruction, malrotation can exactly mimic duodenal atresia. A classic "double-bubble" sign may be present on plain x-rays of the abdomen in both of these instances. Toxic megacolon can present with vomiting

and constipation. Upper and lower GI contrast studies should allow its differentiation from malrotation.

In older children, malrotation should be considered in the differential diagnoses of "functional" abdominal pain syndromes and cyclic vomiting. Again, UGI studies should confirm the diagnosis; these exams can be deferred to an outpatient setting if symptoms are chronic and non-emergent.

EMERGENCY DEPARTMENT CARE AND DISPOSITION

Patients who present in severe distress and are suspected to have dead bowel may require airway management and vigorous fluid resuscitation. In the less acute patient with malrotation, intravenous fluids are usually required. When volvulus is suspected, surgical consultation or transfer to an appropriate facility should not be delayed while waiting for laboratory and radiologic tests to be completed. In the rare older child where malrotation is found incidentally or as a suspected cause for chronic symptoms, patients may be discharged to home with appropriate referral for close follow-up.

PITFALLS

- Neonates with malrotation and volvulus may not appear ill. Bilious emesis may be the only sign.

- Do not rely on plain x-rays or contrast enema. These may be normal in cases of malrotation. Upper GI is mandatory for any stable patient with suspected malrotation.

- Do not delay pediatric surgical referral or consultation while waiting for x-rays or lab tests in a patient with suspected volvulus.

REFERENCES

1. Torres AM, Ziegler MM. Malrotation of the intestine. *World J Surg.* 1993;17:326.
2. Spigland N, Brandt ML, Yazbeck S. Malrotation presenting beyond the neonatal period. *J Pediatr Surg.* 1990;25:1139–.
3. Lin JN, Lou CC, Wang KL. Intestinal malrotation and midgut volvulus: A 15-year review. *J Formos Med Assoc.* 1995;94:178.
4. Prasil P, Flageole H, Shaw KS, et al. Should malrotation in children be treated differently according to age? *J Pediatr Surg.* 2000;35:756.
5. Dilley AV, Pereira J et al. The radiologist says malrotation: Does the surgeon operate? *Ped Surg Int.* 2000;16:45–49.
6. Bonadio WA, Clarkson T, Naus J. The clinical features of children with malrotation of the intestine. *Ped Emerg Care.* 1991;7:348.
7. Berdon WE, Baker DH, Bull S, et al. Midgut malrotation and volvulus: which films are most helpful? *Radiology.* 1970;96:375.
8. Patino M, Munden M. Utility of the sonographic whirlpool sign in diagnosing midgut volvulus in patients with atypical clinical presentations. *J Ultrasound Med.* 2004;23:397.

36

Henoch-Schönlein Purpura

Douglas K. Holtzman

HIGH YIELD FACTS

- The cutaneous purpuric lesions of Henoch-Schönlein purpura (HSP) are 2 to 10 mm in diameter, are concentrated on the legs and buttocks, and may be preceded by urticarial lesions.

- Other manifestations of HSP include arthritis, which is typically polyarticular, abdominal pain, occult and gross gastrointestinal (GI) bleeding, intussusception, orchitis, and renal involvement; all nondermatologic symptoms may precede the purpura.

- Average age at presentation is 6 years, but HSP has occurred in patients as young as 6 months of age and up to 86 years old.

- Therapy is controversial and while no prospective controlled studies have been done, corticosteroids are effective in treating the arthritis and abdominal pain of HSP.

- The disease may recur multiple times in up to one half of patients, and long-term prognosis is dependent on the presence and severity of nephritis.

EPIDEMIOLOGY

Henoch-Schönlein purpura has been noted in patients as young as 6 months and up to 86 years of age. The mean age at presentation is 6 years with 75% of patients ≤8 years and 90% ≤10 years of age.[1] The mean age for adults is 50 years.[2] Clinical features may be atypical in age extremes such that infants less than 2 years tend to have milder disease and adults have more severe symptoms and have more numerous recurrences with a longer duration of illness.[3]

Henoch-Schönlein purpura typically presents in the fall or winter months and may follow an upper respiratory infection. Multiple pathogens have been speculated including group A beta-hemolytic streptococcus, but no single pathogen has been identified.[3]

Incidence of HSP in children is approximately 10 cases per 100,000 children per year.[1,2] In adults, the incidence is 10 cases per 1 million per year. The male:female ratio is 2:1 in children and 1:1 in adults. Henoch-Schönlein purpura is found in a wide geographic and ethnic distribution but is relatively uncommon in people of African descent.[4]

PATHOPHYSIOLOGY

Henoch-Schönlein was once referred to as an "anaphylactoid purpura" because of the initial appearance of an urticarial rash, which was followed by palpable purpura. Henoch-Schönlein purpura is now known to be a leukocytoclastic process involving granular deposits of IgA, C3, and fibrin.[4] The antigens implicated in this process are numerous and include: upper respiratory infections, measles, parvovirus B19, streptococcus, vancomycin, enalapril, leukemias, breast cancer, small cell lung cancer, and others.[5] Henoch-Schönlein purpura presenting in adults should especially alert the clinician to search for malignancy, systemic necrotizing vasculitis, or connective tissue disease as it is often the first manifestation.[6]

The associated renal disease ranges from minimal change, focal or diffuse mesangial proliferation, and crescentic glomerulonephritis. The histopathology is indistinguishable from IgA nephropathy.[4] There is evidence to suggest the two diseases may be pathogenetically linked.[5] Current research is focusing on abnormalities involving the glycosylation of the hinge region of IgA1.[3]

Although HSP has been recognized as a distinct entity for nearly 200 years, its true cause and pathogenesis remain unknown.

CLINICAL FEATURES

In 1837, Johann Schönlein described an association of arthralgia and purpura. His former student, Eduard Henoch noted GI involvement with these patients in 1874, and noted that renal involvement was an important component in 1899.[1] It is typically a disease of childhood but may occur in adults. In 90% of patients, there is evidence of an infection and/or fever either prior to or at onset of symptoms.[7] Associated symptoms may precede the purpura often leading to extensive workups and delayed diagnosis. Arthritis may occur 1 to 2 weeks before the rash in 20% of cases. Nephritis rarely precedes the purpura and may in fact be delayed for weeks to months.[2]

The dominant clinical features are: purpura (100%), arthritis (75%), abdominal pain (65%), occult and gross

GI bleeding (35%), and nephritis (40%).[2] The cutaneous purpura, 2 to 10 mm in diameter and concentrated in crops on the legs and buttocks is the sine qua non of HSP (Figure 36-1). It is often preceded by a rash that is urticarial or maculopapular in nature. The rash is variable in age extremes with facial edema being common in children younger than 1 year and presenting as bullous or necrotic skin lesions in 60% of adults.[4] In 10% of patients, the lower extremities are not involved. The purpura tends to resolve with bed rest, but recurs when the patient resumes ambulation. Arthritis is the second most common finding. The knees and ankles are typically involved. The arthritis is typically acutely incapacitating but is self-limited.

Colicky abdominal pain and vomiting are the most frequent GI complaints. Occult GI bleeding is seen in approximately 25% of patients and gross bleeding in 10%.[2] Gastrointestinal bleeding does not appear to occur in the absence of abdominal pain.[1] Intussusception is the

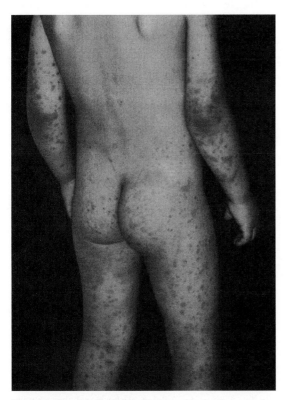

Fig. 36-1. Henoch–Schönlein Purpura. Used with permission se from Knoop KJ, Stack LB, Storrow AB. *Atlas of Emergency Medicine.* 2nd ed. McGraw-Hill. 381.

most common surgical complication. The overall incidence is 3.5% with ranges reported from 1.3 to 13.6%. Katz et al. found 8% of the children they studied had a serious potentially life-threatening GI complication.[8] The average age is 6 years, thus distinguishing it from idiopathic intussusception. The other differentiation is 70% of HSP intussusceptions are ileoileal. The jejunum is involved in approximately 7% of cases and there are reports of colocolic intussusception.[9] Mural edema and hemorrhage in the small bowel are thought to serve as lead points for the intussusception.

Nephritis is the typical renal manifestation of HSP. Microscopic hematuria in 60% of patients has been reported. No cases of hematuria were seen prior to the onset of other HSP symptoms.[7] Approximately 75% of patients will manifest nephritis within 4 weeks of purpura presentation and 95% occur within 3 months of presentation.[2] Most children recover from the nephritis; however, 2% to 10% will progress to renal failure. While most children recover, 40% of adults have persistent hematuria and 10% of them progress to chronic renal failure. On average, chronic renal failure is seen in 18% of children and 28% of adults with HSP.[6]

In males, scrotal and glans edema and hemorrhage are seen. Orchitis is seen and frequently mistaken as a possible testicular torsion. Central nervous system symptoms include headache, irritability, altered mental status, seizures, and ataxia. These are commonly seen but are frequently under reported. Other such complications include myocarditis, myocardial infarction, plural effusions, and pulmonary hemorrhage.

Henoch-Schönlein purpura typically lasts 4 weeks with ranges of 1 to 3 days to 2 years reported.[7] Up to one half will have recurrences. The symptoms, typically the purpura and abdominal pain, are similar but usually milder and shorter. The average onset is 2 months after the initial resolution of symptoms. The average number of recurrences is 2.[4]

DIAGNOSIS AND DIFFERENTIAL

In 1992, Michel et al.,[10] using the American College of Rheumatology's data comparing hypersensitivity vasculitis and HSP established criteria for identifying HSP. The presence of three of more of the following criteria yields a correct classification in 87% of the cases. The criteria are: (1) palpable purpura, (2) bowel angina, (3) GI bleeding, (4) hematuria, (5) age at onset ≤20 years, and (6) no medications.

Laboratory evaluation typically includes a complete blood count (CBC), urinalysis (UA), and creatinine (CR).

The white blood cell (WBC) count is typically normal or shows a modest leukocytosis. Hemoglobin and hematocrit are utilized for a baseline reference or may demonstrate anemia with the presence of GI bleeding. Other laboratory evaluations to consider include fibrin split products (may be elevated), fibrinogen (decreased levels), and factor XIII. Studies have found an association between HSP and decreased concentrations of factor XIII as one of the risk factors for the progression of renal involvement.[11] Also in a recent study, Brendel-Muller et al. found elevated D-dimer levels without evidence of disseminated intravascular coagulopathy.[12] Of the HSP patients, 50% had D-dimer values ≥10 times normal range and levels correlated well with disease activity.[12]

Radiography studies are primarily done to evaluate GI complications. Plain abdominal x-rays are nonspecific and may show signs of obstruction. Ultrasound is the study of choice for intussusceptions involving small bowel only. Barium enema is used to diagnose and potentially treat ileocolic intussusception.[8]

In infants ≤2 years, the differential for HSP includes acute hemorrhagic edema (Finkelsteins disease). Infants with acute hemorrhagic edema present with ecchymotic lesions of the limbs and trunk, edema of head and limbs, and a leukocytoclastic vasculitis of dermal vessels. The difference is that it occurs without IgA deposits.

Other diagnoses to consider include clotting disorders, infectious diseases (syphilis, rickettsia, meningococcemia, Epstein-Barr virus), lupus, rheumatoid arthritis, and drug-induced hypersensitivity vasculitides.

EMERGENCY DEPARTMENT CARE AND DISPOSITION

Treatment of HSP remains controversial and is linked primarily to supportive measures. Acetaminophen is preferred, as nonsteroidal anti-inflammatory drugs or acetylsalicyclic acid (ASA) may exacerbate GI symptoms. Ranitidine is effective for moderate GI involvement.

The use of corticosteroids continues to be debated. Most agree that their use has beneficial effects on abdominal pain, articular involvement, subcutaneous edema, and scrotal involvement.[4,7,13] The typical dose of oral prednisone used is 1 mg/kg/day × 1 to 2 weeks. While debate continues about the prevention of nephritis, several studies have found corticosteroids beneficial. Mollica et al. noted that of patients treated with prednisone 0 of 84 developed nephritis compared to control patients, of whom 10 of 84 developed nephritis.[14]

Kaku et al. found corticosteroids decreased the risk of renal involvement independently, and recommended their use in patients with the risk factors of severe abdominal pain, persistent purpura, decreased factor XIII activity, or any patient older than 7 years.[11]

Other therapies such as the use of IVIG, plasmaphoresis, dapsone, administration of factor XIII, or high dose methylprednisolone combined with immunosuppressive agents remain investigational.

Because nephritis can occur weeks to months after the initial presentation, all HSP patients should have careful, long-term follow up. It is recommended that a urinalysis (UA) be performed at least every 7 days while the disease is active and if there remains no evidence of nephritis, a UA once a month for 3 months.[1] Women with a history of HSP nephritis as children should be closely monitored during pregnancy as they may develop renal complications.

PITFALLS

- The presenting rash is often urticarial in appearance, thus HSP may be mistaken as an allergic reaction or a drug eruption.
- Abdominal pain with or without GI bleeding often occurs prior to the rash and is confused with acute appendicitis, intussusception, or inflammatory bowel disease.
- Orchitis may be confused with testicular torsion.
- Arthritis may also occur prior to the rash, thus confusing the practitioner.
- Failing to warn patients/parents that hematuria may follow the rash and should prompt seeking medical reevaluation.

REFERENCES

1. Saulsbury FT. Henoch-Schönlein purpura in children report of 100 patients and review of the literature. *Medicine.* 1999;78:395.
2. Saulsbury FT. Epidemiology of Henoch-Schönlein purpura. *Cleve Clin J Med.* 2000;69:87.
3. Saulsbury FT. Henoch-Schönlein purpura. *Curr Opin Rheumatol.* 2001;13:35.
4. Sells LL, Mihalov LK, Mellick LB. Approaching the child with a vasculitis: Piecing together an accurate diagnosis. *Ped Emerg Med Reports.*2003;8:1.
5. Rai A, Nast C, Adler S. Henoch-Schönlein purpura nephritis. *J Am Soc Nephrol.* 1999;10:2637.

6. Ilan Y, Naparstek Y. Henoch-Schönlein purpura in children and adults: It is one entity? *Semin Arthritis Rheum.* 2002; 32:139.

7. Allen DM, Diamond LK, Howell DA. Anaphylactoid purpura in children (Schönlein-Henoch syndrome). *Am J Dis Child.* 1960;99:833.

8. Katz S, Borst M, Seekri I, et al. Surgical evaluation of Henoch-Schönlein purpura. *Arch Surg.* 1991;126:849.

9. Choong CK, Kimble RM, Pease P, et al. Colo-colic intus-susception in Henoch-Schönlein purpura. *Pediatric Surg Int.* 1998;14:173.

10. Michel BA, Hunder GG, Block DA, et al. Hypersensitivity vasculitis and Henoch-Schönlein purpura: A comparison between the two disorders. *J Rheumatol.* 1992;19:721.

11. Kaku Y, Nohara K, Honda S. Renal involvement in Henoch-Schönlein purpura: A multivariate analysis of prognostic factors. *Kidney Int.* 1998;53:1755.

12. Brendel-Müller K, Hahn A. Schneppenheim R, et al. Laboratory signs of activated coagulation are common in Henoch-Schönlein purpura. *Pediatr Nephrol.* 2001;16: 1084.

13. Rostoker G. Schönlein-Henoch purpura in children and adults. *BioDrugs.* 2001;15:99.

14. Mollica F, LiVolti S, Garozzo R, et al. Effectiveness of early prednisone treatment in preventing the development of nephropathy in anaphylactoid purpura. *Eur J Pediatr.* 1992; 151:140.

37

Colic in Infants

Kim Askew
Milan Nadkarni

HIGH YIELD FACTS

- Despite years of research, no true etiology or treatment of colic has been identified.
- Colic is defined by Wessel criteria of crying for more than 3 hours a day, 3 or more days a week, for more than 3 weeks.
- Colic remains one of the leading causes for health care visits in infants less than 3 months of age.
- Parents often feel anxious and overwhelmed when caring for a child with colic, requiring the physician to reassure parents while caring for the child.

EPIDEMIOLOGY

Colic in infants remains an area with little understanding of etiology and pathophysiology despite many hours of research and treatment by clinicians and parents alike. Suggested etiologies include gastrointestinal (GI), psychosocial, and developmental causes. First described by Wessel in the early 1950s, colic is defined as excessive, inconsolable crying for 3 hours or more per day, for 3 or more days a week, persisting for at least 3 weeks in an otherwise normal, healthy infant.[1] The incidence of colic is between 9% and 30%, depending on the definition of colic and the study mechanism. However, colic appears to be the second most common GI presentation in neonates after reflux, causing 1 in 6 families to seek medical attention.[2,3]

PATHOPHYSIOLOGY

The first proposed theory of colic's origin lies in the GI tract. Investigators suggested that a patient's allergy to cow's milk/protein initiated the symptoms of colic.[4–6] Others have suggested increased peristalsis, increased gas formation, or lactose intolerance as the cause of colic.[4–6] However, treatment modalities based on these theories have shown limited benefit. Introducing a nonallergenic diet in select patients has shown benefit,[7,8] but other studies looking at medication treatment have shown little to no effect, leading others to propose non-GI causes.[4,5,7]

The second proposed theory of colic's origin is based on a psychosocial/behavioral model. Proponents of this model have suggested that there is a higher frequency of colicky children from parents with higher education, with nonmanual labor jobs, and older maternal age at first gestation.[8] Others have suggested a poor parent-child interaction, sometimes as a result of a difficult temperament of the infant, as a causative agent for colic. However, studies have shown no correlation between a parent's anxiety and the presence of colic.[5] Studies investigating parental behavior modification (increased carrying times, avoidance of overstimulation, etc.) have shown mixed results, with the majority demonstrating no improvement in symptoms when compared to no interaction or simply educating parents about colic.[3,4,7]

The third proposed theory of colic concerns child development. According to this theory, colic is a manifestation of the child's emotional development. Data supporting this theory show that children with colic have the same crying patterns as noncolicky children, but the episodes are of longer duration.[5,9] Also, children with colic have been shown to respond to some of the same regulators of crying (i.e., feeding) as children without colic, but shortened response durations.[9] Therefore, a child with colic may just be the normal progression of the child's emotional development. Other investigators have pointed to maternal smoking during pregnancy as a potential associated cause, but further research is needed to control for the effect of delivery associated variables that also may affect the frequency of observed colic.[10,11]

CLINICAL FEATURES

A child with colic typically develops symptoms around 2 weeks of life and resolves by the 4th to 5th month of life. The crying episodes usually occur in the late afternoon and evening hours,[1] and are unpredictable and unrelated to surrounding environmental triggers. The episodes do not respond to soothing techniques by parents or other care providers. The child may have associated symptoms such as clenched fists, flexed legs over the abdomen, arching back, flushing, flatus, and a hard distended abdomen.[1,6] When not crying, the child does not look ill, and otherwise has completely normal function. The child interacts with caretakers normally outside of these episodes, grows well, and meets all developmental milestones.

DIAGNOSIS AND DIFFERENTIAL

The diagnosis of colic is a diagnosis of exclusion. No confirmatory tests exist for the diagnosis of colic. Therefore, the physician should consider and rule out the organic causes of excessive crying in infants (Table 37-1). The physical exam and history provide clues to the diagnosis of colic, as well as the exclusion of other diagnoses. The physician must do a head to toe exam of the undressed child to look for signs of organic pathology. Exam findings to investigate include poor skin perfusion, lethargy, poor muscle tone, presence of corneal abrasions or hair tourniquets, etc. Vital signs should be within normal range for a child with colic. A colicky child should be gaining weight despite the fact that feeding does not quiet the colic episodes and should otherwise appear healthy.

EMERGENCY DEPARTMENT CARE AND DISPOSITION

After a thorough examination of the child and historical findings to rule out more serious causes of excessive crying, the physician's most important responsibility is acknowledging the parent's difficulty with the child. The physician should be supportive. The physician must also inquire into the parent's emotional status, due to the fact that excessive crying of an infant is a risk factor for child abuse.

Parents and physicians alike have investigated numerous techniques and treatments for the child with colic based on the described theories of origin. However, not one treatment has been found to be the cure for colic. Regarding the GI theory, a hypoallergenic diet has been suggested for the breast-feeding mother or the bottle-fed

Table 37-1. Differential Diagnosis of Colic

Corneal abrasion
Hair tourniquet
Child abuse
Subdural hematoma
Constipation
Gastroesophageal reflux
Protein intolerance
Urinary tract infection
Fracture
CNS malformation
Sepsis
Otitis media
Meningitis

Abbreviation: CNS, central nervous system.

child. A recent metaanalysis showed a beneficial effect of a hypoallergenic diet; however, this may not work in all children and may be unacceptable to the breast-feeding mother.[3,4,7,8] The same therapeutic effect was not seen in soy or low lactose diets as with hypoallergenic diets, and the American Association of Pediatrics does not recommend changing to soy formula for a child with colic.[3,4,7,12] One randomized controlled trial showed a benefit of using whey hydrolysate formula in the child with colic.[13] Therefore, diet change may be useful in the child with colic if signs and symptoms support a potential allergy. Several medications have been used to treat colic. Simethicone has not been shown to be effective for treatment of colic.[3,4,7] Dicyclomine has been shown to be effective for the treatment of excessive crying; however, reports of apnea and other adverse events have resulted in the manufacturer's recommendation to stop using the medication for the treatment of colic.[3-5,7]

Regarding the psychosocial/behavioral theory, several treatments have been investigated. Trials have shown that carrying an infant, soothing techniques, car riding, vibration, and avoidance of overstimulation were no more beneficial than educating the parents about the colic.[3-5,7] Therefore, general education and support of the parents are indicated in all instances.

Colic has no long-term associated morbidity. Symptoms usually resolve by 4 to 5 months of age. However, the associated anxiety that families feel with the excessively crying infant is enormous. Therefore, after truly identifying the child with colic, the primary goal is to help reduce family anxiety and prevent further degradation of the parent-child relationship.

PITFALLS

- The physician fails to consider other causes of excessive crying other than colic.

- The physician fails to perform a complete exam looking for other causes of excessive crying.

- The physician fails to discuss the characteristics of colic with parents and does not address their thoughts of anxiety or fears of being poor parents.

REFERENCES

1. Wessel MA, Cobb JC, Jackson EB, et al. Paroxsymal fussing in infancy, sometimes called colic. *Pediatrics.* 1954;14:421.
2. Iacono G, Merolla R, D'Amico D, et al. Gastrointestinal symptoms in infancy: A population-based prospective study. *Dig Liver Dis.* 2005;37:432.

3. Wade S, Kilgour T. Infantile colic. *BMJ.* 2001;323:437.

4. Lucassen PLBJ, Assendelft WJJ, Gubbels JW. Effectiveness of treatments for infantile colic: A systematic review. *BMJ.* 1998;316:1563.

5. Roberts, DM Ostapchuk M, O'Brien J. Infantile colic. *Am Fam Physician.* 2004;70:735.

6. Reasi C, Blake RL. Diagnostic work-up before diagnosing colic. *Arch Fam Med.* 2000;9:282.

7. Garrison MM, Christakis DA. Early childhood: Colic, child development, and poisoning prevention. *Pediatrics.* 2000; 106:184.

8. Hill DJ, Roy N, Heine RG, et al. Effect of a low-allergen maternal diet on colic among breastfed infants: a randomized, controlled trial. *Pediatrics.* 2005;116:e709.

9. Barr RG. Colic and crying syndromes in infants. *Pediatrics.* 1998;102:1282.

10. St James-Roberts I, Conroy S. Do pregnancy and childbirth adversities predict infant crying and colic? Findings and recommendations. *Neurosci Biobehav Rev.* 2005;29:313.

11. Shenassa ED, Brown MJ. Maternal smoking and infantile gastrointestinal dysregulation: the case of colic. *Pediatrics.* 2004;114:e497.

12. AAP Committee on Nutrition. American Academy of Pediatrics. Committee on Nutrition. Soy protein-based formulas: recommendations of use in infant feeding. *Pediatrics.* 1998;101:148.

13. Lucassen PLBJ, Assendelft WJJ, Gubbels JW, et al. Infantile colic: Crying time reduction with a whey hydrolysate: A double-blind randomized placebo-controlled trial. *Pediatrics.* 2000;106:1349.

38

Pyloric Stenosis

David Magilner

HIGH YIELD FACTS

- Ninety-five per cent of cases occur between 3 and 12 weeks of age, and boys are affected 4 times more often than girls.
- A palpable "olive," dehydration, and classic electrolyte abnormalities are only seen late in the disease process.
- Ultrasound (US) has replaced upper gastrointestinal (UGI) x-rays as the study of choice for diagnosis.

EPIDEMIOLOGY

The overall incidence of hypertrophic pyloric stenosis (HPS) is 2 to 5 cases per 1000 live births.[1,2] Ninety-five per cent of cases present between 3 and 12 weeks of life,[3] but rare cases have presented as late as two years of age.[4] In all series, about 80% of cases occur in males.[3–6] Historically, it had been thought that first-born children are at significantly increased risk; however, first born children only seem to have a very slight predilection for HPS,[3,4] and the majority of cases do not occur in first-born children.[7] White and Hispanic infants are about three times more likely as Black and Asian infants to have the condition.[5] There is a strong familial predisposition to HPS. If the mother had HPS, an infant's risk increases approximately 100-fold; this statistic is approximately 20-fold if the infant's father had HPS.[6] The mean time from the onset of vomiting to diagnosis is 8 days[3]; this has decreased from 12 days over the course of the past 35 years.[8]

PATHOPHYSIOLOGY

The cause of HPS, hypertrophy, and stenosis of the pylorus leading to gastric outlet obstruction remains unknown. Recently, it has been found that there are multiple histological and biochemical abnormalities of the pylorus in infants with HPS, the most important of which seems to be inadequate enervation of the muscular layer of the pylorus.[9] It has been hypothesized that inadequate enervation leads to an increase in local growth factors and subsequent hypertrophy and stenosis.[10] It is unclear, however, whether these findings indicate a cause or a result of gastric outlet obstruction. Since the disease is not present at the time of birth, it is hypothesized that stimuli which are present after birth may lead to HPS in genetically predisposed infants. Recently, an increase in HPS has been noted in infants given erythromycin; it is hypothesized that the effects of this drug on gastric motility may lead to pyloric hypertrophy and stenosis.[11]

CLINICAL FEATURES

The diagnosis of HPS should be considered in any patient who presents with nonbilious vomiting in the first 3 months of life. Typically, the vomiting is initially noted to be mild in volume, force, and frequency; it may then progress in all of these aspects to the point where there is voluminous projectile vomiting after every feed. Because HPS is being diagnosed earlier in the course of illness,[8] projectile vomiting is present in only two thirds of patients at the time of diagnosis.[3] Vomiting is usually within 15 minutes of feeding. Patients typically continue to exhibit normal or even increased appetite, and, unless vomiting has progressed to the point where gastritis or esophagitis is present, there are no symptoms of pain associated with the condition.

Most infants with HPS appear well on physical examination, although, physical signs of dehydration should be assessed. Palpation of an "olive," a firm mass in the right epigastrium, is highly specific for the presence of HPS. In the past, this finding was reported to be present in up to 90% of patients with HPS.[3] However, in more recent studies, an olive was palpated in only 25% to 70% of patients.[8,9] This decline is attributed to the use of early radiologic studies (and diagnosis),[3] when the olive is smaller in size.[12] It has also been proposed that the clinician's ability to palpate the olive has declined as the ease of obtaining radiologic studies has increased.[13] Palpation of the olive may be facilitated by gastric decompression with a nasogastric tube or by calming the infant with a small sucrose feed.

DIAGNOSIS AND DIFFERENTIAL

Every patient with suspected or confirmed HPS should have laboratory evaluation of electrolytes. Electrolyte abnormalities may be present if there has been prolonged vomiting of stomach contents prior to diagnosis.

Classically, infants with HPS present with a hypochloremic, hypokalemic, metabolic alkalosis. Recent studies have shown that less than one quarter of patients have any electrolyte abnormalities on presentation.[14–16] Those with symptoms longer than one week or clinical signs of dehydration are most likely to have electrolyte abnormalities.[16] No other laboratory examinations have been found to be helpful.

In a patient with a typical presentation and a palpable olive on physical examination, the diagnosis of HPS can be made clinically and the patient should be referred for surgery. When HPS is suspected but an olive is not palpated, surgical consultation should be obtained if readily available. An experienced surgeon may palpate an olive and obviate the need for radiologic studies. If a surgeon is not readily available, a radiologic study should be obtained. Plain films of the abdomen may show an air-filled stomach with a paucity of gas distally (Figure 38-1). Historically, an UGI x-ray with swallowed barium has been the modality of choice (Figure 38-2). This study, when viewed in real time, has a sensitivity of 95%, but the error rate has been reported to be as high as 11%.[17] More recently, US has been used to make the diagnosis, and it has been reported to have a sensitivity and specificity approaching 100%. Pyloric stenosis is confirmed on US when the pyloric muscle width is 4 mm or greater or the length is 18 mm or greater[18] (Figure 38-3).

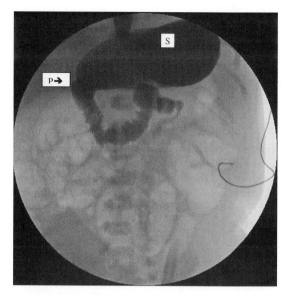

Fig. 38-2. Upper GI contrast study showing stomach (S) a thickened pylorus (P) and poor gastric emptying. (Courtesy of Dr. Craig Barnes.)

Ultrasound has the advantages of being faster than UGI, and it spares the infant exposure to radiation. Ultrasound, where available, has therefore replaced UGI as the study of choice when HPS is suspected.[19]

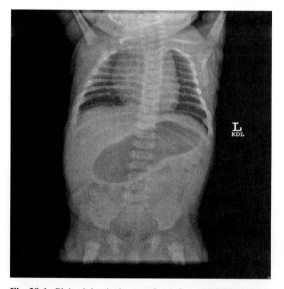

Fig. 38-1. Plain abdominal x-ray of an infant with HPS showing an air-filled stomach with a paucity of gas in the small and large intestines.

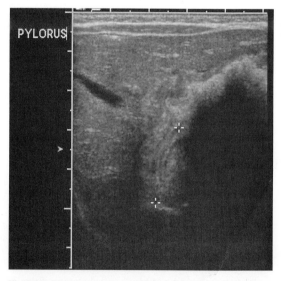

Fig. 38-3 Ultrasound image of HPS. A long, thickened pylorus is seen between the cursors. The length measured 20.1 mm. (Courtesy of Dr. Craig Barnes.)

The differential diagnosis of HPS includes all causes of vomiting early in life. Malrotation, with or without volvulus, usually presents earlier than HPS and has bilious emesis as its cardinal feature. In these patients, an UGI study is indicated if the patient is stable. If the infant presents early in the course of HPS, clinical features may mimic gastroesophageal reflux disease (GERD). In these infants, a trial of feeding under the observation of a clinician may be helpful. If vomiting is forceful and voluminous, further evaluation for HPS is warranted. If vomiting is mild and the child appears well, expectant observation is indicated. Reliable parents may observe the infant at home with careful instructions to return if symptoms progress.

EMERGENCY DEPARTMENT CARE AND DISPOSITION

The emergency clinician has two important tasks in the care of a patient with HPS. The first is accurate assessment and treatment of dehydration. Patients who present late in the course of illness may be significantly dehydrated and require fluid resuscitation. The second task is the accurate and timely diagnosis of the condition, as outlined above. If radiologic studies are not readily available, it may be appropriate to admit the patient to the hospital or observation unit overnight, ensure adequate hydration, and obtain ultrasonography as soon as it becomes available. All patients who are found to have HPS require surgical consultation for pyloromyotomy, a procedure which relaxes the pylorus using a small incision through the anterior pyloric wall to the layer of the submucosa (Figure 38-4). Once the diagnosis has been established, there is no urgency to surgical correction as long as adequate hydration is ensured.

PITFALLS

- Most patients with HPS appear well and lack any abnormalities on either physical or laboratory tests.

- Hypertrophic pyloric stenosis is an urgent but not an emergent condition; if the infant is adequately hydrated, diagnosis and surgery may be safely postponed as long as an appropriate plan is initiated.

- Patients who present with bilious emesis should be presumed to have a more serious condition than HPS.

REFERENCES

1. Applegate MS, Druschel CM. The epidemiology of infantile hypertrophic pyloricstenosis in New York State, 1983 to 1990. *Arch Pediatr Adolesc Med.* 1995;1491123.
2. Jedd M, Melton LJ, Griffin M, et al. Factors associated with infantile hypertrophic pyloric stenosis. *Am J Dis Child.* 1988;142:334.
3. Shaoul R, Enav B, Steiner Z, et al. Clinical presentation of pyloric stenosis: the change is in our hands. *Isr Med Assoc J.* 2004;6:134.
4. Reyna TM, Otero C, Weir MR. Epidemiological survey of 6 years' federal health service experience of pyloric stenosis: case report of presentation in a 26-month male. *Clin Pediatr (Phila).* 1987;26:412.
5. Schechter R, Torfs CP, Bateson TF. The epidemiology of infantile hypertrophic pyloric stenosis. *Paediatr Perinat Epidemiol.* 1997;11:407.
6. Carter CO, Evans KA. Inheritance of congenital pyloric stenosis. *J Med Genet.* 1969;6:233.
7. Okazaki T, Yamataka A, Fujiwara T, et al. Abnormal distribution of nerve terminals in infantile hypertrophic pyloric stenosis. *J Ped Surg.* 1994;29:655.
8. Hulka F, Campbell T, Campbell J, et al. Evolution in the recognition of infantile hypertrophic pyloric stenosis. *Pediatrics.* 1997;100:9.
9. Ohshiro K, Puri P. Increased insulin-like growth factor and platelet-derived growth factor system in the pyloric muscle in infantile hypertrophic pyloric stenosis. *J Pediatr Surg.* 1998;33:378.
10. Honein MA, Paulozzi LJ, Himelright IM, et al. Infantile hypertrophic pyloric stenosis after pertussis prophylaxis with erythromycin: a case review and cohort study. *Lancet.* 1999;354:2101.
11. White MC, Langer JC, Don S, DeBaun MR. Sensitivity and cost minimization analysis of radiology versus olive palpation for the diagnosis of hypertrophic pyloric stenosis. *J Pediatr Surg.* 1998;33:913.

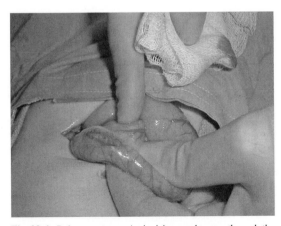

Fig. 38-4. Pyloromyotomy. An incision can be seen through the anterior wall of the thickened pylorus. (Courtesy of Dr. Thomas Pranikoff.)

12. Ozsvath R, Poustchi-Amin M, Leonidas J, et al. Pyloric volume: An important factor in the surgeon's ability to palpate the pyloric "olive" in hypertrophic pyloric stenosis. *Ped Rad.* 1997;27:175.

13. Macdessi J, Oates RK. Clinical diagnosis of pyloric stenosis: A declining art? *Br Med J.* 1993;306:553.

14. Bell MJ. Infantile pyloric stenosis: Experience with 305 cases at Louisville Children's Hospital. *Surgery.* 1968;64:983.

15. Touloukian RJ, Higgins E. The spectrum of serum electrolytes in hypertrophic pyloric stenosis. *J Pediatr Surg.* 1983;18:394.

16. Beasley SW, Hudson I, Yuen HP, et al. Influence of age, sex, duration of symptoms and dehydration on serum electrolytes in hypertrophic pyloric stenosis. *Aust Paediatr J.* 1986; 22:193.

17. Hernanz-Schulman M, Sells LL, Ambrosino MM, et al. Hypertrrophic pyloric stenosis in the infant without a palpable olive: Accuracy of sonographic diagnosis. *Radiology.* 1994;193:771.

18. Cohen HL, Zinn H, Haller J, et al. Ultrasonography of pylorospasm: Findings may simulate hypertrophic pyloric stenosis. *J Ultrasound Med.* 1998;17:705.

19. Hernanz-Schulman M. Infantile hypertrophic pyloric stenosis. *Radiology.* 2003;227:319.

39

Chronic Abdominal Pain

Alan Heins

The presentation of a patient with chronic abdominal pain is a particular challenge for the clinician in emergency, urgent, and primary care settings. First, the patient often describes acute, severe symptoms that suggest any number of the abdominal emergencies presented in other chapters of this book. Without a careful history, physical examination, and judicious diagnostic testing, the clinician may miss the positive diagnosis of a chronic abdominal pain syndrome and subject the patient to excessive, and potentially harmful, testing and interventions in search of an emergency condition that is not present. On the other hand, several serious and/or treatable conditions, such as inflammatory bowel disease, peptic ulcers, gastroesophageal reflux disease (GERD), and mesenteric ischemia, cause chronic or recurrent abdominal pain and may not be discovered if the clinician prematurely assumes that a more benign chronic pain condition exists when it does not. Finally, a patient with a known chronic pain syndrome may experience a new, acute emergency.

The focus of this chapter is to describe the clinical features and treatment options for some of the most common disorders causing chronic or recurrent abdominal pain, with emphasis on a systematic approach to history, physical examination, and diagnostic testing. After reading this chapter, the clinician will have a clearer understanding of chronic abdominal pain and be able to provide more accurate, compassionate, and cost-effective care to patients with these conditions.

HIGH YIELD FACTS

- Alarm symptoms and signs, including gastrointestinal (GI) bleeding, involuntary weight loss, protracted severe vomiting or diarrhea, family history of inflammatory bowel disease (IBD), localized tenderness, or other signs of organic disease, require investigation and are not likely to be due to a chronic, functional pain problem.

- The chronic abdominal pain syndromes are highly prevalent and result in billions of dollars in spending for medical care that is often unnecessary and not helpful in relieving symptoms, distress, and disability.

- Irritable bowel syndrome (IBS) is characterized by continuous or recurrent abdominal pain or discomfort, for at least 12 weeks in the past 12 months, that has two out of three of the following features: relieved by defecation, associated with change in frequency of stooling, or associated with change in consistency of stool.

- Functional constipation is characterized by no evidence of organic cause and by long-standing, symptomatic experience of abnormal defecation including two or more of the following features: straining, hard stools, sensation of incomplete evacuation, and/or two or fewer bowel movements in a week.

- In population-based studies of endometriosis, the prevalence in women is 6% to 10% and among women with pelvic pain and/or infertility, the prevalence approaches 35% to 50%.

EPIDEMIOLOGY

Patients with chronic abdominal pain syndromes often experience multiple symptoms in overlapping and variable combinations. In addition, the pathophysiologic basis of these conditions is far from clear and definitions and diagnostic terminology are inconsistent, adding to the difficulty of studying and understanding these illnesses. Only those conditions with the most consistent definitions and most extensive literature will be discussed here: recurrent abdominal pain in children, IBS, functional dyspepsia, constipation, and endometriosis. Estimates of prevalence of the various conditions are widely variable depending on the definition and population studied, but it is clear that women suffer much more frequently than men from the functional GI disorders and only women have endometriosis. Frequent health care-seeking behavior is described for a subset of patients with chronic abdominal pain.[1] Chronic pain patients in a large health maintenance organization suffered from more anxiety, depression, and somatization than nonpain patients.[2] No description of emergency department (ED) patients with chronic abdominal pain has been published, but an observational study of 2333 frequent ED users ($\geq$5 ED visits) found that 30.6% of the study patients presented to the ED with abdominal pain. In this study, no distinction between acute, recurrent, or chronic pain was made.[3]

RECURRENT ABDOMINAL PAIN (RAP) OF CHILDHOOD

Epidemiology

Childhood RAP is defined in most research by criteria of Apley and Naish from 1958, as $\geq$3 episodes of abdominal pain, over a period of $\geq$3 months, severe enough to affect activities.[4] This definition describes patients with both functional (meaning not associated with definite objective pathophysiologic correlates of symptoms) and organic disorders, though, in current usage, RAP refers to chronic functional abdominal pain, which is often more specifically diagnosed as functional dyspepsia, IBS, constipation, etc. A systematic review found the prevalence of RAP to range from 0.3% to 19% (median 8.4%: interquartile range 2.3% to 14.7%), with higher prevalence in females and peaks between 4 and 6 years and in early adolescence. Childhood RAP was also correlated with psychological comorbidity among children and as they become adults.[5] The American Academy of Pediatrics and the North American Society for Pediatric Gastroenterology, Hepatology and Nutrition conducted a comprehensive, systematic review of chronic abdominal pain in children and prepared a report on the relative value of clinical features, diagnostic tests, and specific therapies in the evaluation and management of these patients. A summary of these results is in Table 39-1.[6]

IRRITABLE BOWEL SYNDROME

Epidemiology

Irritable bowel syndrome is most commonly and reliably defined by the Rome II diagnostic criteria: characterized by continuous or recurrent abdominal pain or discomfort, for at least 12 weeks in the past 12 months, that has two out of three of the following features: relieved by defecation, associated with change in frequency of stooling, or associated with change in consistency of stool.[1] Exploring the epidemiology of IBS is difficult since most people with symptoms of IBS do not seek medical care, symptoms fluctuate over time, and multiple diagnostic criteria have been used. Incidence rates from population studies range from 0.2% to 6.6%, but higher numbers may include recurrence.[8,9] Prevalence of IBS has been estimated to range from 0.8% to 28%.[1] To add to

the difficulty in understanding IBS, sufferers frequently also have other chronic pain disorders, such as functional dyspepsia, fibromyalgia, chronic pelvic pain, interstitial cystitis, and temporomandibular joint disorder.[9,10] Clinical features, differential diagnosis and treatments are summarized in Table 39-1.

FUNCTIONAL DYSPEPSIA

Epidemiology

Functional dyspepsia is characterized by persistent or recurrent pain or discomfort centered in the upper abdomen, with no evidence of organic disease or typical gastroesophageal reflux symptoms, and not consistent with characteristics IBS. In this definition, discomfort is further described as a subjective negative feeling that is nonpainful and may incorporate a sense of fullness or early satiety. Upper abdominal symptoms are described by about 40 % of the population in a given 6-month period and account for about 50% of gastroenterologist's work load.[12] The prevalence of dyspepsia is about 25% if those with typical GERD symptoms are excluded and somewhat lower if all with any refluxlike symptoms are excluded. In addition, billions of dollars are spent annually on medications for dyspepsia and medical evaluation.[13] Clinical features, differential diagnosis, and treatments are included in Table 39-1.

FUNCTIONAL CONSTIPATION

Epidemiology

Functional constipation is characterized by no evidence of organic cause and by long-standing, symptomatic experience of abnormal defecation including two or more of the following features for at least 12 weeks out of the past 12 months: straining, hard stools, sensation of incomplete evacuation, and/or two or fewer bowel movements in a week.[1] Prevalence rates of self-reported constipation range from 20% to 27%, and it is more frequent with older age and female sex. Using Rome diagnostic criteria, the prevalence of functional constipation ranges from 3.0% to 16.7%. Clinical features, differential diagnosis, and treatments are described in Table 39-1. Also see Chapter 8.

ENDOMETRIOSIS

Epidemiology

Endometriosis is a chronic, estrogen-dependent disorder associated with deposits of endometrial tissue outside

Table 39-1. Summary of Common Chronic Abdominal Pain Syndromes

Disorder	Recurrent Abdominal Pain (RAP) in Children	Irritable Bowel Syndrome	Functional Dyspepsia	Functional Constipation	Endometriosis
Clinical features	≥3 episodes of abdominal pain, over a period of ≥3 months, severe enough to affect activities, but without demonstrable evidence of a pathologic condition and without the characteristics of dyspepsia, chronic constipation, IBS, or abdominal migraine.[7]	Continuous or recurrent abdominal pain or discomfort, for at least 12 weeks in the past 12 months, that has two out of three of the following features: relieved by defecation, associated with change in frequency of stooling, or associated with change in consistency of stool.[1]	Persistent or recurrent pain or discomfort centered in the upper abdomen, with no evidence of organic disease or typical gastroesophageal reflux symptoms, and not consistent with characteristics of IBS.	Characterized by no evidence of organic cause and by long-standing, symptomatic experience of abnormal defecation including two or more of the following features: straining, hard stools, sensation of incomplete evacuation, and/or two or fewer bowel movements in a week.[1]	Endometriosis is a chronic, estrogen-dependent disorder associated with deposits of endometrial tissue outside of the uterus, usually in the pelvis, and frequently characterized by cyclic and noncyclic pelvic pain and infertility. Pain complaints may include dysmenorrhea, dyspareunia, and pressure-like sensations.
Diagnosis and differential	RAP may be diagnosed if clinical features above and no alarm symptoms or signs are present, such as involuntary weight loss, GI bleeding, bilious, protracted, or cyclical vomiting, chronic severe diarrhea, family history of IBD, localized tenderness, mass, organomegaly or perianal lesions.[7] Alarm symptoms and signs suggest organic disease and require investigation.	IBS may be diagnosed if above clinical features are present and no alarm symptoms or signs are discovered. Alarm symptoms or signs require additional evaluation.	Functional dyspepsia may be diagnosed if above clinical features are present and no alarm symptoms or signs are discovered. Alarm symptoms or signs require additional evaluation. In the emergent or urgent care setting, distinguishing functional dyspepsia from reflux disease may be difficult.[12]	Constipation may be diagnosed if above clinical features are present and no alarm symptoms or signs are discovered. Alarm symptoms or signs require additional evaluation.	Endometriosis may be considered if above clinical features are present and no alarm symptoms or signs are discovered. Definitive diagnosis is made at laparoscopy with visualization of endometrial deposits. Alarm symptoms or signs require additional evaluation.

(Continued)

Table 39-1. Summary of Common Chronic Abdominal Pain Syndromes (*Continued*)

Disorder	Recurrent Abdominal Pain (RAP) in Children	Irritable Bowel Syndrome	Functional Dyspepsia	Functional Constipation	Endometriosis
ED care and disposition	RAP requires no specific therapy in the ED and should require no diagnostic testing unless alarm symptoms or signs of organic conditions exist. Reassurance that serious disease is very unlikely and referral to primary care for continued care is indicated.	IBS requires no specific therapy in the ED and should require no diagnostic testing unless alarm symptoms or signs of organic conditions exist. Reassurance that serious disease is very unlikely and referral to primary care for continued care is indicated. Studies suggest that use of alosetron in diarrhea-predominant IBS may be effective in relieving some symptoms.[11]	Functional dyspepsia requires no specific therapy in the emergency department and should require no diagnostic testing unless alarm symptoms or signs of organic conditions exist. Since exclusion of reflux or ulcer disease is not likely in the emergent or urgent care setting, an appropriate trial of antisecretory therapy with H2 blockade or PPI is acceptable. Referral to primary care for continued care is indicated.	Functional constipation requires no specific therapy in the emergency department and should require no diagnostic testing unless alarm symptoms or signs of organic conditions exist. Reassurance that serious disease is very unlikely and referral to primary care for continued care is indicated. Tegaserod, previously recommended on the strength of controlled trials showing benefit,[14,15] has been pulled from the market due to concerns over heart attack and stroke risk.	Endometriosis requires no specific therapy in the emergency department and should require no diagnostic testing unless alarm symptoms or signs of organic conditions exist. Referral to an obstetrician-gynecologist for continued care, especially for infertility is indicated. Studies suggest that hormonal treatments with danazol, medroxy-progesterone, gestrinone, and gonadotrophin releasing hormone analogues are effective in treating chronic pain from endometriosis, but treatment of infertility requires OB/GYN surgical intervention.[16-18]

Abbreviations: IBD, inflammatory bowel disease; IBS, irritable bowel syndrome; PPI, proton pump inhibitor; RAP, recurrent abdominal pain in children.

of the uterus, usually in the pelvis, and frequently characterized by cyclic and noncyclic pelvic pain and infertility. The etiology and pathophysiology of the condition is not well known and quantity and location of endometrial tissue is not related to symptoms.[16–18] In population-based studies, the prevalence in women is 6% to 10% and among women with pelvic pain and/or infertility, the prevalence approaches 35% to 50%. Clinical features, differential diagnosis, and treatments are described Table 39-1.

REFERENCES

1. Corazziari E. Definition and epidemiology of functional gastrointestinal disorders. *Best Pract Res Clin Gastroenterol.* 2004;18:613.
2. Van Korff M, Dworkin SF, LeResche L, et al. An epidemiologic comparison of pain complaints. *Pain.* 1988:32:173.
3. Sun BC, Burstin HR, Brennan TA. Predictors and outcomes of frequent emergency department users. *Acad Emerg Med.* 2003;10:320.
4. Apley J, Naish N. Recurrent abdominal pains: A field survey of 1,000 school children. *Arch Dis Child.* 1958;33:165.
5. Chitkara DK, Rawat DJ, Talley NJ. The epidemiology of childhood recurrent abdominal pain in Western countries: A systematic review. *Am J Gastroenterol.* 2005;100:1868.
6. Subcommittee on Chronic Abdominal Pain: Chronic Abdominal Pain in Children. *Pediatrics.* 2005;115:370.
7. Subcommittee on Chronic Abdominal Pain: Chronic Abdominal Pain in Children. *Pediatrics.* 2005;115:812.
8. Talley NJ, Weaver AL, Zinmeister AR, Melton LJ. Onset and disappearance of gastrointestinal and functional gastrointestinal disorders. *Am J Epidemiol.* 1992;136:165.
9. Agreus L, Swarsdudd K, Nyren O, Tibblin G. Irritable bowel syndrome and dyspepsia in the population: overlap and lack of stability over time. *Gastroenterology.* 1995;109:671.
10. Heitkemper M, Jarrett M. Overlapping conditions in women with irritable bowel syndrome. *Urol Nurs.* 2005;25:25.
11. Chey WD, Chey WY, Heath AT, Dukes GE, Carter EG, Northcutt A, et al. Long-term safety and efficacy of alosetron in women with severe diarrhea predominant irritable bowel syndrome. *Am J Gastroenterol.* 2004;99:2195.
12. Moayyedi P, Talley NJ, Fennerty MB, Vakil N. Can the clinical history distinguish between organic and functional dyspepsia. *JAMA.* 2006;295:1566.
13. Talley NJ, Vakil N, and the Practice Parameters Committee of the American College of Gastroenterology. Guidelines for the Management of Dyspepsia. *Am J Gastroenterol.* 2005;100:2324.
14. Johanson JF, Wald A, Tougas G, Chey WD, Novick JS, Lembo AJ et al. Effect of tegaserod in chronic constipation: a randomized, double-blind, controlled trial. *Clin Gastroenterol Hepatol.* 2004;2:796.
15. Kamm MA, Muller-Lissner S, Talley NJ, Boeckxstaens G, Minushkin ON, Kalinin A, et al. Tegaserod for the treatment of chronic constipation: a randomized, double-blind, placebo-controlled multinational study. *Am J Gastroenterol.* 2005;100:362.
16. Farquhar CM. Endometriosis. *BMJ.* 2000;320:1449.
17. Winkel CA. Evaluation and management of women with endometriosis. *Obstet Gynecol.* 2003;102:397.
18. Giudice LC, Kao LC. Endometriosis. *Lancet.* 2004;364:1789.

40

Conditions Presenting with Abdominal Wall Pain

M. Fernanda Bellolio

HIGH YIELD FACTS

- Abdominal wall pain (AWP) can be considered only when intraabdominal pathology has been reasonably ruled out.
- Most of the time it is self-limited and rarely life-threatening.
- Always consider rectus sheath hematoma and complicated hernias in distressed patients referring pain to the abdominal wall.
- Accentuated localized tenderness with abdominal wall tensing (Carnett test) is a helpful sign to diagnose abdominal wall etiology.
- Abdominal computed tomography (CT) scanning permits evaluation of both abdominal wall and intraabdominal etiologies.

EPIDEMIOLOGY

The prevalence of AWP in the general population and in the emergency department (ED) is largely unknown. It represents between 10% and 15% of patients with abdominal pain seen in gastroenterological practices.[1,2] The most common etiologies are neuropathies, such as entrapment of an anterior cutaneous branch of the thoracic intercostal nerves, herpes zoster, and scar related entrapments.[3] Other causes include radiculopathies, space occupying lesions such as hernias and hematomas, and myofascial pain.[4–7] This entity usually coexists with other disorders, such as an increased body mass index (greater than 25 kg/m^2) in 84%, chronic low back pain (30%), gastroesophageal reflux (27%), irritable bowel syndrome (22%), and depression (22%).[8]

PATHOPHYSIOLOGY

Abdominal wall pain corresponds to a somatic type of pain due to the activation of Aδ-nociceptors in soft tissues, that activate fibers to the dorsal horns in the spinal cord.[6] These translate clinically to a typical exquisitely sharp and well localized pain that helps differentiate it from the visceral type of pain seen with intraabdominal pathology.

CLINICAL FEATURES

Clinical characteristics of AWP constitute a myriad of subtle presentations depending on the etiology. However, there are general features that help in the diagnostic approach (Table 40-1). Classically the pain is not related to meals or bowel movements. The most important factors triggering or worsening the pain are changes in posture, abdominal wall tension, or direct pressure. Rarely, AWP is accompanied by severe nausea, vomiting, or diarrhea.[6] Radiation may be widespread, sometimes extending posteriorly over the dermatome. When severe, the pain may be described as diffuse.[4] The presence of systemic symptoms, with the exception of those attributable to the pain itself, should rouse suspicion for visceral pathology.

During the evaluation of a patient with abdominal pain, the presence of an exquisitely localized point of tenderness less than 2.5 cm diameter[1] ("one-finger-pain"), directs us towards a wall etiology. Clinically, one may look for a trigger point with Carnett test (Figure 40-1); the patient is asked to lift his head and shoulders a few inches off the table to flex the rectus abdominalis and pyramidalis muscles, isolating the abdominal wall from intrapelvic organs as well as tensing the muscles. A one finger search is performed along the wall to palpate muscle twitches, taut band, or elicit a painful response from the patient.[3,4,8] The Carnett test has a sensitivity of 78% to 85% and specificity of 88% to 97%.[1]

DIAGNOSIS AND DIFFERENTIAL

The evaluation of AWP depends entirely on history and physical examination findings. A diagnosis of abdominal wall pathology should only be made after intraabdominal causes for pain have been ruled out. A trigger point of pain is diagnostic.

The etiology for AWP is broad; however, frequent causes are described below. **Rectus sheath hematoma** results from sudden disruption of epigastric vessel with or without muscle tear into the rectus sheath. Can occur spontaneously or after minor trauma (e.g., subcutaneous injections), surgery, or increased intraabdominal pressure (coughing, straining, or pregnancy). Most of these patients present with abdominal pain (84%)[7]; it is more

Table 40-1. Characteristics of Abdominal Wall Pain

Constant or fluctuating pain

Affected by abdominal wall muscle tensing

Pain is unrelated to bowel function or meals

Absence of symptoms suggestive of intraabdominal process (diarrhea or constipation, vomiting, weight loss, fever, rectal bleeding, or anemia)

Localized tenderness

Compression of trigger may result in referred pain to distant site

prevalent in women (64%) and patients of an older age group.[7,9,10] Anticoagulation is a major risk factor; 69% of the patients with rectus sheath hematoma were on anticoagulation in one series.[7] It is more commonly seen in the lower abdominal wall.[9,11]

Hernias constitute protrusions of the abdomen content through the fascial planes. Severe pain can be produced even in the absence of bowel obstruction when only the omentum becomes incarcerated. Hernias can cause pain along a nerve distribution by traction of the associated nerve. A surgical scar predisposes to a hernia, so physical

examination should always be performed with the patient both standing and supine.[3,4,12]

Anterior cutaneous nerve entrapment and **compressive sensory radiculopathy** probably represent the most common etiologies of AWP seen in patients without a clearly identifiable cause during evaluation. Oral contraceptives and pregnancy have been associated with AWP secondary to entrapment syndromes, perhaps from tissue edema due to estrogen and progesterone.[2,13] The pain is secondary to nerve ischemia and radiates along sensory dermatomes.[6,8,13]

Herpes zoster can be caused by the reactivation of latent Varicella zoster virus from within the dorsal root ganglia of sensory nerves. It has a prodrome with pain distributed in a dermatomal pattern, causing cutaneous hyperesthesia, followed by a vesicular rash which develops 2 to 7 days afterward (Figure 40-2). Postherpetic neuralgia can also occur, and it is seen mostly in patients over 60 years of age.[5]

Other causes of AWP[2,3,5,14–17] are listed in Table 40-2.

When there is laboratory evidence of inflammation (leukocytosis, elevated sedimentation rate, or C-reactive protein level), anemia, or abnormal liver function tests, an intraabdominal cause of pain should be sought.[8]

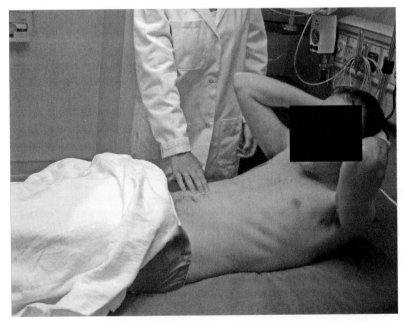

Fig. 40-1. Carnett test. The patient is asked to lift his head and shoulders a few inches off the table to flex the rectus abdominalis and pyramidalis muscles, isolating the abdominal wall from intrapelvic organs as well as tensing the muscles. A one finger search is performed along the wall to palpate muscle twitches, taut bands, or elicit a painful response from the patient.

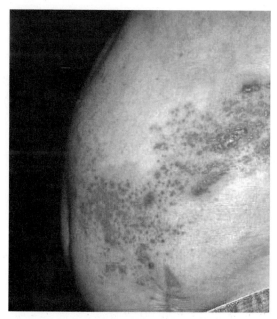

Fig. 40-2. Herpes Zoster This eruption consists of a dermatomal distribution of umbilicated vesicles on an erythematous base. Tzank smear is positive. (Courtesy of the Department of Dermatology, Wilford Hall USAF Medical Center and Brooke Army Medical Center, San Antonio, TX.)

Table 40-2. Etiology of Abdominal Wall Pain

Trauma related	Tumors
Hematomas	Lipoma, desmoid tumor,
Muscle tears	hemangiomas
Rib fractures	Lymphatic malformations
Foreign bodies	Metastases
Spontaneous hematomas	Primary malignant tumors
Abscesses (Figure 40-3)	of the wall
Myofascial pain	Lymphoma, melanoma,
syndrome	fibrous histocytoma
Compressive sensory	(adults) and sarcoma
radiculopathy	(children)
Cutaneous nerve	Herpes zoster infection
entrapment	Endometriosis,
Mononeuritis multiplex	endometriomas
Vasculitis	Abdominal wall neuroma
Diabetic radiculopathy	Related to surgical
Slipping rib syndrome	interventions
Hernia	Transfascial sutures
Inguinal (direct	Scar nerve entrapment
and indirect)	Neuroborreliosis
Midline	Trichinosis
Umbilical	
Femoral	
Scrotal	
Spigelian	
Incisional	
Richter	

Computed tomography scanning is useful in the evaluation of most causes and complications of AWP, especially in obese patients.[12,18] It can also help us to rule out intraabdominal pathologies. However, it is important to alert the radiologist regarding relevant history and physical examination findings, as it is not unusual for abdominal wall defects to be overlooked on CT scans. Sonography can also be useful to differentiate causes of AWP such as abscesses or hematomas, as well as distinguish intraabdominal pathologies.[17,18]

Abdominal wall pain may arise from other sources, including referred pain from abdominal or thoracic viscera due to neural convergence in the spinal cord from somatic and visceral sites, and peritoneal wall lesions.[1] Acute appendicitis is the most common intraabdominal source that can be confused with AWP.[8] Other less common intraabdominal pathologies such as mesenteric adenitis or epiploic appendangitis can also be confused with AWP.

The course and complications will depend on the underlying cause. Usually causes of AWP have a benign natural history. There are a few clinical scenarios where the AWP can become life-threatening, such as can be seen with a massive rectus sheath hematoma or an ischemic bowel secondary to an incarcerated or strangulated hernia. Chronic AWP may also develop subsequent to neuropathies.

EMERGENCY DEPARTMENT CARE AND DISPOSITION

Patients who look ill, have unstable vitals, are immunocompromised or elderly, must be admitted for further careful evaluation and an intraabdominal pathology ruled out. Proper patient education about AWP prevents further ED visits, unnecessary testing, and helps alleviate concerns.[8] Failure to recognize AWP is costly in terms of unnecessary testing and generating further anxiety in the patient and physician.[8,20] The probability of missing

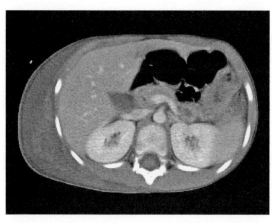

Fig. 40-3. Abdominal CT demonstrating multiple collections in the right side of the abdominal wall consistent with abscess. (Courtesy of Dimitri A. Parra, MD. Departament of Diagnostic Imaging. The Hospital For Sick Children. Toronto, Ontario, Canada.)

visceral disease is small (3% to 7%), with strict adherence to diagnostic criteria and diligent observation of patients.[1,8]

Treatment depends upon the etiology and severity of the symptoms. The majority of patients with rectus sheath hematoma are treated conservatively. Only a small group needs embolization or surgical management.[7,9–12,19] To prevent incarcerated bowel strangulation in a hernia, immediate reduction may be necessary, and if it cannot be reduced, surgical consultation should be sought.[12] Massage, physical therapy with stretching, cooling topical anesthetic sprays, warm soaks, heat application, and other local methods are often useful.[4,8] Modification of identified precipitating activities and an abdominal binder are useful if gentle hand pressure alleviates the pain. Nonspecific treatments, such as nonsteroidal anti-inflammatory drugs, analgesics, and antidepressants have been effectively used in chronic AWP.[1,8] Injections of local anesthetics and steroids, give substantial pain relief to 60% to 90% of patients, often for prolonged periods, but their long term benefit is yet to be proven.[1,3,4,6,8,13] Avoid injection of steroids into fascia, as they can predispose to hernia formation.

When the AWP becomes chronic, referral to a subspecialist is necessary.

PITFALLS

- Failure to consider intraabdominal pathology mimicking wall pain.
- Failure to consider the serious AWP etiologies.

- Failure to educate the patient about the etiology and when to look for further evaluation.
- AWP may be confused with visceral pain because superficial innervations from the lower thoracic roots enter the spinal cord via the same dorsal horn as the deeper visceral afferents.
- Visceral disease with involvement of the local parietal peritoneum may give a false positive Carnett test, but generally tenderness is not as distinctly localized.

REFERENCES

1. Srinivasan R, Greenbaum DS. Chronic abdominal pain: a frequently overlooked problem. Practical approach to diagnosis and management. *Am J Gastroenterol.* 2002; 97:824.
2. Peleg R. Abdominal wall pain caused by cutaneous nerve entrapment in an adolescent girl taking oral contraceptive pills. *J Adolesc Health.* 1999;24:45.
3. Suleiman S, Johnston DE. The abdominal wall: An overlooked source of pain. *Am Fam Physician.* 2001;64:431.
4. Gallegos NC, Hobsley M. Recognition and treatment of abdominal wall pain. *J R Soc Med.* 1989;82:343.
5. Roy S, Weimersheimer P. Nonoperative causes of abdominal pain. *Surg Clin North Am.* 1997;77:1433.
6. Sharp HT. Myofascial pain syndrome of the abdominal wall for the busy clinician. *Clin Obstet Gynecol.* 2003; 46:783.
7. Cherry WB, Mueller PS. Rectus sheath hematoma: Review of 126 cases at a single institution. *Medicine.* 2006;85:105.
8. Costanza CD, Longstreth GF, Liu AL. Chronic abdominal wall pain: Clinical features, health care costs, and long-term outcome. *Clin Gastroenterol Hepatol.* 2004;2:395.
9. Holmes SJ, Yale SH, Mazza JJ. Rectus sheath hematoma as a cause of acute abdominal pain. *Am Fam Physician.* 2001; 64:1681.
10. Edlow JA, Juang P, Margulies S, Burstein J. Rectus sheath hematoma. *Ann Emerg Med.* 1999;34:671.
11. Siu WT, Tang CN, Law BK, et al. Spontaneous rectus sheath hematoma. *Can J Surg.* 2003;46:390.
12. Mensching JJ, Musielewicz AJ. Abdominal wall hernias. *Emerg Med Clin North Am.* 1996;14:739.
13. Peleg R, Gohar J, Koretz M, Peleg A. Abdominal wall pain in pregnant women caused by cutaneous nerve entrapment. *Eur J Obstet Gynecol Reprod Biol.* 1997;74:169.
14. Rosson GD, Dellon AL. Abdominal wall neuroma pain after breast reconstruction with a transverse abdominal musculocutaneous flap: Cause and treatment. *Ann Plast Surg.* 2005;55:330.
15. Blanco RG, Parithivel VS, Shah AK, et al. Abdominal wall endometriomas. *Am J Surg.* 2003;185:596.
16. Mormont E, Esselinckx W, De Ronde T, et al. Abdominal wall weakness and lumboabdominal pain revealing

neuroborreliosis: A report of three cases. *Clin Rheumatol.* 2001;20:447.

17. Meuwly JY, Gudinchet F. Sonography of the thoracic and abdominal walls. *J Clin Ultrasound.* 2004;32:500.

18. Moreno Gallego A, Aguayo JL, Flores B, et al. Ultrasonography and computed tomography reduce unnecessary surgery in abdominal rectus sheath haematoma. *Br J Surg.* 1997;84:1295.

19. Zack JR, Ferral H, Postoak D, et al. Coil embolization of rectus sheath hemorrhage. *J Trauma.* 2001;51:793.

20. Greenbaum DS, Greenbaum RB, Joseph JG, et al. Chronic abdominal wall pain: Diagnostic validity and costs. *Dig Dis Sci.* 1994;39:1935.

41

Cardiac Disease Presenting as Abdominal Pain

Howard K. Mell

HIGH YIELD FACTS

- Patients with cardiac pathology may present with a primary complaint of abdominal pain.
- Some abdominal pathology (e.g., acute pancreatitis, duodenal perforation) may mimic the electrocardiogram (ECG) and echocardiographic findings of a myocardial infarction (MI).
- While the location, character, onset, and nature of the pain may provide important diagnostic clues, there are no specific findings in the history or on physical examination that can reliably exclude cardiac pathology in the abdominal pain patient.
- A high index of suspicion for cardiac pathology should be maintained in abdominal pain patients, especially in those patients with significant risk factors for cardiac disease (e.g., smoking, diabetes, strong family history, hypertension [HTN], known cardiovascular disease, etc.).

EPIDEMIOLOGY

Cardiovascular disease can complicate the diagnoses of patients presenting with abdominal pain in one of three ways. First, patients with MIs or vascular disasters, such as aortic dissection, may present with abdominal pain or associated symptoms, such as nausea. Second, abdominal pathology, such as pancreatitis or duodenal perforation, may cause a patient to display electrocardiographic and echocardiographic symptoms that closely mimic a MI. Third, significant abdominal pathology may precipitate a hypoperfusion state that precipitates or unmasks cardiac pathology.

Nearly 50% of patients with an acute MI present to the emergency department without a primary complaint of chest pain.[1,2] Research indicates that between 2% and 15% of these patients will present with abdominal pain.[1,3,4] Older patients and female patients are more likely to present with symptoms other than chest pain; however, men are more likely than women, on a percentage basis, to present with abdominal (epigastric) pain.[3] Multiple studies suggest that non-Caucasian patients with acute MI have a greater likelihood of presenting with a primary complaint other than chest pain.[5,6] It should be noted that patients with significant cardiovascular pathology other than acute MI, such as acute aortic dissection[7,8] or unstable angina[9], might also present with abdominal pain.

While patients with acute MI who present with abdominal pain most often complain of epigastric pain, the location of the abdominal pain is neither sensitive nor specific enough to be diagnostic. Additionally, research suggests that slightly more than half of all patients diagnosed with an acute MI in the emergency department (ED) will have complained of nausea during the course of their emergency department visit.[3]

Patients with significant abdominal pathology, such as perforated duodenal ulcers,[10] intestinal obstruction,[11] cholecystitis,[12] dissecting hematoma of the esophagus,[13] and pancreatitis,[14–17] have demonstrated electrocardiographic changes consistent with MI (see Table 41-1). Transient electrocardiographic changes mimicking MI have been particularly well described in pancreatitis. Interestingly, there are case reports of regional wall motion abnormalities on echocardiography[15] and cardiac specific enzyme deran-gements[14] associated with pancreatitis.

Critically ill patients often suffer myocardial injury as a result of their illnesses. Research suggests that nearly one third of all patients admitted to intensive care units with diagnoses other than acute coronary syndrome or cardiac injury have cardiac specific enzyme deran-gements.[18] Interestingly, this proportion (nearly one third) has also been described as the rate of cardiac complications in the intensive care unit in patients presenting with severe gastrointestinal bleeding.[19] Advanced age is consistently described as a risk factor for development of these complications.[18,19] While the literature is silent as to the rate of these complications occurring while the patient is in the emergency department, the physician should maintain a high index of suspicion for cardiac injury occurring as a result of significant abdominal pathology. Likewise, the significant rate of these complications should guide the emergency physician towards an intensive care disposition of patients with significant abdominal pathology, especially in the elderly.

Table 41-1. Conditions Reported to Cause ECG Changes Mimicking Myocardial Infarction

Pancreatitis
Acute cholecystitis
Esophageal hematoma
Intestinal obstruction
Duodenal ulcer perforation
Peptic ulcer perforation

Abbreviation: ECG, electrocardiogram.

PATHOPHYSIOLOGY

The tendency of diabetic patients with acute coronary syndromes to present without pain or with atypical pain, including abdominal pain, has been well established. It is believed that this results from autonomic neuropathy secondary to their diabetes. In nondiabetic patients various psychological and neuropsychiatric factors have been postulated as the cause of impaired pain perception.[20]

Patients with abdominal pathology who display electrocardiographic changes that mimic MI may do so as a result of mechanical displacement of the heart, electrolyte derangement, coronary vasospasm, or a vagally mediated reflex.[11,15] Additionally, pancreatitis may precipitate cardiac myonecrosis from pancreatic proteolytic enzymes.[15]

CLINICAL FEATURES

Abdominal pain may be a symptom of cardiac or cardiovascular pathology. While epigastric pain is commonly described, other locations of abdominal pain are also associated with cardiac or cardiovascular pathology. No specific feature (i.e., location, quality, severity) of abdominal pain is specific or sensitive enough to reliably predict or exclude cardiac or cardiovascular pathology in all patients. The presence of cardiac risk factors, advanced age, and diabetes may reasonably increase the suspicion of cardiac disease presenting as abdominal pain.

While nausea and vomiting are associated with many abdominal complaints, they are also strongly associated with acute coronary syndromes. Research suggests that more than half of all patients with an acute MI complain of nausea.[3] Nearly one quarter of all acute coronary syndrome patients who present without chest pain complain of nausea and vomiting.[21] Therefore the presence of nausea and/or vomiting concurrently with abdominal pain should not diminish the clinical suspicion of cardiac disease.

DIAGNOSIS AND DIFFERENTIAL

Cardiac and cardiovascular disease may present as abdominal pain. Specific entities include MI, unstable angina, and aortic dissection.

EMERGENCY DEPARTMENT CARE AND DISPOSITION

Patients presenting with abdominal pain should be assessed for cardiac pathology. A 12-lead ECG and cardiac specific enzyme assays should be routine components of the assessment of abdominal pain patients. If alterations are detected by these tests, echocardiography is warranted.

If evidence of an acute coronary syndrome is detected in a patient in whom clinical suspicion of abdominal pathology remains high, and treatment for the acute coronary syndrome is initiated, preference should be given toward percutaneous angiography over thrombolytic therapy in order to prevent bleeding complications.

Patients with pancreatitis or other abdominal pathology, who develop electrocardiographic changes consistent with myocardial injury, should be treated with nitroglycerin to reduce coronary artery vasospasm. Formal echocardiography is warranted in these patients. Percutaneous coronary angiography may be necessary to exclude concurrent acute coronary syndrome in these patients, as cardiac injury is a possible complication of significant illness.

Patients with significant pathology, advanced age, and/or hemodynamic instability should be considered for intensive care unit admission.

PITFALLS

- Cardiac disease may present as abdominal pain. This may delay or prevent accurate diagnosis.

- Abdominal pathology may cause a patient to display electrocardiographic, echocardiographic, and/or laboratory values that mimic cardiac injury.

- Cardiac injury is a potential complication of any illness capable of causing hemodynamic instability, including significant abdominal pathology.

REFERENCES

1. Gupta M, Tabas JA, Kohn MA. Presenting complaint among patients with myocardial infarction who present to an urban, public hospital emergency department. *Ann Emerg Med.* 2002;40:180.
2. Coronado BE, Pope JH, Griffith JL, et al. Clinical features, triage, and outcome of patients presenting to the ED with

suspected acute coronary syndromes but without pain: a multicenter study. *Am J Emerg Med.* 2004;22:568.

3. Kudenchuk PJ, Maynard C, Martin JS, et al. Comparison of presentation, treatment, and outcome of acute myocardial infarction in men versus women (the Myocardial Infarction Triage and Intervention Registry). *Am J Cardiol.* 1996;78:9.

4. Clark LT, Adams-Campbell LL, Maw M, et al. Clinical features of patients with acute myocardial infarction presenting with and without typical chest pain: an inner city experience. *J Assoc Acad Minor Phys.* 1989;1:29.

5. The International Study Group. In-hospital mortality and clinical course of 20,891 patients with suspected acute myocardial infarction randomised between alteplase and streptokinase with or without heparin. *Lancet.* 1990; 336:71.

6. Ayanian JZ, Epstein AM. Differences in the use of procedures between women and men hospitalized for coronary heart disease. *N Engl J Med.* 1991;325:221.

7. Kasher JA, El-Bialy A, Balingit P. Aortic dissection: a dreaded disease with many faces. *J Cardiovasc Pharmacol Ther.* 2004;9:211.

8. Armstrong WF, Bach DS, Carey LM, et al. Clinical and echocardiographic findings in patients with suspected acute aortic dissection. *Am Heart J.* 1998;136:1051.

9. Pope JH, Ruthazer R, Beshansky JR, et al. Clinical features of emergency department patients presenting with symptoms suggestive of acute cardiac ischemia: A multicenter study. *J Thromb Thrombolysis.* 1998;6:63.

10. Thomas I, Mathew J, Kumar VP, et al. Electrocardiographic changes in catastrophic abdominal illness mimicking acute myocardial infarction. *Am J Cardiol.* 1987;59:1224.

11. Mixon TA, Houck PD. Intestinal obstruction mimicking acute myocardial infarction. *Tex Heart Inst J.* 2003;30:155.

12. Ryan ET, Pak PH, DeSanctis RW. Myocardial infarction mimicked by acute cholecystitis. *Ann Intern Med.* 1992; 116:218.

13. Amott DH, Wright GM. Dissecting haematoma of the oesophagus masquerading as acute myocardial infarction. *Med J Aust.* 2006;184:182.

14. Albrecht CA, Laws FA. ST segment elevation pattern of acute myocardial infarction induced by acute pancreatitis. *Cardiol Rev.* 2003;11:147.

15. Ro TK, Lang RM, Ward RP. Acute pancreatitis mimicking myocardial infarction: evaluation with myocardial contrast echocardiography. *J Am Soc Echocardiogr.* 2004;17:387.

16. Khairy P, Marsolais P. Pancreatitis with electrocardiographic changes mimicking acute myocardial infarction. *Can J Gastroenterol.* 2001;15:522.

17. Patel J, Movahed A, Reeves WC. Electrocardiographic and segmental wall motion abnormalities in pancreatitis mimicking myocardial infarction. *Clin Cardiol.* 1994;17:505.

18. Quenot JP, Le Teuff G, Quantin C, et al. Myocardial injury in critically ill patients: relation to increased cardiac troponin I and hospital mortality. *Chest.* 2005;128:2758.

19. Prendergast HM, Sloan EP, Cumpston K, Schlichting AB. Myocardial infarction and cardiac complications in emergency department patients admitted to the intensive care unit with gastrointestinal hemorrhage. *J Emerg Med.* 2005;28:19.

20. Torosian T, Lumley MA, Pickard SD, Ketterer MW. Silent versus symptomatic myocardial ischemia: the role of psychological and medical factors. *Health Psychol.* 1997; 16:123.

21. Brieger D, Eagle KA, Goodman SG, et al. GRACE Investigators. Acute coronary syndromes without chest pain, an underdiagnosed and undertreated high-risk group: insights from the Global Registry of Acute Coronary Events. *Chest.* 2004;126:461.

42

Nonabdominal Infectious Disorders Presenting with Abdominal Pain

Kim Ryan Schutterle
Larry F. Vukov

HIGH YIELD FACTS

- Gender and age stratification may help narrow the differential diagnosis quickly.
- Certain risk groups are more likely to present with abdominal pain associated with infectious disorders (i.e., patients with immunocompromise presenting with herpes zoster).

INTRODUCTION

In creating a differential diagnosis for nonabdominal infectious disorders presenting with abdominal pain, dividing patients into three categories may facilitate the task (Table 42-1). Cystitis is covered in Chapter 26; female reproductive tract infections are covered in Chapters 30 and 31.

EPIDIDYMITIS

Epidemiology

Epididymitis is the most common cause of inflammation within the scrotum and affects less than 1 per 1000 men per year. Epididymitis usually affects adult males accounting for more than 600,000 physician visits per year. Inflammatory lesions are much more common in the epididymis than in the testes proper. After puberty, epididymitis accounts for approximately 75% of acute scrotal pain.

Pathophysiology

Epididymitis is an inflammation of the epididymis. The epididymis is the tubelike structure that lies along the posterior testicular border that is attached to the scrotum posteriorly (anterior attachment in 7% of patients).

Epididymal function includes storage, transport, and maturation of spermatozoa.

Infections of the epididymitis can be divided into three major categories: Sexually transmitted diseases (STDs), non-STD infections associated with prostatitis and urinary tract infections (UTIs), and hematologic seeding (rare). Epididymitis in a prepubescent child is generally associated with congenital urinary tract malformations (47%); coliform bacteria predominate as the causative agent. In men under the age of 35, the most common pathogens are *Chlamydia* and *Gonorrhea*. The preceding urethral infection due to *Gonorrhea* and *Chlamydia* is asymptomatic in up to 50% of cases, and the exposure can occur months before symptoms develop. In men over the age of 35, bacteriuria from functional urinary obstruction is often the cause. Infectious organisms such as *Escherichia coli*, enterococci, *Pseudomonas*, and *Proteus* predominate. Acute infections develop over a couple of days, tend to be severe and usually resolve with treatment. Chronic infections may result from repeated episodes of untreated acute epididymitis and treatment may fail to provide complete resolution.

Clinical Features

The history and clinical findings that are suggestive of epididymitis are outlined in Table 42-2.[1] Patients with three or more of the findings are likely to have epididymitis. The abdominal pain associated with epididymidis is often vague, cramplike, located in the lower abdomen, and worse on the affected side. Abdominal pain is more common in severe or prolonged infections. The typical history for acute epididymitis is gradual onset of scrotal pain and swelling that peaks over a period of 3 to 48 hours. Other features may include testicular swelling on one or both sides, dysuria, painful intercourse or ejaculation, fever, discharge, hematospermia, and pain in the inguinal canal, scrotum, or testicle.

Physical examination of acute epididymitis will reveal an acutely inflamed epididymis that is tender and swollen. Elevation of the testicle (Prehn sign) may yield some relief of the pain, but this sign in unreliable and should not be used to differentiate epididymitis from torsion.

Diagnosis and Differential

Diagnosis is made by careful history and physical examination. Suggested laboratory studies include urinalysis (pyuria or bacteriuria seen in only 50% of patients), urine culture, urethral gram stain, and testing for gonorrhea and chlamydia. Complete blood count may be considered in acutely ill patients.

Table 42-1. Nonabdominal Infectious Disorders Presenting with Abdominal Pain

Male	Female	Male and Female
Epididymitis	Pelvic inflammatory	Pneumonia
Prostatitis	disease	Herpes zoster
	Tuboovarian	Cystitis
	abscesses	Lyme disease
		Streptococcal
		pharyngitis

The differential diagnosis includes testicular torsion, testicular appendage torsion, inguinal hernia, scrotal abscess, hydrocele, varicocele, viral orchitis, testicular neoplasm, Fournier gangrene, Henoch-Schönlein purpura, and renal colic.

Emergency Department Care and Disposition

Supportive measures include scrotal support such as a soft athletic supporter, ice packs (10 minutes, 3 times per day), analgesics such as nonsteroidal anti-inflammatory agents (NSAIDS) and/or opioids, and stool softeners. Antibiotic therapy is divided by age groups. If less than 13 years old, trimethoprim-sulfamethoxazole one double strength orally twice daily for 14 days or ciprofloxacin 500 mg PO twice daily for 14 days. For heterosexual males <35 years old, ceftriaxone 250 mg IM × 1 plus doxycycline 100 mg orally twice daily for 10 days. For patients allergic to cephalosporins and/or tetracyclines: ofloxacin 300 mg orally twice a day for 10 days or levofloxacin 500 mg orally once daily for 10 days. Heterosexual males >35 males, bisexual males, and homosexual males Levofloxacin

500 mg PO twice daily for 10 days or ofloxacin 400 mg orally twice daily for 10 days. Refer to urology or primary care provider for follow up in 5 to 7 days. Admission criteria for intravenous (IV) antibiotic therapy includes toxic-appearing patients, immunosuppressed patients, or patients who cannot tolerate oral therapy.

Pitfalls

- Epididymitis is the most common misdiagnosis in cases of testicular tumor and torsion.
- Failure in treating both partners if a sexually transmitted infection is suspected.
- Delayed diagnosis can result in testicular ischemia from inflammation.
- Pain can be mistaken for appendicitis or diverticulitis.
- Bladder outlet obstruction and urinary retention must be considered in the older patient with epididymitis.

PROSTATITIS

Epidemiology

Prostatitis can occur at any age, but is more common between the ages of 20-and-50 years old. Prostatitis is the most common urologic diagnosis in men younger than 50 years of age and the third most common in men above 50.[2] Prostatitis is difficult to diagnose, categorize, and treat despite how common it is.

Pathophysiology

Prostatitis is defined as the inflammation of the prostate. The main function of the prostate is to store and secrete a clear, slightly basic fluid that constitutes up to one third of the volume of semen. Semen is composed of spermatozoa and seminal fluid; about 10% to 30% of the

---

Table 42-2. Clinical Findings Suggestive of Epididymitis[1]

1 Gradual onset of pain
2 Dysuria, urethral discharge, or recent genitourinary instrumentation
3 History of UTI, imperforate anus, neurogenic bladder, or genitourinary surgery
4 Fever of more than 38.3°C
5 Tenderness and induration at the epididymis
6 Urinalysis showing 10 or more WBCs or red blood cells per high-power field

Patients with 3 or more of these findings are likely to have epididymitis

Abbreviations: UTI, urinary tract infection; WBC, white blood cell.

seminal fluid is produced by the prostate gland—the rest is produced by the two seminal vesicles. The prostate also contains some smooth muscles that help expel semen during ejaculation. The fluids produced by the prostate have innate antibacterial properties. Despite this, the prostate can become infected usually via direct invasion from the urethra or bladder. The prostate is normally sterile and is poorly penetrated by antibiotics.

Clinical Features

Clinical features of acute bacterial prostatitis may include abrupt onset of fever, chills, low back pain, and perineal pain with irritative urinary tract symptoms, pain in the rectum, testicles, hematuria, pain with ejaculation, hematospermia, and abdominal pain that is located in the lower abdomen and is vague in character. Urinary retention may occur. Symptoms may be worsened with defecation. Recent Foley catheterization or instrumentation of the urethra is a risk factor. On physical examination, the prostate is typically "boggy" (diffuse enlargement), and tender to palpation. The digital rectal exam (DRE) should not be too vigorous as to prevent bacteremia. Although urinalysis and culture are necessary, other labs are of little benefit unless the patient is suspected to be toxic or immunocompromised (acute bacterial prostatitis occurs more often in human immunodeficiency virus [HIV] infected patients). Acute prostatitis is usually caused by the same microbes responsible for other acute urinary tract infections (UTIs) (*E. coli* [65% to 85%], *Pseudomonas*, *Klebsiella*, and *Proteus*, but *Chlamydia*, *Neisseria gonorrhoeae*, and *Treponema pallidum* must be considered and treated appropriately). Most patients with acute prostatitis have concomitant urethrocystitis.

Clinical features of chronic bacterial prostatitis may include mild irritative symptoms (frequency, urgency, and dysuria), urethral discharge, painless hematuria, painful ejaculation, hematospermia, recurrent UTIs, perineal discomfort, frequency, urgency, dysuria, asymptomatic bacturia, and abdominal pain, but it may also be asymptomatic. Fever is uncommon except during acute exacerbations. The prostate is sometimes irregular and mildly tender, but examination is often unremarkable. Chronic bacterial prostatitis may occur after an acute bacterial prostatitis or without any antecedent infection. Common organisms include *E. coli*, *Enterococcus*, *Proteus*, and *Klebsiella*. Prostatic calculi may act as a nidus for these organisms complicating the treatment as antibiotics do not readily penetrate the chronically inflamed prostate.

Diagnosis and Differential

Cultures may be collected after prostatic massage, which may produce a thick discharge with leukocytes that grows large numbers of pathogens on culture. Urinalysis and Gram stain usually shows abnormal sediment and the pathogenic bacteria (usually gram-negative enteric rods). Cultures are the most accurate way of establishing diagnosis. The gold standard of culture diagnosis is the Meares-Stamey 4 glass test, but it is not used in the emergency department.

Differential diagnoses include cystitis, urethritis, epididymitis/orchitis, seminal vesiculitis, benign prostatic hyperplasia, prostatic cancer, proctitis, perirectal/perianal/peroneal abscess, pyelonephritis, urolithiasis, vesicular calculi, sacroiliitis, discitis, osteomyelitis, and pyriformis muscle strain.

Emergency Department Care and Disposition

Supportive treatments include hydration, antipyretics/analgesics (often opioids), spasmolytic drugs to alleviate pain, stool softeners, sitz baths, anticholinergic agents, or α-adrenergic blocking agents for patients with irritative urination symptoms. Antibiotic therapy includes fluoroquinolones, such as levofloxacin 500 mg IV daily or orally, or ciprofloxacin 500 mg orally twice a day, or ofloxacin 300 mg orally twice a day, for up to 30 days. If drug cost is an issue, trimethoprim-sulfamethoxazole (TMP/SMX) double strength, one tablet orally BID for 30 days is an alternative, although cure rates are lower for TMP/SMX than for ciprofloxacin. Follow-up with urology is recommended. Admission should be considered for toxic appearing patients or suspected sepsis or patients with urinary retention.

Pitfalls

- Chronic prostatitis may be asymptomatic and should be suspected in men with recurrent UTIs.
- In the setting of acute prostatitis, there may be elevated prostate specific antigen (PSA) levels, which may need to be followed after resolution.
- Failure to schedule follow up with urology.
- In immunocompromised patients (e.g., diabetics) with persistent fever, computed tomography (CT) scan or transrectal ultrasound (US) of prostate may reveal a prostatic abscess(es).
- Failure to place a suprapubic catheter in the setting of bladder outlet obstruction from acutely inflamed prostate.

STREPTOCOCCAL PHARYNGITIS

Epidemiology

The majority of cases of pharyngitis are viral in nature and the infection is of short duration and usually self-limited. Streptococcal bacteria (mostly group A beta-hemolytic streptococcus [GABHS] species) account for approximately 5% to 15% of cases. Peak age is 4 to 11 years. Because of the sequelae of *Streptococcus* infection, it must be determined whether the pharyngitis is caused by this bacterium. It occurs most commonly in the winter and spring months and has higher rates in those who have close, regular contact with children.

Pathophysiology

The cause of strep throat is GABHS, which infects the pharynx. Transmission is by direct, close contact with an infected person via respiratory droplets. Casual contact and contaminated food are rare causes.

Clinical Features

The incubation period for GABHS is 2 to 4 days after exposure followed by abrupt onset of sore throat, malaise, fever, and headache. There is often associated dysphagia and odynophagia, neck stiffness, palatal petechiae, and gastrointestinal symptoms including abdominal pain. Twenty-seven percent of patients with GABHS have abdominal pain, typically diffuse and vague in character.[3] Physical exam may reveal tender anterior cervical and tonsillar lymph nodes (at the jaw angle), and enlarged, erythematous tonsils with exudates. Abdominal tenderness when present is diffuse, and rebound tenderness is uncommon. Cough, hoarseness and rhinorrhea, laryngitis, stridor, conjunctivitis, and diarrhea are not usually present in patients with strep throat.[3,4]

Scarlet fever (a clinical diagnosis) is an exotoxin-mediated dermatologic manifestation of strep throat. A scarlatiniform rash associated with pharyngitis is almost always GABHS. The rash characteristically appears 12 to 48 hours after the fever and begins on the upper body and may spread to all areas. Scarlet fever is *not* rheumatic fever, but may progress to the autoimmune mediated disease. Scarlet fever is characterized by a diffuse red blush that usually starts on the trunk (may also start in the axilla or postauricularly) that spreads centrifugally with circumoral pallor. The rash blanches and acquires a sandpaper texture. The rash begins to fade 3 to 4 days after onset, with desquamation with flakes of skin peeling from the face and palms and can last up to a month.

Diagnosis and Differential

Clinical prediction rules have been developed, such as the Centor and McIsaac criteria; however, these criteria perform poorly.[5] Diagnosis is usually dependent on throat culture or rapid antigen tests.

Emergency Department Care and Disposition

Antibiotic therapy[4] may include: benzathine penicillin 1.2 million U IM (or 600,000 U IM for patients less than 27 kg), (the only therapy proven to prevent rheumatic fever), penicillin V 1 g orally twice daily for 10 days (500 mg orally twice daily for patients less than 27 kg), amoxicillin 20 mg/kg orally 3 times daily for 10 days, erythromycin ethylsuccinate 13 to 16 mg/kg orally 3 times daily for 10 days, cefprozil 15 mg/kg orally twice daily for 10 days, cefuroxime 15 mg/kg twice daily for 10 days, or azithromycin 12 mg/kg daily for 5 days. Supportive care includes antipyretics and sometimes analgesics, encouraging increased fluid intake; intravenous fluid may be required.

Pitfalls

- A negative rapid strep test does not exclude GABHS and should be verified with a throat culture.
- Obtaining a proper throat culture can often be difficult, but necessary in guiding therapy.

LYME DISEASE

Lyme disease is a vector-borne, multisystem inflammatory disease caused by the spirochete *Borrelia*.

Epidemiology

Lyme disease (*Lyme borreliosis*) is the most common tick-borne disease in North America where the white-footed mouse and the white-tailed deer are the preferred animal reservoirs. Lyme disease is caused by a spirochete from the genus *Borrelia* with several species that have been identified as insect vectors. The vector is an infected Ixodes tick. The disease incidence is greatest in the midspring through the late fall corresponding with tick populations. Lyme disease is most frequently reported in the northeast, Midwest, and western United States, although it has been reported in all states. The reported incidence is 4.4 cases per 100,000 persons.

Pathophysiology

The Ixodes tick has 4 stages of development: egg, larva, nymph, and adult. The larvae, nymphs, and adult female ticks require blood meals as part of their life cycle. The risk of disease transmission from tick to human is directly proportional to the time of tick attachment. There have been case reports that biting flies have successfully transmitted Lyme disease, and indeed Lyme spirochetes have been found in biting flies and mosquitos.[6]

Clinical Features

The disease has great variability in its presentation and often is not on the differential diagnosis due to its non-specific findings.[7,8] The incubation period from infection to the onset of symptoms is usually within 2 weeks (with a range from a couple of days to years). Lyme disease is divided into 3 stages based on clinical manifestations; however, most patients lack characteristic progression from one stage to the next. Seventy percent to 85% of patients present during the first month after the bite, when abdominal pain is most likely to be present. The abdominal pain is diffuse, vague, and mild to moderate in severity. Early localized disease often includes a rash. The classic rash is erythema migrans (EM) (or erythema chronicum migrans [ECM]) with the "bull's-eye" lesion, but homogenous red rashes are more common.[9] The rash

starts at the site of the bite with common sites including the axillae, groin, and waistline. Erythema migrans begins as an erythematous macule or papule, which expands outwards with a sharply demarcated, warm, and nontender border.

Early localized disease can progress to hematogenous dissemination within a month. Symptoms can be broken down into neurologic, cardiac, musculoskeletal, dermatologic, and ophthalmic symptoms. See Table 42-3, for a complete listing of early symptoms.

Diagnosis and Differential

Lyme disease is diagnosed based on history (may include exposure), symptomatology, and physical findings. Serology testing may be beneficial in some cases, specifically antibodies to *B. burgdorferi* in the serum (enzyme immunoassay and Western blot). A history of tick bite is often unnoted secondary to the size of tick and the painless bites. Culture of the organism is extremely difficult. Clinical suspicion is crucial since laboratory testing can often be false positive. An electrocardiogram should be considered for patients with suspected cardiac manifestations.

Table 42-3. Lyme Disease Symptoms by Stage

		Stage 1 (1 to 30 days after bite)	
System	**% Affected in Untreated (approx.)**	**Symptoms**	**Notes**
Constitutional	50	Rash, fever, chills, flulike symptoms (malaise, fatigue, headache) muscle pain, joint pain, abdominal pain, stiff neck, lymphadenopathy	Signs and symptoms often resolve without treatment
Dermatologic	50	Multiple, smaller, disseminated annular lesions	Resolve with therapy
Neurologic	15	Meningitis, cranial neuropathy, radiculoneuropathy	Usually within 2 months after EM resolution Bell palsy may be bilateral in 25% of patients Most cases resolve within one month regardless of treatment
Cardiac	10	From first to complete atrioventricular block, cardiomyopathy, pericarditis, myocarditis	Manifestations usually resolve within 8 weeks Heart block usually resolves with treatment

Abbreviation: EM, erythema migrans.

The differential diagnosis is expansive because of the multisystemic manifestation of Lyme disease and includes (but is hardly limited to) many autoimmune and neurologic diseases such as multiple sclerosis, rheumatoid arthritis, fibromyalgia, chronic fatigue syndrome, syphilis and other tick-borne illnesses, acute disseminated encephalomyelitis, Alzheimer disease, ankylosing spondylitis, aseptic meningitis, atypical facial pain, bell palsy, fibromuscular dysplasia, prion-related diseases, toxic neuropathy, and trigeminal neuropathy.

Emergency Department Care and Disposition

Antibiotic therapy is outlined in Table 42-4. Admission should be considered for patients with abnormal vital signs. Referral should be made to the patient's primary care doctor or an infectious disease specialist.

Pitfalls

- False-positive serology testing can be due to patients with syphilis, rheumatologic diseases, or infectious mononucleosis.

- Tics should not be removed by "burning" or "unscrewing" the tick, as this may cause the tick to regurgitate and thus increase risk for transmission. Proper removal involves using a tweezer and grabbing the head of the tick and pulling it straight out, then disinfecting with rubbing alcohol or hydrogen peroxide.

PNEUMONIA

Pneumonia is an inflammation of the lung parenchyma characterized by consolidation of the affected part, the alveolar air spaces being filled with exudates, inflammatory cells, and fibrin. Causes of pneumonia range from infectious etiologies, chemicals, or trauma.

Distribution may be lobar, segmental, or lobular. The subject of pneumonia could fill tomes, and that is not the purpose of this chapter. The most common bacterial etiologies of community-acquired pneumonia (CAP) will primarily be discussed.

Epidemiology

There are an estimated 4 million cases of pneumonia per year in the United States, a rate of 12 cases per 1000 persons per year. Pneumonia is the 6th leading cause of death in the United States and the most common cause of death from infectious disease. In the United States, over 3 million people contract CAP annually resulting in 500,000 to 600,000 hospital admissions. Pneumonia is usually the result of a single bacterial species.

Pathophysiology

Bacterial pneumonia, depending on the causative organism, can have different effects on the host. The host's immune status also plays a large role on the severity of the pneumonia. Risk factors include impaired cough or gag reflex, impaired mucociliary clearance, chronic disease, immunocompromise, underlying lung pathology, chest wall dysfunction, and altered upper respiratory tract flora. Aspiration of oropharyngeal secretions is the primary mechanism of acquisition as 50% of normal healthy individuals aspirate in their sleep.

Pneumonia has several classifications, depending upon how the examiner wishes to categorize the disease. Often pneumonia is broken into "typical and atypical" and "community and health care acquired." Community acquired pneumonia is defined as an infection that begins outside the hospital or is diagnosed within 48 hours after admission to the hospital in a person who has not resided in a long-term care facility for 14 days or more before admission. Although the classification of typical

Table 42-4. Recommended Antimicrobial Regimens for Treatment of Patients with Lyme Disease

Drug	Dosage for Adults	Dosage for Children
Amoxicillin	500 mg 3 times per day[*]	50 mg/kg per day in 3 divided doses (maximum, 500 mg per dose)[*]
Doxycycline	100 mg twice per day[†]	Not recommended for children aged <8 years
		For children aged ≥8 years, 4 mg/kg per day in 2 divided doses (maximum, 100 mg per dose)
Cefuroxime axetil	500 mg twice per day	30 mg/kg per day in 2 divided doses (maximum, 500 mg per dose)

[*]Although a higher dosage given twice per day might be equally as effective, in view of the absence of data on efficacy, twice-daily administration is not recommended.
[†]Tetracyclines are relatively contraindicated in pregnant or lactating women and in children <8 years of age.

(pyogenic bacterial) and atypical are somewhat artificial, "typical" pneumonia is associated with the abrupt onset of fever and chills followed by cough that is productive of purulent sputum and pleuritic chest pain. "Atypical" is associated with a subacute onset of systemic complaints associated with a nonproductive cough.

Clinical Features

The typical history from a patient with bacterial pneumonia consists of a combination of fever, dyspnea, cough, pleuritic chest pain, and sputum production.[10] There is usually an associated tachypnea and tachycardia.[11] Some typical historical features stratified by organism are outlined in Table 42-5. When abdominal pain occurs in association with pneumonia, typically the pain is dull, constant, located in the upper abdomen, and made worse with deep inspiration.

Diagnosis and Differential

The diagnosis of pneumonia is based on history, physical, and chest radiograph. Further investigation may include complete blood count (CBC) with differential, pulse oximetry, blood cultures, arterial blood gas, and pleural fluid examination. The white blood cell (WBC) count may or may not be helpful in making the diagnosis of pneumonia. In a healthy patient, a WBC >15,000 is highly suggestive of bacterial pneumonia. In elderly and septic patients, the WBC becomes less reliable.

The chest radiograph may help suggest a specific causative organism (see Table 42-6), but patients should

Table 42-5. Clinical Findings in Community Acquired Pneumonia

Community Acquired Pneumonia in Adults	
Organism	Clinical findings
*Streptococcus pneumoniae**	Abrupt fever, rigors and rusty brown sputum, pleuritic chest pain. Pleural effusion in 25% of patients
*Haemophilus influenzae**	More common in smokers, COPD patients, malnourished patients, malignancy, diabetes, and elderly. Rales and rhonchi without signs of consolidation
*Staphylococcus aureus**	Frequently follows viral illness, IV drug users
*Legionella pneumophilia**	Nonproductive cough and commonly GI symptoms. Patchy bronchopneumonia to frank consolidation. Relative bradycardia and confusion. Often will have hyponatremia, hypophosphatemia, elevated liver enzymes. Alcoholics, diabetic, institutionalized or intubated patients are at risk
Mycoplasma pneumoniae†	Fine rales, rhonchi, or normal breath sounds. Bullous myringitis is pathognomic for mycoplasma
Chlamydia pneumoniae†	Fine rales, rhonchi, or normal breath sounds
*Klebsiella pneumoniae**	Alcoholism, diabetes, chronic illnesses. Currant jelly sputum. Lobar pneumonia with consolidation. Bronchial breath sounds, egophony, increased tactile and vocal fremitus, dullness to percussion, pleural friction rub, cyanosis
Anaerobic organisms	History of aspiration (alcoholics, seizures, stroke, neuromuscular disease). Right lower lobe is most common due to anatomy
Pneumocystitis jiroveci (previously *carinii*)	Common in HIV patients
*Pseudomonas aeruginosa**	Rare, underlying lung disease, CF
Aspiration pneumonia	Immediate suction and bronchoscopy for large particles. Oxygen should be administered, but steroids and prophylactic antibiotics should be withheld
*Escherichia coli**	Rare
Group A streptococci*	Rare
*Moraxella catarrhalis**	Rare

*Typical (80%–90%).
†Atypical (10%–20% of cases).
Abbreviations: CF, cystic fibrosis; COPD, chronic obstructive pulmonary disease; GI, gastrointestinal; HIV, human immunodeficiency virus; IV, intravenous.

Table 42-6. Chest Radiograph Findings in Community Acquired Pneumonia by Causative Organism

Organism	Chest Radiograph Findings
S. pneumoniae	Most common cause of lobar pneumonia
	Singular lobe infiltrate in LLL, RLL, or RML
	Small pleural effusion
	Abscess formation
Group A strep	Patchy, multilobar infiltrates (usually lower)
	Large pleural effusion
H. influenza	Patchy (frequently basilar) infiltrates
	Occasional pleural effusion
Klebsiella pneumoniae	Upper lobe infiltrates
	Bulging fissure
	Abscess formation
Staph. aureus	Patchy, multicentric infiltrates
	Abscess formation
	Emphysema
	Pneumothroax
Pseudomonas aeruginosa	Patchy, mid or lower lobe infiltrates
	Abscess formation
E. coli	Patchy, bilateral lower lobe infiltrates

Abbreivations; LLL, left lower lobe; RLL, right lower lobe; RML, right middle lobe.

be treated empirically until the organism is known. When pneumonia is the cause of abdominal pain, typically the infiltrate is in contact with the diaphragm.

The differential diagnosis should include tracheobronchitis, pulmonary embolus or infarction, chronic obstructive pulmonary disease (COPD) exacerbation, pulmonary vasculitides (Goodpasture disease and Wegener granulomatosis) bronchiolitis obliterans and endocarditis, silicosis, chemical pneumonitis, toxic drugs, radiation, thermal injury, and oxygen toxicity.

Emergency Department Care and Disposition

Disposition can be a complicated matter.[10] Many hospitals use a pneumonia severity index to determine whether the patient should be treated as an outpatient, inpatient, or ICU patient. Hospital admission should be considered in immunocompromised patients, pregnant patients, and those with clinical signs of toxicity (RR >30, HR >125, systolic BP <90, hypoxemia, altered mental status (AMS), dehydration) or serious comorbid disease (neoplastic disease, renal failure, diabetes, cardiac disease, debilitated state).[11,12] Because most patients do not require identification of the organism, most cases of CAP are treated empirically.[12] Treatment options are outlined in Table 42-7.[11]

Pitfalls

- Most patients do not require identification of organism.
- Sputum Gram stain rarely changes therapy.
- Being unaware of the hospital's antibiotic resistance data.
- A normal WBC does not rule out pneumonia.
- Leukopenic or dehydrated patients may have normal-appearing x-rays.
- Failure to recognize pneumonia in patients with exacerbation of underlying lung disease (COPD, asthma).
- Delay of initiation of antibiotics in seriously ill.
- Failure to ask about HIV risk factors or consideration of tuberculosis (TB) in high-risk individuals.
- Failure to administer pneumococcal and influenza vaccine to high risk patients.

HERPES ZOSTER

Herpes zoster (shingles) is the reactivation or latent herpes zoster virus infection. There is a lifetime incidence of almost 20%, with the majority of cases being among the elderly.

Clinical Features

The lesions of shingles are identical to those of chickenpox, but are limited to a single dermatome in distribution. Thoracic and lumber dermatomes are most common. The disease begins with a prodrome of pain in the affected area for 1 to 3 days, followed by the outbreak of a maculopapular rash that quickly progresses to a vesicular rash. The course of the disease is usually around 2 weeks, but may persist for a full month. Rash involving more than a single dermatome or crossing the midline should raise suspicion of disseminated disease.

Involvement of thoracic nerve 5 (xiphoid) through thoracic nerve 12 (pubis) could be associated with abdominal pain. The abdominal pain associated with zoster can be severe, and described as sharp or knifelike or shocklike. Abdominal exam rarely reveals tenderness.[13]

Table 42-7. Treatment Options for CAP

Therapy for Outpatient Treatment of Uncomplicated Patients

Class	Example	Comments
Macrolide	Clarithromycin XL 1000 mg orally each day for 7 days or Azithromycin 500 mg orally on day 1 and 250 mg on days 2–5	Respiratory fluoroquinolones could also be used but the CDC recommends other agents except under some circumstances.
Tetracyline	Doxycycline 100 mg bid for 10–14 days	

Therapy for Outpatient Management: Patients with Significant Comorbidities

Class	Example	Comments
Fluoroquinolone	Levofloxacin 750 mg orally daily for 5 days or Moxifloxacin 400 mg daily for 7–14 days	Other respiratory fluoroquinolones may also be used
Penicillin +β-lactamase inhibitor with a macrolide	Amoxicillin-clavulanate 2 gm twice daily with Azithromycin 500 mg orally on day 1 and 250 mg on days 2–5	A 3rd generation cephalosporin may be used instead of the amino-penicillin

Inpatient Therapy for Non-ICU Patients

Class	Example	Comments
Fluoroquinolone	Levofloxacin 750 mg IV or Moxifloxacin 400 mg IV	Other respiratory fluoroquinolones may also be used
Cephalosporin + Macrolide	Ceftriaxone 1 g IV with azithromycin 500 mg IV	Other 3rd generation cephalosporins may also be used in combination with other macrolides or doxycycline.

Inpatient Therapy for ICU Patients

Class	Example	Comments
Cephalosporin with a Macrolide	Ceftriaxone 1 gm IV with azithromycin 500 mg IV	Other beta lactams may also be used
Cephalosporin with a Fluoroquinolone	Ceftriaxone 1 gm with either moxifloxacin 400 mg IV or with levofloxacin 750 mg IV	
Fluoroquinolone with either a monobactam or a lincosamide	Moxifloxacin 400 mg IV or with levofloxacin 750 mg IV with either aztreonam 1–2 g IV or clindamycin 600 mg IV	Aztreonam is generally well tolerated in penicillin allergic patients
Note that for patients with MRSA risk or HCAP patients add additional coverage to the above	Vancomyin 10–15 mg/kg IV or linezolid 600 mg	To be added to one of the above regimens for patients with MRSA or HCAP risk

Patients with Pseudomonas Risk

Class	Example	Comments
Beta-lactam/beta lactamase inhibitor+ quinolone	Piperocillian-tazobactam 3.375 mg IV plus ciprofloxacin 400 mg IV	Other anti-pseudomonal cephalosporins or quinolones may be used. Carbapenems are also appropriate. Consider adding an aminoglycoside if using a macrolide
Other fluoroquinolone	Aztreonam 1 g IV plus either moxifloxacin 400 mg IV or levofloxacin 750 mg IV	May be used for patients with penicillin allergy. Carbapenems and aminoglycosides may also be appropriate
Note that for patients with MRSA risk or HCAP patients add additional coverage to the above	Vancomyin 10–15 mg/kg IV or linezolid 600 mg	To be added to one of the above regimens for patients with MRSA or HCAP risk

Abbreviations: CDC, Centers for Disease Control and Prevention; IV, intravenous; MRSA, methicillin-resistant *Staphylococcus aureus*; HCAP, health care acquired pneumonia.

The most common complication of shingles is postherpetic neuralgia (PHN). Postherpetic neuralgia occurs in 10% to 20% of all patients after an episode of acute zoster, but in up to 70% of patients aged 70 years or older. It generally resolves in 1 to 2 months, but may last longer than a year in some patients.

Emergency Department Care and Disposition

The treatment of herpes zoster in the normal host is aimed at decreasing the risk of PHN, since the antivirals have a clinically small, but statistically significant, effect on the duration of the acute disease. Treatment should begin as soon as possible, and within 72 hours of disease onset for maximal benefit. There is a suggestion that both famciclovir (500 mg 3 times a day for 7 days) and valacyclovir (1000 mg 3 times a day for 7 days) may be more effective than acyclovir (800 mg 5 times a day for 7 days), but this has not been shown to be clinically significant.

Patients with evidence of disseminated disease should be admitted for IV acyclovir. Treatment with antiherpes agents has been shown to decrease the duration of PHN but not to reduce its incidence. Initial treatment of patients with PHN is typically systemic analgesia, often narcotics. Patients should be referred back to their primary care provider, because first-line agents often fail, and a trial of gabapentin 300 mg to 600 mg PO TID, or carbamazepine may be tried as second-line therapy.

Pitfalls

- Failing to consider the diagnosis.

REFERENCES

1. Knight PJ, Vassy LE. The diagnosis and treatment of the acute scrotum in children and adolescents. *Ann Surg.* 1984;200:664.
2. Moon TD, Hagen L, Heisy DM. Urinary symptomatology in younger men. *Urology.* 1997;50:700.
3. Kreher NE, Hickner JM, Barry HC, et al. Do gastrointestinal symptoms accompanying sore throat predict streptococcal pharyngitis? *J Fam Pract.* 1998;46:159.
4. Bisno AL. Acute pharyngitis. *N Engl J Med.* 2001;344:205.
5. Bonner AB, Johnson SE, Rajab MH, et al. Should the Centor and McIsaac criteria be used to predict the probability of group a streptococcal pharyngitis in children aged 2–12 years? *Acad Emerg Med.* 2005;12:S108.
6. Magnarelli L, Anderson J. Ticks and biting insects infected with the etiologic agent of Lyme disease, Borrelia burgdorferi. *J Clin Microbiol.* 1988;26:1482.
7. Wormser GP, Dattwyler RJ, Shapiro ED, et al. The Clinical assessment, treatment, and prevention of Lyme Disease, human granulocytic anaplasmosis, and babesiosis: Clinical Practice Guidelines by the Infectious Diseases Society of America. *Clin Inf Dis.* 2006;43:1089.
8. Smith RP, Schoen RT, Rahn DW, et al. Clinical characteristics and treatment outcome of early Lyme disease in patients with microbiologically confirmed erythema migrans. *Ann Intern Med.* 2002;136:421.
9. Edlow JA. Erythema migrans. *Med Clin North Am.* 2002; 86:239.
10. Halm EA, Teirstein AS. Management of community acquired pneumonia. *N Engl J Med.* 2002;347:2039.
11. Metlay JP, Kapoor WN, Fine MJ. Does this patient have community-acquired pneumonia? Diagnosing pneumonia by history and physical examination. *JAMA.* 1997;278;1440.
12. ACEP Clinical Policy for the Management and Risk Stratification of Community Acquired Pneumonia in Adults in the Emergency Department. *Ann Emerg Med.* 2001; 38:107.
13. Vinzio S, Lioure B, Enescu I, et al. Severe abdominal pain and inappropriate antidiuretic hormone secretion preceding varicella-zoster virus reactivation 10 months after autologous stem cell transplantation for acute myeloid leukemia. *Bone Marrow Trans.* 2005;35:525.

43

Metabolic and Toxicologic Disorders Presenting with Abdominal Pain

M. Fernanda Bellolio

HIGH YIELD FACTS

- Pain perceived as originating in the abdomen may arise from extraabdominal sites or from acute systemic illness.
- In a patient with unknown etiology of abdominal pain, look for signs and symptoms of extraabdominal illness.
- Suspect an unusual cause of abdominal pain in patients with severe abdominal pain with negative abdominal physical examination findings.

EPIDEMIOLOGY

Symptoms referable to the digestive system are very common and abdominal pain is the most common reason for emergency department (ED) visits in the United States.[1,2] Metabolic and toxicologic disorders are considered extraabdominal causes of abdominal pain and are uncommon. The true incidence of metabolic and toxicologic disorders presenting with acute abdominal pain in the ED is not known.

PATHOPHYSIOLOGY

The pathophysiology depends on the cause of abdominal pain. In metabolic acidosis, nausea and vomiting have been attributed to either a central neurogenic response to increased ketone bodies and acidosis, or to gastric atony and generalized ileus.[3] Delayed gastric emptying secondary to gastroparesis is a direct effect of acute hyperglycemia.[3] In vasculitis, abdominal visceral arterial involvement has been suspected as a cause of pain. This is seen in 60% to 70% of cases of polyarteritis nodosa.[4] In hematologic diseases, the abdominal pain is attributed to microvessel occlusion and infarcts of mesentery and abdominal viscera.[5]

In toxicologic causes, severe gastroenteritis and esophageal or gastric perforation are seen when corrosives are ingested; ileus or intestinal obstruction when anticholinergics and opiates are ingested; and ischemic bowel injury when vasoconstrictors and cocaine ingestion. Direct injury to organs such as the liver and pancreas is seen secondary to toxic metabolites.[6]

CLINICAL FEATURES

Extraperitoneal diseases may present with abdominal pain as a prominent symptom. In order to make a diagnosis, a high index of suspicion must be maintained for unusual causes of abdominal pain.

The history and the physical examination are the greatest tools in suspecting and identifying the unusual cause of abdominal pain.[7] Inquiry into prior similar episodes, exacerbating features, and constitutional and extraabdominal symptoms is needed. Family, occupational, and travel histories may be clues to the possibility of a less common cause for the patient's complaint. Physical examination of the abdomen is essential, and it is important to include pulmonary, cardiac, genitourinary, and back examinations. In addition, clues to unusual diagnoses are often found on careful evaluation of the skin, head, and neck, as well as the musculoskeletal, vascular, and nervous systems.[4]

Pursuit of an unusual cause of abdominal pain might be suggested by any of the following[4]:

1. Repeated visits to the ED for the same chief complaint without definitive diagnosis.
2. Ill-appearing patient with minimal or nonspecific findings on abdominal examination.
3. Abdominal pain out of proportion to physical findings.
4. Unusual systemic symptoms for intraabdominal pathology (e.g., neurologic deficits, dysrhythmias, or arthralgias).

DIAGNOSIS AND DIFFERENTIAL

Metabolic Causes

Metabolic Acidosis

Metabolic acidosis results from increased production or decreased excretion of acids, or loss of alkali.[8] Elevated anion-gap metabolic acidosis is a common cause of abdominal pain, particularly in diabetic (DKA) and alcoholic (AKA) ketoacidosis. Other causes of metabolic acidosis with elevated anion gap are: lactic acidosis,

Table 43-1. Metabolic Causes of Abdominal Pain

Metabolic Acidosis	Hematologic
Diabetes, alcoholic,	Sickle cell disease
starvation ketoacidosis	Porphyria
Lactic acidosis	Hemolytic anemia
Uremia	Acute leukemia
Vasculitis	Lymphoma
Rheumatoid vasculitis	Cyclic neutropenia
Systemic lupus	Hemochromatosis
erythematosus	Thrombocytosis
Polyarteritis nodosa	Others
Eosinophilic enteritis	Inflammatory bowel
Henoch-Schönlein	disease
purpura	Familial Mediterranean
Endocrine	fever
Hypercalcemia	Chronic angioedema
Acute adrenal insufficiency	Hyperlipidemia
Pheochromocytoma	Heat stroke
Hyperparathyroidism	Glaucoma
Thyrotoxicosis	

chronic renal insufficiency, intoxications with methanol, ethylene glycol, isoniazid, iron, salicylates, and paraldehyde, (see Table 43-1).[8,9] There is a direct correlation between the severity of metabolic acidosis and the presence of abdominal pain.[3]

Diabetic ketoacidosis is a common complication of diabetes. It presents with hyperglycemia, ketonemia, and acidemia. The incidence is 4.6 to 8.0 per 1000 person-years among diabetic patients.[10] Current mortality is 4% to 10%.[3,9] The most common precipitating factor is infection. Other precipitating factors are omission or undertreatment with insulin, surgery, myocardial infarction, trauma, or drugs.[3,9] New onset diabetics account for up to 30% of patients presenting in DKA.[10]

Patients with DKA may complain of nonspecific symptoms such as fatigue and malaise. Polyuria, polydipsia, polyphagia, and weight loss are more characteristic of DKA. Nausea, vomiting, and abdominal pain are also common complaints and are caused by either the acidosis itself or decreased mesenteric perfusion.[9]

Abdominal manifestations occur in 40% to 75% of cases of DKA.[3] The abdomen is often diffusely tender.[9] Diabetic ketoacidosis can mimic an acute abdomen, especially in children.[3] The abdominal pain usually resolves with correction of hyperglycemia, metabolic acidosis, and electrolyte disturbances.[3,9] In one study,[3] abdominal pain was reported in 86 of 189 (46%) patients with DKA. Pain was associated with abdominal

tenderness in all patients, and rebound tenderness was present in 12% of patients. Nausea and vomiting were reported in 66% of DKA patients with abdominal pain. In 35% of DKA patients with abdominal pain, the etiology of the pain was considered to be secondary to the precipitating cause of metabolic decompensation.[3] Fewer than 10% of patients with DKA have no identifiable precipitant of the disease.[9] If the acidosis is resistant to standard treatment, or the pain persists after normalization of the pH, intraabdominal disease should be suspected.[3]

Hyperglycemic hyperosmolar nonketotic syndrome (HHNS) In contrast to DKA, abdominal pain in HHNS is much less common; significant acidosis is absent, and therefore nausea and vomiting may not be present. In one study, no patient with HHNS complained of abdominal pain on admission.[3] When the abdominal pain is a predominant symptom, it should be investigated as a precipitating cause of HHNS, rather than a manifestation of it.[11]

Alcoholic ketoacidosis is seen in patients with chronic alcoholism. Clinical presentation is remarkable for vomiting, abdominal pain, and dehydration. In contrast to DKA, serum glucose levels are most often low to normal.[8] Alcohol levels are negligible. In this population, other life-threatening causes such as withdrawal and pancreatitis should be considered.

Emergency department management of ketoacidosis consists of intravenous fluid hydration, insulin administration, and electrolyte replacement. The presence of infection or other precipitating factors will determine whether other specific treatments are necessary. Care of patients with DKA requires frequent and intensive monitoring.[9] The cause of death in patients with DKA and HHNS rarely results from the metabolic complications of hyperglycemia or metabolic acidosis, but relates to the underlying medical illness that precipitated the ketoacidosis.[3]

Uremia: Clinical manifestations appear with glomerular filtration rates reduced 15% to 20% of normal. Anorexia, nausea, and vomiting are frequently seen in uremic patients. These symptoms are caused by accumulation of nitrogenous wastes. Gastritis and pancreatitis are associated with acute renal failure. Gastrointestinal (GI) hemorrhage is seen in 10% to 30% of patients,[12] but severe GI symptoms are usually seen only in advanced disease.

Vasculitides

Several systemic vasculitides may involve the GI tract to varying degrees, ranging from mild transient pain to life-threatening complications such as bowel infarction or hemorrhage.[13] These include systemic lupus erythematosis, Henoch-Schönlein purpura, polyarteritis nodosa, eosinophilic enteritis, dermatomyositis, microscopic polyangiitis, Wegener granulomatosis, Churg-Strauss syndrome, or rheumatoid arthritis-associated vasculitis.[13]

Abdominal pain is the most frequent finding in systemic necrotizing vasculitis (97% in one report).[13] The pain varied widely in intensity and location. Nausea and vomiting were present in one third of the patients, and 27% had diarrhea. For 18% patients, mild abdominal pain was the sole manifestation of GI involvement, and another 18% presented with abdominal tenderness due to peritonitis.[13]

Rheumatoid arthritis related vasculitis: Rheumatoid vasculitis is a necrotizing arteritis that affects only a subset of patients with articular rheumatoid disease. It often manifests with constitutional symptoms and skin infarction or ulceration. Gastrointestinal involvement occurs in 1% to 10%, affecting multiple visceral vascular beds, producing bowel infarction, ulceration, perforation, colitis, stricture, aneurysm, or hemorrhage.[13]

Systemic lupus erythematosus (SLE): Young women are most commonly afflicted.[14] Systemic lupus erythematosus involves the cutaneous and musculoskeletal systems, and can involve the GI tract in multiple ways. Abdominal pain is reported in up to 37% of patients.[15] Patients rarely present with isolated GI manifestations.[14] Causes of SLE-related abdominal pain are serositis, intestinal vasculitis, malabsorption, intestinal pseudoobstruction, protein-losing enteropathy, ischemic bowel disease, mesenteric or hepatic vein thrombosis, hepatitis, pancreatitis, and acalculous cholecystitis.[15] Also there are treatment-related causes of abdominal pain, like gastritis, peptic ulcer, and entero-colonic infections. Corticosteroid therapy may mask classical clinical presentations.[15]

Henoch-Schönlein purpura is a self-limited systemic vasculitis, usually nonsevere. It primarily affects children And is characterized by palpable purpura, arthralgias, nephritis, and colicky abdominal pain. Gastrointestinal involvement occurs in 50% to 75% of patients.[16] According to one report, abdominal pain occurs in 63% of patients and GI bleeding in 33%.[16] Arthritis or abdominal pain preceded the onset of the purpura by 1 to 14 days in less than 50% of patients. Nausea, vomiting, and transient paralytic ileus can occur. Intussusception and bowel ischemia or perforation, are less common.[16]

Polyarteritis nodosa is characterized by generalized inflammation of medium and small arteries. It usually presents as a chronic disease with fever, weight loss, malaise, anorexia, myalgia, and asymmetric arthritis.

Abdominal pain, nausea, vomiting, diarrhea, and GI bleeding are attributable to abdominal visceral arterial involvement, occurring in 40% to 60% of cases.[13] Acute surgical abdominal events, such as bowel infarction, perforation, and life-threatening hemorrhage occur in as many as 31% of patients, but they are rarely the initial manifestation of disease.[17]

Endocrine

Acute adrenal insufficiency: Without a history of similar prior episodes following reduced intake or absorption of adrenal steroids, these patients may be indistinguishable from those with an intraabdominal catastrophe. Clinically patients present weakness, confusion, anorexia, nausea, vomiting, diarrhea, fever, myalgia, craving for salt, headache, and abdominal pain.[18] Patients can be in shock and have diffuse peritoneal signs.[18] Even with adequate fluid resuscitation hemodynamic instability can be present; this can occur in the setting of systemic inflammation without an obvious source and which has not responded to empirical treatment. These patients must receive stress dose steroids.[18]

Pheochromocytoma is a rare catecholamine-secreting tumor. The classical symptoms are present in half of all patients. They consist of attacks of severe hypertension, headache, palpitations, and sweating caused by intermittent release of catecholamines.[19] Pheochromocytma is often associated with other symptoms such as nausea (35% to 65% of cases) and epigastric pain.[4] Also the tumor itself may produce localized pain because of mass effect or local invasion and may cause circulatory collapse following rupture and hemorrhage.[4] Approximately half of all patients have persistent, labile hypertension that is difficult to manage; however, up to one third of patients are normotensive.[19]

Thyrotoxicosis: Gastrointestinal symptoms include nausea, vomiting, frequent bowel movements, abdominal pain, and weight loss. The pain is generally crampy, and frank tenderness is absent. More intense pain is seen in acute hepatomegaly and distension of the liver capsule secondary to the hyperthyroid state. In one report, 25 patients with thyrotoxicosis were evaluated, 44% reported vomiting, 28% reported nausea, and 20% complained of abdominal pain during hospital admision.[20] One or more of these abdominal symptoms was included as a chief complaint in 36% of the cases.[20]

Hypercalcemia: Constipation is the most common GI complaint in patients with hypercalcemia of any etiology, Hypercalcemia secondary to hyperparathyroidism can result in calcifications in the pancreatic ducts, blocking secretions and resulting in acute pancreatitis.[21]

Hematologic

Sickle Cell Disease: (See Chapter 45)
Porphyria: (See Chapter 44)

Others

Familial Mediterranean fever is characterized by recurrent episodes of fever and serosal inflammation of the peritoneum, pleura, or synovium. It is most commonly seen in Sephardic Jews, Armenians, Egyptians, Lebanese, and Turks.[4,22] Attacks resemble the clinical presentation of acute abdomen, with severe abdominal pain and rigidity.[22] Onset is sudden and acute, leading to rapid development of symptoms within 1 to 2 hours. The pain is usually diffuse throughout the entire abdomen, and it may be very severe in intensity. Episodes are self-limited, and usually resolve over 48 hours and misdiagnosis as acute appendicitis is common. A family history of familial Mediterranean fever is often absent.[22]

Chronic angioedema frequently causes abdominal pain and pseudoobstruction. Nausea, vomiting, and cramping abdominal pain are secondary to complement activation and increased vascular permeability, resulting in submucosal edema.[23] A diagnosis of chronic angioedema of the GI tract should prompt an evaluation for underlying lymphoproliferative malignancy.[23]

Toxicological Causes

Toxicologic causes of abdominal pain are secondary to poisoning and overdose (see Table 43-2). Hypersensitivity reactions and opiate withdrawal will also be discussed here.

Mueller and Benowitz[6] propose a classification of causes of abdominal disorders based on five mechanisms of injury:

a. Corrosives, e.g., aspirin, iron, mercury, acids, and alkali produce severe gastroenteritis and may result in esophageal or gastric perforation.

b. Ileus or obstruction by pharmacologic actions, e.g., anticholinergics and narcotics, or by mechanical obstruction, e.g., charcoal and drug bezoars.

c. Ischemic bowel injury from vasoconstriction, e.g., amphetamines, ergotamines, and cocaine.

d. Direct injury to intraabdominal organs such as the liver and pancreas, e.g., acetaminophen.

e. Abdominal pain as a component of systemic effects of black widow spider envenomation or heavy metal poisoning.

Table 43-2. Toxicologic Causes of Abdominal Pain

Caustics	Ischemic bowel
Salicylates (Aspirin)	(vasoconstrictors)
Iron	Ergotamines
Mercury	Amphetamines
Acid and alkali	Cocaine
Ileus	Mushroom poisoning
Anticholinergics	Direct injury in liver or
Narcotics	pancreas
Heavy metals	Hypersensitivity reactions
Lead	Insect bites
Arsenic	Black widow spider bite
Thallium	Reptile venoms
Cadmium	Scorpion bite
	Alcohol, methanol
	Narcotic withdrawal

Corrosives or Caustics

Corrosives or caustics may produce mucosal or transmucosal injury to the GI tract with resultant pain, ulceration, bleeding, perforation, mediastinitis, or peritonitis. Aspirin impairs the gastric mucosal barrier, frequently leading to abdominal pain, vomiting, and hematemesis as an early component of acute overdose with dehydration, electrolyte, acid-base, and neurologic disturbances to follow.[6] Metals, including iron and mercury, are corrosive when ingested. Although presentation may be similar when caustic agents are ingested, the degree of symptoms and severity of complications depend on the type of substance (volume, concentration, liquid vs. solid), form of material (acid vs. alkali), and duration of contact with the mucosa.[4] Findings include oropharyngeal burns, drooling, stridor, nausea, vomiting, hematemesis, chest pain, odynophagia, dysphagia, abdominal pain, and esophageal or gastric perforation with attendant complications.[4]

Heavy Metals

The American Association of Poison Control Centers (AAPCC) data for 2004 lists 12,968 calls for heavy metal exposures. Thirty percent of these victims sought medical attention. There were 6 deaths reported that year.[24] Usually related to occupational exposures, poisoning with inorganic lead, arsenic, thallium, or cadmium may produce a variety of intestinal symptoms. In the setting of acute oral exposure, plain abdominal radiographs may be useful in demonstrating radiopaque metallic densities in the GI tract.[4]

In most patients heavy metal intoxication causes esophageal and abdominal pain, nausea, and vomiting. Patients may present diarrhea (e.g., bloody rice water diarrhea in arsenic intoxication), constipation (e.g., oral thallium intoxication)[25] or crampy abdominal pain and tenesmus (e.g., cadmium intoxication).[4] Acute mercury ingestion produces corrosive gastroenteritis, and patients report a metallic taste in the mouth, gingivostomatitis, loose teeth, an oral burning sensation, hypersalivation, and they may have a grayish discoloration of the mucous membranes.[25] Iron exhibits a direct toxicity into the vascular walls, resulting in GI cell necrosis and hemorrhage.[26] Clinically, iron poisoning takes place in five stages: Stage 1 consists of GI symptoms ranging from abdominal pain and vomiting to life-threatening GI hemorrhage, and symptoms begin 1 to 6 hours after ingestion. Stage 2 represents a period of relative stability. Stage 3 is characterized by reoccurrence of GI symptoms, hypoperfusion, severe metabolic acidosis, altered mental status, and coagulopathy. Progression to Stage 4 is rare, but it is marked by acute hepatic failure;[26] stage 5 presents with bowel obstruction 2 to 8 weeks after ingestion.

The general management of the patients with heavy metal poisoning relies on the provision of basic and advanced life support, decontamination, fluids, and chelation therapy. Patients should have continuous cardiac monitoring. Other specific therapies are available for specific toxicities, such as Prussian blue in thallium poisoning.

Latrodectus mactans (Black Widow Spider) Envenomation

The AAPCC data for 2004 lists 19,349 calls for spider bites, and 14% of these calls involved a black widow spider. Thirty-two percent of the black widow victims sought medical attention, but no deaths were related to the bites.[24] The black widow spider is found worldwide, and only the female is able to envenomate humans. Its bite yields a neurotoxin that stimulates release of acetylcholine peripherally and centrally.

The onset of symptoms occurs 1 to 8 hours following the bite. Local symptoms at the site of the bite are rare. Systemic toxicity generally produces diaphoresis, tachycardia, nausea, abdominal cramping, and painful muscle spasms. Severe abdominal pain with rigidity simulates an acute surgical abdomen or renal colic. Associated symptoms include dizziness, restlessness, ptosis, nausea, vomiting, headache, pruritus, dyspnea,

conjunctivitis, diaphoresis, weakness, difficulty in speaking, anxiety, and cramping pain in all muscle groups. The patient is usually hypertensive. There may be electrocardiogram changes similar to those produced by digitalis. In adults the signs and symptoms disappear in 2 to 3 days. A child bitten by a black widow spider, however, may not survive.[27,28]

The management of the patient with a suspected black widow bite consists of applying an ice pack to the area after cleaning the site with soap and water. Tetanus immunization should be instituted. The patient should be observed for about 4 to 6 hours, and all patients with severe progressive symptoms of envenomation should be admitted to the hospital.[27,28] Intravenous benzodiazepines are useful for relieving muscle spasms. Intravenous calcium initially was touted to be efficacious to alleviate the pain associated with cramps, but subsequent studies have not found it to be of significant benefit.[27,28] Latrodectus antivenin is derived from horse serum and it is indicated for victims who have severe unrelenting systemic symptoms. Allergic reactions occurring 7 to 14 days after administration of the antivenom is seen in 75% of patients who receive it.[27] Consultation with a poison control center may be of benefit.

Alcohol Poisoning

The AAPCC data for 2004 lists 74,268 alcohol exposures. Fifty-three percent of these victims sought medical attention. There were 114 deaths related to alcohol exposure in the report.[24] Methanol, ethylene glycol, and isopropyl alcohol can produce potentially fatal intoxication causing metabolic acidosis. Its toxicity predominantly affects the neurologic, ophthalmologic, and GI systems. Gastrointestinal effects are often limited to nausea and vomiting, but may include severe abdominal pain, GI hemorrhage, diarrhea, liver function abnormalities, and pancreatitis.[8]

Mushroom Poisoning

The AAPCC data for 2004 lists 8601 calls for mushrooms exposure. Unknown mushroom types were seen in 81% of them. Forty-one percent of these victims sought medical attention. There were 5 deaths related to mushrooms in the AAPCC report.[24] The most common type of mushroom exposure is hallucinogenic (62% of the known mushroom types).[24] The majority of deadly mushroom poisonings are related to consumption of the genus Amanita.[29]

Symptoms develop within a few hours of ingestion and include nausea, vomiting, and diarrhea, which may be bloody with accompanying severe abdominal cramping pain out of proportion to tenderness.[29] Significant dehydration can occur, and supportive management with fluid therapy is necessary.

If Amanitas intoxication is suspected, hepatic and renal failure may ensue within several days of ingestion. Gastric aspiration of remaining mushroom fragments, followed by activated charcoal is recommended. Other therapeutic maneuvers include protection of the liver from the toxic effect of amanitin. Penicillin G and silibinin may be beneficial.[29]

Food Allergy

Most of the allergy food reactions include nausea, vomiting, abdominal distension, and diarrhea. **Immediate GI hypersensitivity** manifestations include nausea, abdominal pain, and vomiting within 1 to 2 hours, and subsequent diarrhea. **Allergic eosinophilic gastroenteropathy** is characterized by postprandial nausea and vomiting, abdominal pain, diarrhea, steatorrhea, early satiety, and weight loss. **Protein intolerance or protein enterocolitis** is seen in patients 1 day to 1 year of age; clinically, they have diarrhea with bleeding, anemia, abdominal distension, and vomiting.[30,31] **Eosinophilic gastroenteritis** presents with postprandial nausea, abdominal pain, vomiting and diarrhea, protein losing enteropathy, and weight loss.[31] The general treatment for food allergies is eliminating the specific allergen, often a protein, from the diet.[31,32]

Opiate Withdrawal

Opiate withdrawal produces crampy abdominal pain, and is associated with anxiety, restlessness, insomnia, rhinorrhea, lacrimation, diaphoresis, and mydriasis. Later, tremor, muscle spasms, vomiting, diarrhea, hypertension, tachycardia, fever, chills, diaphoresis, and piloerection are seen. In some individuals, the abdominal skin is dyesthetic, but significant tenderness should not be present.

Emergency Department Care and Disposition

Systemic or extraperitoneal disease processes may present with abdominal pain as the main clinical manifestation. Usually abdominal pain is not the only complaint, so one should look for further clues to aid in arriving at the diagnosis.

Initial resuscitation and stabilization of the patient is the first priority. Serial evaluations over several hours are useful to improve the diagnostic accuracy in patients with unclear causes of abdominal pain.[2,32] Consider elderly and immunocompromised patients as high risk patients; they have atypical presentations and increased morbidity and mortality.[2]

Pitfalls

- Failure to consider that an underlying abdominal problem may have triggered ketoacidosis.

- Failure to consider coexistent critical conditions presenting with acute abdominal pain (e.g., alcohol withdrawal and pancreatitis).

- Failure to recognize early stages of heavy metal poisoning presenting with vague abdominal pain.

REFERENCES

1. McCaig LF, Nawar EW: National Hospital Ambulatory Medical Care Survey: 2004 emergency department summary. Adv Data, 2006;372:1.
2. Clinical policy: critical issues for the initial evaluation and management of patients presenting with a chief complaint of nontraumatic acute abdominal pain. *Ann Emerg Med.* 2000;36:406.
3. Umpierrez G, Freire AX. Abdominal pain in patients with hyperglycemic crises. *J Crit Care.* 2002;17:63.
4. Pearigen PD. Unusual causes of abdominal pain. *Emerg Med Clin North Am.* 1996;14:593.
5. Ahmed S, Shahid RK, Russo LA. Unusual causes of abdominal pain: Sickle cell anemia. *Best Pract Res Clin Gastroenterol.* 2005;19:297.
6. Mueller PD, Benowitz NL. Toxicologic causes of acute abdominal disorders. *Emerg Med Clin North Am.* 1989 7:667.
7. Purcell TB. Nonsurgical and extraperitoneal causes of abdominal pain. *Emerg Med Clin North Am.* 1989;7:721.
8. Casaletto JJ. Differential diagnosis of metabolic acidosis. *Emerg Med Clin North Am.* 2005;23:771.
9. Charfen MA, Fernandez-Frackelton M. Diabetic ketoacidosis. *Emerg Med Clin North Am.* 2005;23:609.
10. Fishbein H, Palumbo PJ. Acute metabolic complications in diabetes. In: Anonymous, National Diabetes Data Group (eds.): *Diabetes in America.* 2nd ed. Washington, DC: U.S. Department of Health and Human Services, National Institutes of Health, National Institute of Diabetes and Digestive and Kidney Diseases. NIH Publication No. 95–1468;1995:283.

11. Nugent BW. Hyperosmolar hyperglycemic state. *Emerg Med Clin North Am.* 2005;23:629.

12. Wolfson AB. Renal failure. In: Marx JA, Hockberger RS, Walls RM, et al. (eds.) *Rosen's Emergency Medicine: Concepts and Clinical Practice.* 6th ed. Philadelphia: Mosby;2006:1532.

13. Pagnoux C, Mahr A, Cohen P, Guillevin L. Presentation and outcome of gastrointestinal involvement in systemic necrotizing vasculitides: Analysis of 62 patients with polyarteritis nodosa, microscopic polyangiitis, Wegener granulomatosis, Churg-Strauss syndrome, or rheumatoid arthritis-associated vasculitis. *Medicine (Baltimore).* 2005; 84:115.

14. Roy S, Weimersheimer P. Nonoperative causes of abdominal pain. *Surg Clin North Am.* 1997;77:1433.

15. Mok CC. Investigations and management of gastrointestinal and hepatic manifestations of systemic lupus erythematosus. *Best Pract Res Clin Rheumatol.* 2005;19:741.

16. Saulsbury FT. Henoch-Schönlein purpura in children: Report of 100 patients and review of the literature. *Medicine (Baltimore).* 1999;78:395.

17. Zizic TM, Classen JN, Stevens MB. Acute abdominal complications of systemic lupus erythematosus and polyarteritis nodosa. *Am J Med.* 1982;73:525.

18. Gibson SC, Hartman DA, Schenck JM. The endocrine response to critical illness: update and implications for emergency medicine. *Emerg Med Clin North Am.* 2005; 23:909.

19. Elder EE, Elder G, Larsson C. Pheochromocytoma and functional paraganglioma syndrome: No longer the 10% tumor. *J Surg Oncol.* 2005;89:193.

20. Harper MB. Vomiting, nausea, and abdominal pain: unrecognized symptoms of thyrotoxicosis. *J Fam Pract.* 1989; 29:382.

21. Dahan M, Chang RJ. Pancreatitis secondary to hyperparathyroidism during pregnancy. *Obstet Gynecol.* 2001;98:923.

22. Simon A, van der Meer JW, Drenth JP. Familial Mediterranean fever—a not so unusual cause of abdominal pain. *Best Pract Res Clin Gastroenterol.* 2005;19:199.

23. Eck SL, Morse JH, Janssen DA, Emerson SG, et al. Angioedema presenting as chronic gastrointestinal symptoms. *Am J Gastroenterol.* 1993;88:436.

24. Watson WA, Litovitz TL, Rodgers GC, et al. 2004 Annual Report of the American Association of Poison Control Centers Toxic Exposure Surveillance System. *Am J Emerg Med.* 2005;23:589.

25. Ibrahim D, Froberg B, Wolf A, et al. Heavy metal poisoning: clinical presentations and pathophysiology. *Clin Lab Med.* 2006;26:67.

26. Mills KC, Curry SC. Acute iron poisoning. *Emerg Med Clin North Am.* 1994;12:397.

27. Saucier JR. Arachnid envenomation. *Emerg Med Clin North Am.* 2004;22:405.

28. Singletary EM, Rochman AS, Bodmer JC, et al. Envenomations. *Med Clin North Am.* 2005;89:1195.

29. Broussard CN, Aggarwal A, Lacey SR, et al. Mushroom poisoning—from diarrhea to liver transplantation. *Am J Gastroenterol.* 2001;96:3195.

30. Scurlock AM, Lee LA, Burks AW. Food allergy in children. *Immunol Allergy Clin North Am.* 2005;25:369.

31. Sampson HA, Sicherer SH, Birnbaum AH. AGA technical review on the evaluation of food allergy in gastrointestinal disorders. American Gastroenterological Association. *Gastroenterology.* 2001;120:1026.

32. Graff LG, Robinson D. Abdominal pain and emergency department evaluation. *Emerg Med Clin North Am.* 2001; 19:123.

44

Neurosychiatric Disorders Presenting with Abdominal Pain

Sara R. Shimmin

CYCLIC VOMITING SYNDROME

High Yield Facts

- Up to 2% of the pediatric population may experience cyclic vomiting syndrome (CVS).
- Cyclic vomiting syndrome is a diagnosis of exclusion and one that should be made with caution in the emergency setting.
- A combination of antiemetic, analgesic, and anxiolytic medications with intravenous (IV) therapy will cease most attacks.

Epidemiology

Cyclic vomiting syndrome is closely related to, and is commonly referred to as abdominal migraine. The disorder most typically occurs in children,[1,2] although it can occur in adults.[2,3] Studies have estimated that approximately 2% of the pediatric population is affected with CVS.[2,4] Girls experience CVS more commonly than boys at a ratio of about 1.3:1.[1,2] There are 2 peaks of onset in childhood; the first occurring at age 5 and the second at age 10.[1] Adult median age of onset is 35 years.[2]

Children with CVS are more than twice as likely to have migraine headaches as the general population (24%).[1] Likewise, children with migraine headaches have abdominal migraines at just over twice the rate of the general population (9%).[1] Estimates of 28% to 75% of children who experience cessation of their CVS symptoms go on to experience migraine headaches.[2]

Pathophysiology

By definition, CVS is characterized by recurrent bouts of abdominal pain for which no organic cause can be found. These attacks usually last from 1 to 72 hours.[1] Attacks may be triggered by stress (either physical or emotional), lack of sleep or tiredness, travel, missing a meal, menstruation,

or infection.[1,2] Positive emotional stress (excitement) is twice as likely to trigger an attack as negative stress.[2]

The cause of most cases of CVS is unknown. There has been some recent suggestion that certain cases may be due to disorders in mitochondrial DNA that predispose the individual to the condition.[5] Others have advocated for a role from ion channelopathies.[4]

Clinical Features

The hallmark of abdominal migraines is recurrent attacks of abdominal pain with or without vomiting that last hours to a few days and begin and end relatively abruptly.[1] The vomiting is of high intensity and low frequency with peak average of 12.6 episodes of emesis an hour and episodes occurring every 3 weeks to every 3 months.[2] The pain is described as dull or colicky and most commonly occurs near the umbilicus, although it can be diffuse. Pain from abdominal migraine generally does not radiate, but is severe enough to interrupt daily activities.

Typical symptoms that are associated with migraine headache, such as anorexia, nausea and vomiting, flushing, and pallor may occur with abdominal migraines as well. Headaches have also been associated with acute attacks.[1,2] Vomiting may contain blood or bile.[2,3] Fleisher et al. found that 25% of adult patients report a low-grade fever with the attack. He also noted that once the emetic phase has begun, adult patients are sometimes thought to have psychosis as their thought patterns are so disrupted by their physical symptoms. The patient is "irritable, demanding, and unable to think clearly or even give an accurate history."[3] Adults were also found to engage in binging on water and vomiting behaviors, which the patients reported made the intense nausea less prominent. Additionally, adult sufferers reported that diluting the stomach contents with water lessened the pain associated with nausea.[3]

Those who develop vomiting due to CVS are much more likely to experience dehydration than those who vomit for other reasons with 58% of children and 100% of adults presenting for cyclic vomiting requiring IV rehydration.

In between attacks, sufferers are symptom-free.

Diagnosis and Differential

The diagnosis of abdominal migraine is one of exclusion. It can only be made after other etiologies are excluded with normal laboratory, radiographic, and endoscopic examinations.[2] Diagnosis is often delayed in both children and adults, with an average time to diagnosis of 2.7 years in children and 8 years in adults.[2] Differential diagnosis is found in Table 44-1.

Table 44-1. Differential Diagnosis of Cyclic Vomiting Syndrome.[2,4]

Gastrointestinal disorders
   Malrotation
   Appendicitis
   Pancreatitis
   Small bowel obstruction
   Allergies (milk, soy, wheat)
Extraintestinal disorders
   Acute hydronephrosis
   Acute intermittent porphyria
   Brainstem neoplasm
   Metabolic disorders
   Abdominal epilepsy

Emergency Department Care and Disposition

Some success has been achieved at prevention through the use of medications that also help to prevent migraine headaches, with amitriptyline or propranolol[6] offering protection from attacks to half of those who use them.[2] The patient who shows up in the emergency department (ED), however, is in the midst of an attack. If vomiting has not yet commenced, antiemetics as well as anxiolytics and analgesics are the mainstay of management.[3] Ondansetron or triptan medications are much more effective at achieving nausea control than phenothiazines, which only offer relief to 14%.[2] Once the vomiting has begun, termination of the attack may be more difficult. Focus on preventing and correcting dehydration in conjunction with the use of H2 blockers or proton pump inhibitors (PPIs) while administering antiemetics and anxiolytics.[3] Deep sleep will stop the vomiting cycle and often lead to the dissipation of an attack but sedatives may be required to achieve this end. Intravenous hydration alone may be enough to stop the cycle.[2]

Once recovery has started, it may be rapid, with an average of 6 hours to resuming normal activities.[2] Those with significant control of their vomiting and pain may be safely discharged home.

Further complicating emergency management, however, is that many of those who present will not yet have been diagnosed with CVS and symptoms may mimic surgical emergencies such as appendicitis, small bowel obstruction, or intussusception. These emergencies must be satisfactorily ruled out prior to discharge.

Pitfalls

- It is important to remember that even those who carry a diagnosis of CVS can suffer from other causes of abdominal pain as well. One must be sure there is not an appendicitis or pancreatitis masquerading as a slightly atypical CVS attack.
- Delays in diagnosis are frequent, leading to inappropriate management of patients with CVS. An awareness of the process and consideration of the illness is necessary to make the diagnosis.

PORPHYRIA

High Yield Facts

- Acute intermittent porphyria is an uncommon cause of abdominal pain with a potentially fatal outcome if not treated appropriately.
- Maintain a high index of suspicion for porphyria in any patient with hyponatremia and abdominal pain.

Epidemiology

Porphyria is more commonly found in women than in men (5:1), and attacks are most frequent during the second to fourth decades.[7,8]

Genetic mutations in segments coding for enzymes used in the heme biosynthetic pathway cause porphyria. There are more than 90 mutations known to cause acute intermittent porphyria (AIP)[7] with varying degrees of penetrance. Acute intermittent porphyria has its highest incidence in people of Swedish descent.[9] It is estimated that 80% to 90% of those with a mutation that could cause porphyria have a latent form.[8,10] Population studies show that 1 to 2 individuals per 100,000 have clinical porphyria, suggesting that as many as 1 to 2 per 10,000 have the gene mutation.[7,11]

Pathophysiology

Heme is required not only in the synthesis of hemoglobin and myoglobin, but also in catalases, peroxidases, and cytochromes. A breakdown anywhere along the pathway or in the 8 enzymes that are required to produce heme can lead to porphyria. The porphyrias can be divided into types based on symptom manifestation including cutaneous, hepatic, and neuropsychiatric.[11] Neuropsychiatric porphyrias are the most common, with acute AIP being the most common of this category.

Menstruation, calorie restriction, and medications that are unsafe in porphyria are the most common precipitating factors for an acute attack of AIP, although stressful events including infection have been known to incite attacks.[7,10] Medications that induce the P450 system increase the requirement for heme by the liver.[7,12] Medications that have been known to precipitate symptoms include barbiturates, diazepam, phenytoin, spironolactone, chloramphenicol, estrogens, and rifampin.[11] Lorazepam is considered safe. It is as yet unknown how drugs that are not known to use the P450 system can induce an acute attack. Alcohol intake is also often implicated in precipitating attacks.[7,11]

It has been suggested that the symptoms of pain, tachycardia, hypertension, and partial ileus are caused by an autonomic neuropathy. The mechanism, however, has yet to be found. It has been suggested that during acute attacks there is a neurotransmitter deficiency, heme is depleted in nerve cells, or that one of the accumulating byproducts acts as a neurotoxin.[7] The structure of aminolevulinate (ALA), one of the products that accumulates during an attack of AIP, bears similarity to GABA and may act through these receptors.[12] In one study, an MRI scan done 8 days following onset of an attack showed high signal intensity lesions that resolved with treatment.[12]

Clinical Features

An acute attack from AIP is marked by severe, constant abdominal pain that occurs in all or any quadrant and may extend to the back, buttocks, or thighs.[7,8] Other common symptoms include nausea/vomiting (43%), extremity pain/parasthesias (50%), and constipation (48%).[9] Attacks are often precipitated by drugs. The abdominal examination is surprisingly benign given the degree of pain. A useful clue to the diagnosis of acute porphyria is that most cases will demonstrate some neurologic symptoms, such as confusion, hallucinations, or motor weakness. The pain is severe enough to require opiates, often in large amounts. The frequent request for opiates has been known to incorrectly label these patients as drug seekers.[7]

Vomiting is often present in attacks of AIP and dehydration is not uncommon. Hyponatremia is frequently found, likely secondary to syndrome of inappropriate secretion of antidiuretic hormone (SIADH) that develops with the acute attack.[7] The hyponatremia may be profound enough to cause seizures.[7,11] Some individuals with normal sodium levels also have seizures during acute attacks. Constipation, cardiac arrhythmia secondary to catecholamine release, fever, and visual impairment may also be present.[11]

Motor neuropathies resembling Guillain-Barré have been described.[7,8] In fact, in rare cases quadriparesis and respiratory failure has been known to cause death during AIP attacks.[8] Mild sensory disturbances over the trunk and thighs or a distal neuropathy with wrist and foot drop may be seen.[7]

Finally, psychiatric symptoms of hallucinations, confusion, and agitation may be seen during an acute attack incorrectly labeling these patients as histrionic, schizophrenic, or with other psychiatric disorders.[7]

Diagnosis and Differential

Emergency department testing for suspected cases of porphyria can be done by sending a random urine sample for porphobilinogen (PBG), which will be elevated during an acute attack. 5-ALA levels are also increased in the urine, but to a lesser degree.[7,13] While a negative screening test doesn't exclude porphyria as the cause of the abdominal discomfort, a positive screening test should later be confirmed by a quantitative assay.[7] Samples must be protected from light and analyzed shortly after the sample is obtained, otherwise the concentrations of PBG may decrease by 50%, leading to a false negative test.[13]

Differential diagonsis includes lead poisoning, hereditary tyrosinemia, and Guillain-Barré syndrome.

Emergency Department Care and Disposition

Most attacks will require admission for IV hydration, antiemetics, and opiate analgesia. Hyponatremia should be corrected. Intravenous hematin has been tried as a therapy for acute attacks, but trials have shown the efficacy to be only modest at best.[7, 12]

Diets rich in carbohydrates, including IV dextrose containing solutions have been used during attacks with resulting symptomatic improvement.[7,11,12]

Pitfalls

- Neurologic symptoms may develop as the pain remits. Do not send patients home prematurely.
- Avoid unsafe drugs, such as those that induce the P450 system in treating patients with known or suspected porphyria.

REFERENCES

1. Abu-Arafeh I, Russell G. Prevalence and clinical features of abdominal migraine compares with those of migraine headache. *Arch Dis Child.*1995;72:413.
2. Li BU, Misiewicz L. Cyclic vomiting syndrome: a brain-gut disorder. *Gastroenterol Clin North Am.* 2003;32:997.
3. Fleisher DR, Gornouriz B, Adams K, et al: Cyclic vomiting syndrome in 41 adults: the illness, the patients, and problems of management. *BMC Medicine.* 2005;3:20.
4. Li BK, Balint JP. Cyclic vomiting syndrome: Evolution of our understanding of a brain-gut disorder. *Adv Pediatr.* 2000;47:117.
5. Wang Q, Ito M, Adams K, et al. Mitochondrial DNA control region sequence variation in migraine headache and cyclic vomiting syndrome. *Am J Med Genet.* Part A. 2004;131:50.
6. Worawattanakul M, Rhoads JM, Lichtman SN, Ulshen MH Abdominal migraine: Prophylactic treatment and follow-up. *J Pediatr Gastroenterol Nutr.* 1999;28:37.
7. Elder GH, Hift RJ, Meissner PN. The acute porphyries. *Lancet.* 1997;349:1613.
8. James MFM, Hift RJ. Porphyrias. *Br J Anaesth.* 2000; 85:143.
9. Dombeck TA, Satonik RC. The porphyrias. *Emerg Med Clin North Am.* 2005;23:885.
10. Elder GH. Molecular genetics of disorders of haem biosynthesis. *J Clin Pathol..* 1993;46:977.
11. Scarlett YV, Brenner DA. Porphyrias. *J Clin Gastroenterol.* 1998;27:192.
12. Crimlisk HL. The little imitator-porphyria:a neuropsychiatric disorder. *J Neurol Neurosurg Psychiatry.* 1997; 62:319.
13. Deacon AC, Elder GH. Front line tests for the investigation of suspected porphyria. *J Clin Pathol.* 2001;54:500.

45

Hematologic Disorders Presenting with Abdominal Pain—Sickle Cell Disease

Christopher C. Kwon
Johnny J. Vazquez

HIGH YIELD FACTS

- As many as 23% of sickle cell disease (SCD) patients with abdominal pains have acute surgical abdomens.[1]
- An acute surgical abdomen should be considered in SCD patients who fail to respond to conservative management.
- In some cases the only way to differentiate between surgical and nonsurgical abdomen in SCD patients is by the use of laboratory and imaging studies.

EPIDEMIOLOGY

Sickle cell disease is the most common of the hereditary blood disorders. It occurs predominantly among black Americans and black Africans but is also present in the white population.[2] Sickle cell disease in black Americans occurs in 3 of every 1000 live births. Overall, it is estimated that in the United States, some 50,000 African Americans are afflicted with the most severe form of sickle cell anemia. Current estimates are that 1 in 1875 U.S. African Americans is affected with sickle cell anemia.[3,4]

PATHOPHYSIOLOGY

Sickle cell disease is an autosomal recessive genetic disorder that results in the production of defective forms of hemoglobin (HbS), in which valine is substituted for glutamic acid at position 6 of the beta-globin gene.[5] Red blood cells (RBCs) containing structurally defective HbS polymerize secondary to increased hydrophobic interaction with adjacent HbS molecules under deoxygenated conditions; and thus forms the characteristic

sickle shape, which exhibits decreased solubility and stability.[5]

These defective, polymerized RBCs play a critical role in the vasoocclusive crisis. The classic crescent or sickle shaped RBCs (Figure 45-1) are less deformable and have increased adherence to vascular endothelium.[6] However, the actual pathophysiology of vasoocclusive crisis is much more complicated than just a mechanical obstruction by these sickled cells.[7] The primary event in the vasoocclusive cascade is the adhesion of erythrocytes as well as leukocytes to the endothelium of postcapillary venule resulting in heterocellular aggregate formations. These heterocellular aggregates increase hypoxia, further propagating the vasoocclusive cascade–HbS polymerization and endothelial-heterocellular aggregate adhesion. Furthermore, local inflammatory responses, along with neutrophil diapedesis and transmigration through the endothelial gap junctions as well as nitric oxide dysregulation may also play a role.[7–10]

Broadly speaking, acute sickle cell crises may be due to hematologic abnormalities, infectious etiologies, or vasoocclusive phenomena, as outlined above.

Most hematologic crises in SCD patients occur as a result of splenic or hepatic sequestration, with splenic sequestration being more common. This correlates with acute severity of anemia and is accompanied by persistent reticulocytosis and rapid pooling of blood in the engorged organs.[11–13] Parvovirus B19 infection, although classically associated with aplastic crisis, may also be a risk factor for splenic sequestration.[14]

Infectious crises occur as a result of functional asplenia where the patients are more susceptible to encapsulated organisms such as *Haemophilus influenzae* and *Streptococcus pneumoniae* or other organisms such as *Mycoplasma pneumoniae, Salmonella typhimurium, Staphylococcus aureus,* and *Escherichia coli.* Splenic dysfunction, seen as early as 4 months of age, occurs with repeated vasoocclusive crises within the spleen, crippling the spleen's ability to filter microorganisms from the blood stream. There is also evidence suggesting defective phagocytic, IgG, and IgM antibody responses may also contribute to the risk of infections in these patients.[15,16]

CLINICAL FEATURES

The clinical manifestations and the resultant complications of SCD are diverse, affecting multiple organ systems leading to acute problems such as: acute pain crisis, acute chest syndrome, infections, bone marrow necrosis, stroke, splenic/hepatic sequestration crisis, aplastic crisis, and priapism. The severity and frequency

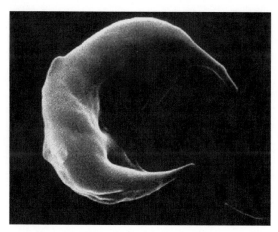

Fig. 45-1. Sickle cell. Scanning electron micrograph of a single red blood cell from a patient with sickle cell disease, illustrating the classical "sickle" shape. (Courtesy of R.L. Nagel, MD)

of these manifestations vary markedly depending on the major genotypes.[17–19]

Acute pain episodes are the first symptoms of the disease in approximately 25% of patients, and it is also the complication for which most SCD patients seek medical attention.[20,21] These episodes most often affect the chest, extremities, and abdomen[22] but can affect any areas of the body and can last between 2 and 7 days.[23] They tend to recur in the same areas of the body for each person.

Sickle cell crisis often manifests with abdominal pain that is clinically indistinguishable from intraabdominal infections or acute surgical abdomens such as appendicitis or acute cholecystitis. One study reveals that as high as 23% of SCD patients with abdominal pains had acute surgical abdomens.[24] Splenic infarcts are common and they are most often small and repetitive, eventually leading to autosplenectomy. Although massive splenic infarcts are extremely rare, they have been reported in some instances.[25] Fulminant ischemic colitis as well as acute pancreatitis due to common bile duct obstruction has also been reported, although it is extremely rare in SCD patients.[26,27]

Though difficult, some clinical parameters may aid in narrowing down the differential of abdominal pains in these SCD patients. Vasoocclusive crises tend to be more diffuse in nature on physical exam when compared to acute surgical abdomens and are more often associated with concomitant pain episodes in the limbs and chest. Furthermore, abdominal vasoocclusive crises tend to mimic prior vasoocclusive episodes when compared to cases of proven surgical abdomens.[24] Other helpful clinical

findings to distinguish abdominal vasoocclusive crisis from surgical abdomens are the presence of precipitating factors for vasoocclusive crisis such as upper respiratory infections or other metabolic/physiologic stressors (e.g., colds, dehydration, alcohol consumption, etc.).[24]

Splenic infarcts often present with left upper quadrant pain on admission, and they may also present with precipitating factors such as high altitude, postoperative, postpartum, septicemia, and strenuous exercise.[25] Splenic sequestration crisis presents with sudden enlargement of the spleen along with a precipitous fall in hematocrit and a rise in the reticulocyte count.[26] It could lead to severe hypotension and circulatory collapse in children.

Because SCD patients undergo chronic hemolysis, they have higher risks of developing pigmented gallstones.[28] Many of these patients will not only exhibit diffuse abdominal pains but will also present with recurrent right upper quadrant pain.[29]

Sickle cell disease patients with right upper quadrant pain may also suffer from various liver abnormalities: hepatic sequestration crisis, acute viral hepatitis, or intrahepatic cholestasis. These patients often present with nausea, hepatomegaly, fever, and jaundice. Hepatic sequestration crisis is most likely secondary to sinusoidal obstruction and resultant hepatocellular ischemia[30] and may often sequester large amounts of red blood cells. These patients exhibit rapidly enlarging livers and a corresponding fall in hematocrit.[30] A severe variant of hepatic sickling/hepatic sequestration crisis is the intrahepatic cholestasis. Above a certain threshold of hepatocellular ischemia and resultant ballooning of hepatocytes intracanalicular cholestasis occurs. Along with right upper quadrant pain, nausea, vomiting, hepatomegaly, and leukocytosis, a significant jaundice develops acutely in these patients.[31]

Some patients with abdominal vasoocclusive crisis may present with respiratory symptoms. In these patients it is important to distinguish a simple upper respiratory infection from an acute chest syndrome. Acute chest syndrome is a clinical diagnosis determined by an acute pulmonary infiltrate on the chest radiograph of a patient with SCD. These syndromes can develop due to infections or infarctions or a combination of both.[32] Infections can be due to gram-negative or gram-positive bacteria, atypical bacteria, and or viruses. Infarctions can be due to *in situ* thrombosis or fat emboli from bone necrosis, which then can lead to acute chest syndromes.[33] In these patients, if acute chest syndrome involves the lower lobes, they might present with upper abdominal pain.

DIAGNOSIS AND DIFFERENTIAL

Diagnosis of SCD varies depending on the age of the patient. For newborns, universal screening, as opposed to targeted or selective screening of newborns of high risk parents, seems to be more effective in preventing deaths.[34–36] Heel stick blood samples are used for electrophoresis and isoelectric focusing. With 44 states providing universal screening, most patients who are presenting to the emergency department will have a history of SCD.

For patients who already have a past medical history of SCD, a differential diagnosis of various acute syndromes is made by history and physical exam and appropriate laboratory and imaging studies. Generally, SCD patients with chronic hemolysis will exhibit mild to moderate anemia—hematocrit of 20% to 30% and reticulocytosis of 3% to 15%, unconjugated hyperbilirubinemia (usually <6 mg/dL), and elevated lactate dehydrogenase. Peripheral blood smears may reveal sickled red cells, polychromasia, and Howell-Jolly bodies.[37]

For hepatic syndromes, unconjugated bilirubins may be >12 mg/dL (but usually <15 mg/dL) and exhibit corresponding lactate dehydrogenase (LDH) and aspartate aminotransferase (AST) elevations.[38,39] AST levels are rarely above 300 IU/L but higher levels have been reported.[39,40] In an aplastic crisis, reticulocyte count maybe <1% and absolute reticulocyte count <10,000/μL.

Computed tomography (CT) scans may reveal hepatic or splenic pathology. The spleen may be small, atrophic, and calcified due to recurrent infarctions, or it may be ruptured or necrotic from repeated hemorrhage and can exhibit splenomegaly from acute sequestrations. Computed tomography scans may also exhibit lung pathology from current or past acute chest syndromes.

Ultrasound may reveal cholelithiasis as well as increased iron deposition from repeated transfusions.

Differential diagnosis of abdominal pain in SCD patients includes: acute pain/vasoocclusive crisis, splenic sequestration crisis, splenic infarction, hepatic sequestration crisis, acute viral hepatitis, intrahepatic cholestasis, cholelithiasis, appendicitis, fulminant ischemic colitis, acute pancreatitis, aplastic crisis, acute chest syndrome, sepsis/infections, and bone marrow necrosis/infarction.

EMERGENCY DEPARTMENT CARE AND DISPOSITION

Emergency department care and disposition must be targeted toward specific acute syndromes. Useful laboratory studies include complete blood count (CBC), reticulocyte count, electrolytes, creatinine, AST, alanine aminotransferase (ALT), unconjugated bilirubin, LDH, urinalysis (UA), blood cultures, and pancreatic enzymes. Computed tomography scans, chest radiographs, and ultrasounds are useful imaging studies though CT scans are preferred over ultrasounds to more accurately delineate splenic infarcts or hepatic pathology.[25]

For typical vasoocclusive/pain episodes, liberal intravenous (IV) fluid administration and pain control with opiates for adolescents and adults, or ibuprofen or acetaminophen with or without codeine in a child less than 6 years of age, is warranted.[41,42] Typically for adults, 2 to 4 mg of hydromorphone can be given over 15 to 20 minutes, followed by another dose in 30 minutes if pain control is inadequate. Following stabilization with IV opiate boluses, the patient should be admitted to the floor for pain control maintenance. For adolescents and adults, opiate administration via patient-controlled analgesia can be advantageous.[43] Intravenous nonsteroidal anti-inflammatory drugs (NSAIDs) such as Ketorolac have been shown to work synergistically with opiates to effectively control pain but not as a stand alone agent.[42]

As mentioned previously, abdominal pain from vasoocclusive crisis can be indistinguishable from acute surgical abdomen. However one study shows that vasoocclusive episodes are usually relieved by IV fluid administration, opiates, and oxygen whereas abdominal pain from surgical abdomens are not readily abated— 97% of vasoocclusive cases resolved within 48 hours versus 0% in proven surgical pathology.[24]

Acute splenic sequestration crisis can be a medical emergency and must be diagnosed early for immediate intervention with intravenously administered fluids and judicious transfusions, both of which can be life saving.[28] One study reveals 50% of survivors of splenic sequestration in children have recurrences and therefore splenectomy may be recommended after the first acute event,[44] although some specialists debate this recommendation. Massive splenic infarctions are rare but do occur, whereas small, repetitive infarctions are more common in these patients. Computed tomography scan can be helpful in differentiating between sequestrations, infarctions, and abscesses but an ultrasound guided biopsy may be necessary for diagnosis in some abscess formations.[25] These patients can be managed conservatively with IV fluids, analgesia, and blood transfusions when necessary.

Patients with SCD are susceptible to overwhelming sepsis and therefore require blood cultures. Therapy with cephalosporins (e.g., cefotaxime, ceftriaxone, cefuroxime) should be initiated in patients with significant temperature elevations. One should also consider the addition of vancomycin in communities with high incidence of PCN resistant pneumococci.[45]

In SCD patients with focal findings in the lower abdomen and in the groin area, one should consider osteomyelitis. These symptoms could be due to sickling in the periosteum but should also raise concerns for osteomyelitis especially if white blood cell counts are greater than 28,000/mm^3 with or without bandemia. Other markers such as sedimentation rate, C-reactive protein, or significant temperature elevations can be helpful in the diagnosis of osteomyelitis. Bone scans may also be helpful in the diagnosis. In children with SCD, *Salmonella* species are the most common cause of osteomyelitis. [46] Patients must be treated with parenteral antibiotics covering for *Salmonella* and *Staphylococcus Aureus* for 2 to 6 weeks.

Treatment for aplastic crisis is purely supportive; however, patients exhibiting symptoms of aplastic crisis require acute transfusions to maintain an acceptable hematocrit level until erythrocyte production is restored. Reticulocyte count usually returns to normal levels within 2 weeks.[47]

Hepatic sequestration crisis will exhibit elevated transaminases and bilirubin levels and may lead to hepatic failure. These patients require IV fluids, oxygen, and analgesia, and may require exchange transfusions to restore blood volumes. Intrahepatic cholestasis may be an extreme variant in the continuum of hepatic sequestration/hepatic sickling crises syndromes. They are marked by elevation of LDH, prolongation of prothrombin and partial thromboplastin time, thrombocytopenia, and lactic acidosis.[31] For these patients, interventions with aggressive exchange transfusions and fresh frozen plasma administrations to correct coagulopathies must be undertaken.[31,48]

As previously mentioned, due to chronic hemolysis, SCD patients are prone to formation of pigmented gallstones. If a patient has been ruled out for hepatic pathology and suffers from severe recurrent right upper quadrant pain, cholecystitis, common duct obstruction, or pancreatitis, one should consider recommending laparoscopic cholecystectomy, which is usually well tolerated.[29]

It is difficult to diagnose and treat acute chest syndromes because of the various etiologies and symptomatology. Classically, the symptoms include fever, dyspnea, cough, and pulmonary infiltrates.[49] Chest radiographs may display lobar distribution and can be bilateral with hazy opacities resembling acute respiratory distress syndromes. Unchecked, acute chest syndromes may lead to cardiovascular collapse and death. Acute chest syndromes are more common in children.[50] Treatment with appropriate antibiotics for any infectious process is important; however, if symptoms progress and arterial oxygen saturation continues to decline, along with worsening chest radiograph, then exchange transfusions must be initiated. Exchange transfusion which is the preferred treatment of choice for acute chest syndromes.[50]

PITFALLS

- A wide differential must be considered when dealing with SCD patients with abdominal pains and not be focused on just pain crisis.

- Sickle cell disease patients may exhibit opiate tolerance. This should be considered when administering analgesia to control vasoocclusive/pain episodes.

- Sickle cell disease patients may present with significant complications from progression of their disease and can present with life threatening emergencies.

REFERENCES

1. Lorey FW, Arnopp J, Cunningham GC. Distribution of hemoglobinopathy variants by ethnicity in a multiethnic state. *Genet Epidemiol.* 1996;13:501.
2. Schiliro G, Samperi P, Consalvo C, et al. Clinical hematological, and molecular features in Sicilians with sickle cell disease. *Hemoglobin.* 1992;16:469.
3. Samperi P, Consalvo C, Romano V, et al. Liver involvement with in white patients with sickle cell disease. *Arch Pediatr Adolesc Med.* 1996;150:1177.
4. Bunn HF: Pathogenesis and treatment of sickle cell disease. *N Engl J Med.* 199711;337:762.
5. Kaul Dk, Fabry ME, Costantini F, et al. In vivo demonstration of red cell-endothelial interaction, sickling and altered microvascular response to oxygen in the sickle transgenic mouse. *J Clin Invest.* 1995;96:2845.
6. Stuart MS, Nagel RL. Sickle-cell disease. *Lancet* 2004;364:1340.
7. Eaton WA, Hofrichter J. Sickle cell hemoglobin polymerization. *Adv Protein Chem.* 1990;40:63.
8. Kaul DK, Fabry ME, Nagel RL. Microvascular sites and characteristics of sickle cell adhesion to vascular endothelium in shear flow conditions: pathophysiological implications. *Proc Natl Acad Sci USA.* 1989; 86:3356.

9. Kaul DK, Tsai HM, Liu XD, et al. Monoclonal antibodies to αβ inhibit sickle red blood cell-endothelial interactions induced by platelet-activation factor. *Blood.* 2000;95:368.

10. Orringer EP, Fowler VGJr, Owens CM, et al. Case report: splenic infarction and acute splenic sequestration in adults with hemoglobin SC disease. *Am J Med Sci.* 1991; 302:374.

11. Emond AM, Collis R, Darvill D, et al. Acute splenic sequestration in homozygous sickle cell disease: Natural history and management. *J Pediatr.* 1985;107:201.

12. Topley, JM, Rogers DW, Stevens MC, Serjeant GR. Acute splenic sequestration and hypersplenism in the first five years in homozygous sickle cell disease. *Arch Dis Child.* 1981;56:765.

13. Smith-Whitley K, Zhao H, Hodinka RL, et al. Epidemiology of human parvovirus B19 in children with sickle cell disease. *Blood.* 2004;103:422.

14. Overturf GD. Infections and immunizations of children with sickle cell disease. *Adv Pediatr Infect Dis.* 1999; 14:191.

15. Bjornson, AB, Lobel, JS. Direct evidence that decreased serum opsonization of Streptococcus pneumoniae via the alternative complement pathway in sickle cell disease is related to antibody deficiency. *J Clin Invest.* 1987; 79:388.

16. Orkin Sh, Kazazian HH Jr, Antonarakis SE, et al. Linkage of betathalassemia mutations and beta-globin gene polymorphisms with DNA polymorphisms in human beta-globin cluster. *Nature.* 1982;296:627.

17. Chui DH, Dover GJ. Sickle cell disease: no longer a single gene disorder. *Curr Opin Pediatr.* 2001;13:1322.

18. Alexander N, Higgs D, Dover G, Serjeant GR. Are there clinical phenotypes of homozygous sickle cell disease? *Br J Haematol.* 2004;126:606.

19. Bainbridge R, Higgs DR, Maude GH, Serjeant GR. Clinical presentation of homozygous sickle cell disease. *J Pediatr.* 1985;106:881.

20. Brozovic M, Davies SC, Brownell AI. Acute admissions of patients with sickle cell disease who live in Britain. *Br Med J* (Clin Res Ed). 1987;294:1206.

21. Ballas SK, Delengowski A. Pain measurement in hospitalized adults with sickle cell painful episodes. *Ann Clin Lab Sci.* 1993;23:358.

22. Jacob E, Beyer JE, Miaskowski C, et al. Are there phases to the vaso-occlusive painful episode in sickle cell disease? *J Pain Symptom Manage.* 2005;29:392.

23. Baumgartner F, Klein S. The presentation and management of the acute abdomen in the patient with sickle-cell anemia. *Am Surg.* 1989;55:660.

24. Jama AH, Salem AH, Dabbous IA. Massive splenic infarction in Saudi patients with sickle cell anemia: a unique manifestation. *Am J Hematol.* 2002;69:205.

25. Karim A, Ahmed S, Rossoff LJ, et al. Fulminant ischaemic colitis with atypical clinical features complicating sickle cell disease. *Postgrad Med J.* 2002;78:370.

26. Ahmed S, Siddiqui AK, Siddiqui RK, et al. Acute pancreatitis during sickle cell vaso-occlusive painful crisis. *Am J Hematol.* 2003;73:190.

27. Lane PA. Sickle cell disease. *Pediatr Clin North Am.* 1996;43:647.

28. Ware RE, Kinney TR, Casey JR, et al. Laparoscopic cholecystectomy in young patients with sickle hemoglobinopathies. *J Pediatr.* 1992;120:58.

29. Hernandez P, Dorticos E, Espinosa E, et al. Clinical features of hepatic sequestration insickle cell anemia. *Haematologia (Budap).* 1989;22:169.

30. Stephan JL, Merpit-Gonon E, Richard O, et al. Fulminant liver failure in a 12-year-old girl with sickle cell anemia: favorable outcome after exchange transfusions. *Eur J Pediatr.* 1995;154:469.

31. Poncz M, Kane E, Gill F. Acute chest syndrome in sickle cell disease: etiology and clinical correlates. *J Pediatr.* 1985;107:861.

32. Vichinsky EP, Styles LA, Colangelo LH, et al. Scute chest syndrome in sickle cell disease: clinical presentation and course. Cooperative study of sickle cell disease. *Blood.* 1997;89:1787.

33. Consensus conference. Newborn screening for sickle cell disease and other hemoglobinopathies. *JAMA.* 1987;258:1205.

34. Tsevat J, Wong JB, Pauker SG, Steinberg MH. Neonatal screening for sickle cell disease: a cost-effectiveness analysis. *J Pediatr.* 1991;118:546.

35. Harris MS, Eckman JR. Georgia's experience with newborn screening: 1981 to 1985. *Pediatrics.* 1989;83:858.

36. West MS, Wethers D, Smith J, et al. Laboratory profile of sickle cell disease: A cross-sectional analysis. The Cooperative Study of Sickle Cell Disease. *J Clin Epidemiol.* 1992;45:893.

37. Johnson CS, Omata M, Tong MJ, et al. Liver involvement in sickle cell disease. *Medicine (Baltimore)* 1985;64:349.

38. Sheehy, TW. Sickle cell hepatopathy. *South Med J* 1977;70:533.

39. Schubert, TT. Hepatobiliary system in sickle cell disease. *Gastroenterology* 1986;90:2013.

40. Dampier CD, Setty BN, Logan J, et al. Intravenous morphine pharmacokinetics in pediatric patients with sickle cell disease. *J Pediatr.* 1995;126:461.

41. Houck CS, Wilder RT, McDermott JS, et al. Safety of intravenous ketorolac therapy in children and cost savings with a unit dosing system. *J Pediatr.* 1996;129:292.

42. Shapiro BS, Cohen DE, Howe CJ. Patient-controlled analgesia for sickle-cell-related pain. *J Pain Symptom Manage.* 1993;8:22.

43. Emond AM, Collis R, Darvill D, et al. Acute splenic sequestration in homozygous sickle cell disease: Natural history and management. *J Pediatr.* 1985;107:201.

44. Chesney PJ, Wilimas JA, Presbury G, et al. Penicillin and cephalosporin-resistant strains of Streptococcus pneumoniae causing sepsis and meningitis in children with sickle cell disease. *J Pediatr.* 1995;127:526.

45. Burnett MW, Bass JW, Cook BA. Etiology of osteomyelitis complicating sickle cell disease. *Pediatrics.* 1998;101:296.

46. Saarinen UM, Chorba TL, Tattersall P, et al. Human parvovirus B19-induced epidemic red cell aplasia in patients with hereditary hemolytic anemia. *Blood.* 1986;67:1411.

47. Betrosian A, Balla M, Kafiri G, et al. Reversal of liver failure in sickle cell vaso-occlusive crisis. *Am J Med Sci.* 1996;311:292.

48. Haynes Jr. J, Kirkpatrick M. The acute chest syndrome of sickle cell disease. *Am J Med Sci.* 1993;305:326.

49. Gill F, Sleeper L, Weiner S, et al. Clinical events in the first decade in a cohort of infants with sickle cell disease. Cooperative Study of Sickle Cell Disease. *Blood.* 1995;86:776.

50. Emre U, Miller S, Gutierez M, et al. Effect of transfusion in acute chest syndrome of sickle cell disease. *J Pediatr.* 1995;127:901.

46

Blunt Abdominal Trauma Presenting with Abdominal Pain

Lekshmi Vaidyanathan
Latha G. Stead

HIGH YIELD FACTS

- Consider early evaluation by a trauma surgeon for patients with evidence of blunt abdominal trauma.
- Focused assessment with sonography for trauma (FAST) to detect free abdominal fluid provides a rapid noninvasive method to evaluate the abdomen in the blunt trauma patient.[1]
- Diagnostic peritoneal lavage (DPL) is a more invasive alternative to the FAST exam, albeit universally available. Diagnostic peritoneal lavage fluid with presence of bile or abnormally high amylase, food fibers, or bacteria indicate requirement of surgical intervention.
- Computed tomography (CT) scans often provide the most detailed images of traumatic pathology and help in determination of methods of management.

EPIDEMIOLOGY

Reviews from adult trauma databases reflect that blunt trauma accounts for two thirds of all injuries and is one of the leading causes of morbidity and mortality. The most common cause of blunt trauma is attributed to motor vehicle collisions or automobile-pedestrian accidents. Although actual incidence of blunt abdominal injury itself is not known, in the United States, the National Center for Injury Prevention and Control detailed that motor vehicle collisions are found to be the 5th most leading cause of death.[2] In 2003, 15.3% of deaths were due to motor vehicle related injuries.[3] This imposes an immense economic burden and more important is a preventable cause of mortality. Other causes of occult trauma include falls, industrial or recreational accidents, and iatrogenic injuries such as a forceful Heimlich maneuver and cardiopulmonary resuscitation. Children are more susceptible than adults to abdominal injury caused by blunt forces. Child abuse also needs to be considered in pediatric abdominal trauma.[4]

PATHOPHYSIOLOGY

Intraabdominal organ injury due to blunt trauma can be caused by various mechanisms.

Rapid deceleration creates shearing forces within the abdomen causing visceral organs and vessels to tear at their attachment (hollow, solid viscera, and large vessels).

Intraabdominal contents can also get crushed between the anterior abdominal wall and the vertebral column or posterior thoracic cage. This mainly affects the larger solid viscera (liver, spleen).

Compression forces increase the intraabdominal pressure rapidly and hence result in rupture of hollow viscera (gut).

CLINICAL FEATURES

History is generally limited due to the serious nature of the presentation. Most blunt abdominal trauma occurs following motor vehicle accidents and, if possible, a thorough history must be acquired from the paramedics and bystanders including the speed of the vehicle, type of collision, types of restraints, deployment of airbag, and status of passengers. Past medical history pertaining to allergies, medications, medical conditions, and last meal taken should be obtained if available for optimal management and potential surgical exploration.

Intraabdominal traumatic injury usually produces symptoms due to blood loss, and patients often develop hypotension. Some patients also develop tachycardia and mental confusion with high amounts of blood loss.[5] Abdominal tenderness and distension in a patient following blunt injury is highly suspicious of internal rupture. Though these symptoms are strongly suspicious for occult trauma they are quite nonspecific. Young patients and pregnant women may lose 50% to 60% of their blood volume and still be asymptomatic.[6] In the presence of hypovolemia, elderly patients may not exhibit tachycardia due to limited cardiac response to catecholamine stimulation or concurrent use of beta-adrenergic blocking agents. The presence of a pacemaker may also limit the ability to increase the heart rate. Trained athletes may not present with a tachycardia due to their slow baseline heart rate.[7] Heart rate also varies with age and the difference in the cut-offs should be kept in mind especially in children (Table 46-1). Abdominal pain or tenderness may not develop at all or until much later in many cases. Hence great care should be taken when evaluating a patient following blunt trauma. Serial examinations should be performed and a high degree of suspicion maintained.

Specific Injury

Solid viscera: The spleen is the organ that is most commonly injured.[4] Patients with splenic injury may present with left upper quadrant or diffuse abdominal tenderness. Left shoulder pain can also occur due to diaphragmatic irritation. The liver is the next most common to get affected. Right upper quadrant pain and tenderness may be a clinical feature and elevation of aspartate aminotransferase (AST) and alanine aminotransferase (ALT) levels can be seen. Both the above injuries in the presence of hemodynamic instability are indications for laparotomy.

Hollow viscera: Hollow visceral injuries are less common in blunt trauma when compared to penetrating wounds. Small bowel perforations are more frequent, followed by colorectal injury, and duodenal and gastric perforation.[8] In addition to hemodynamic instability, peritonitis is seen due to chemical irritation by the acidic gut contents leaking into the abdominal cavity.

Retroperitoneal injury: Injuries of the retroperitoneum are seen in less than 20% of the patients following blunt trauma. Lesions of the pancreas and duodenum are more common while urologic injuries are infrequent. Patients may be deceptively asymptomatic or can develop symptoms days later. Duodenal injuries can be associated with symptoms of bowel obstruction in addition to abdominal pain and pancreatic injuries detected in the presence of a raised amylase. Ureteral injury or avulsion may present along with or without pelvic fracture following trauma. Macroscopic hematuria is often seen,[9] and although more common in children, it has been reported in adults as well.[10]

Table 46-1. Cut-offs for Tachycardia with Respect to Age[7]

Age	Cut-off for Tachycardia
Infant	160
Preschool child	140
School age to puberty	120
Adult	100

Vascular injury: Injuries to the major abdominal arteries and veins are associated with hemorrhage and visceral ischemia.[11] These injuries are more often caused by penetrating injury, but they can also be caused by blunt trauma. The abdominal aorta is rarely injured following blunt trauma but can be seen with seatbelt injury.[12] Other vessels that can be injured are the vena cava, iliac vessels, celiac trunk, and mesenteric vessels.

Complications can arise for unidentified injuries as clinical features are varied and may not typically present on admission. Intraabdominal hemorrhage, infection, sepsis, and death can occur. Delayed rupture or hemorrhage from solid organs, particularly the spleen, has been described. In patients who undergo laparotomy and repair, complications are similar to other conditions requiring surgical intervention. Abruptio placentae should also be considered in pregnant women who present with abdominal pain that may be associated with vaginal bleeding, preterm labor, or trauma.

DIAGNOSIS AND DIFFERENTIAL

Recommended initial lab studies include serum glucose, complete blood count (CBC), serum chemistries, serum amylase, urinalysis, coagulation studies, blood ethanol, urine drug screen, blood type and cross-match (in case of transfusion requirement), and urine pregnancy test for women of childbearing age. Coagulopathy, particularly hypofibrinogenemia, supports a diagnosis of severe abruption, as does the combination of plasma fibrinogen level below 200 mg/dL and thrombocytopenia ($<100,000/\mu L$). Elevated LFTs may indicate liver injury and an elevated white blood cell count may indicate splenic injury.

Radiologic investigations performed for diagnosis include bedside ultrasound (US) and CT. Diagnostic peritoneal lavage (DPL) can also be done to identify presence of free fluid, but it is being used less commonly with the advent of bedside US (Table 46-2). Bedside US in the form of FAST is used in the evaluation of trauma patients and is increasingly gaining acceptance as a non-invasive approach for rapid evaluation of hemoperitoneum[1]. Focused abdominal sonogram for trauma evaluation of the abdomen (Figure 46-1) consists of visualization of the pericardium (from a subxiphoid view), the splenorenal, and the hepatorenal spaces (i.e., Morison pouch), the paracolic gutters, and the pouch of Douglas in the pelvis. The Morison pouch view has been shown to be the most sensitive, regardless of the etiology of the fluid.[13] Free fluid in a hemodynamically unstable patient

Table 46-2. Investigations for Blunt Abdominal Trauma[7]

	Indication	Advantage	Accuracy	Disadvantage
DPL	Document bleeding if hypotensive	Early diagnosis and sensitive	98%	Invasive; misses injury to diaphragm or retroperitoneum
Ultrasound	Document fluid if hypotensive	Early diagnosis, non-invasive and repeatable	86%–97%	Operator dependent; misses diaphragm, bowel, and some pancreatic injuries
CT Scan	Document organ injury if normotensive	Most specific for injury	92%–98%	Cost and time; misses diaphragm, bowel, and some pancreatic injuries

indicates the need for emergent laparotomy (Figure 46-2). Sensitivity and specificity of these studies range from 85% to 95% though the studies demonstrate a degree of operator expertise.[14,15]

Sonographic visualization of a periplacental clot is suggestive of placental abruption, but the absence of a clot does not exclude the diagnosis. The best estimate of sensitivity of US examination for diagnosis of abruption is 25%.[16] Computed tomography scans provide detailed images of intraabdominal trauma and have a high specificity.[17,18] Patient stability required for transport to the scanner is a disadvantage, and CT scanning may miss

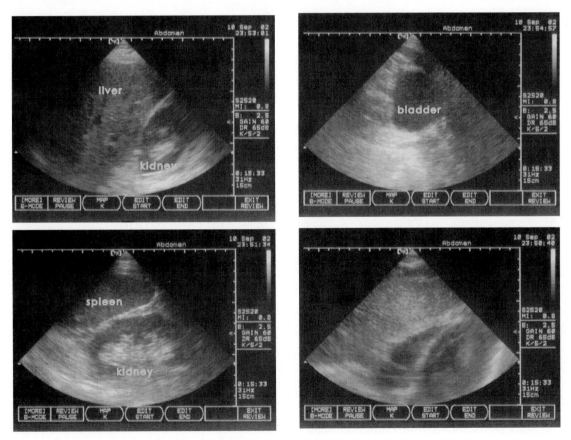

Fig. 46-1. Normal FAST exam.

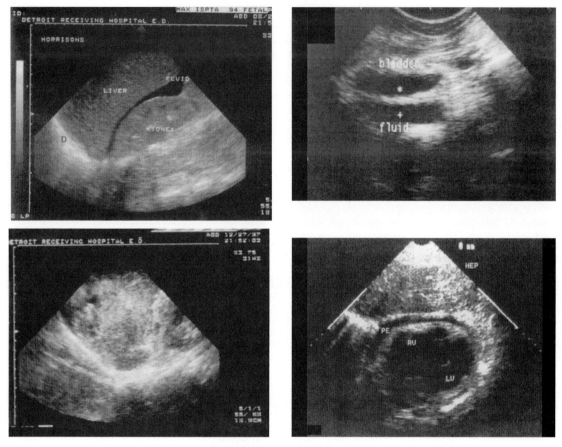

Fig. 46-2. Abnormal FAST exam.

injuries to the diaphragm, pancreas, and perforations of the gastrointestinal (GI) tract if performed soon after the injury.[19] Diagnostic peritoneal lavage helps determine the presence of intraperitoneal fluid or blood. Abdominal exploration is indicated if approximately 10 mL of blood is aspirated upon insertion of the peritoneal catheter (grossly positive) in the unstable patient. If findings are negative, 1 L of crystalloid solution (e.g., lactated Ringer solution) is infused into the peritoneum and allowed to drain. Presence of more than 100,000 RBC/mm^3 or more than 500 WBC/mm^3 is considered a positive finding.[20] Presence of bile, abnormally high amylase, food fibers, or bacteria indicate intraabdominal organ or gut injury.[21] Complications of DPL include bleeding from the incision and catheter insertion, infection (e.g., wound, peritoneal), and injury to intraabdominal structures (e.g., urinary bladder, small bowel, uterus).

EMERGENCY DEPARTMENT CARE AND DISPOSITION

As with all trauma emergencies, stabilizing the patient should be the priority. The Advanced Trauma Life Support (ATLS) protocol should be followed and airway, breathing, circulation, disability, and exposure assessed.[5] Careful history from the patient, bystanders, and paramedics with regards to the mode of injury, extent of vehicle damage, and events leading to the incident must be recorded. Universal precautions should always be taken and a secondary survey completed while resuscitation measures are being carried out. Persisting hypovolemia following fluid resuscitation measures strongly indicates intra abdominal injury and ongoing blood loss. Free abdominal fluid can be identified in the department using bedside DPL[20,21] and FAST.[14,15]

Abdominal CT scans are also performed to assess extent of injury and management options depending on the stability of the patient.[20,21] Placement of a nasogastric tube is routinely done to decompress the stomach and check for presence of blood. Bony pelvic injuries should be ruled out and the patient catheterized in the absence of radiological pelvic fracture. Early involvement and evaluation by the trauma surgeon is advisable in case of the need for surgical intervention.

PITFALLS

- Absence of typical presenting symptoms can make diagnosis a greater challenge. Hence a low threshold must be maintained when dealing with blunt injury patients.

- Since many patients present much after the initial trauma, serial examinations should be performed to ensure that no intraabdominal injury is overlooked.

- Vital signs may not always reflect the true extent of blood loss.

REFERENCES

1. Healey MA, Simons RK, Winchell RJ, et al. A prospective evaluation of abdominal ultrasound in blunt trauma: Is it useful? *J Trauma.* 1996;40:875.
2. Hoyert DL, Heron M, Murphy SL, Kung HC, Deaths: Final data for 2003. *Natl Vital Stat Rep.* 2006;54:1.
3. US Department of Health and Human Services. Centers for Disease Control and Prevention. National Center for Health statistics, Hyattsville, Maryland: 2005.
4. Schafermeyer R. Pediatric trauma. *Emerg Med Clin North Am.* 1993;11:187.
5. American College of Surgeons, Committee on Trauma. Advanced Trauma Life Support Manual. Chicago, IL: American College of Surgeons; 1997.
6. Scalea TM, Holman M, Fourtes M, et al. Central venous blood oxygen saturation: An early, accurate measurement of volume during hemorrhage. *J Trauma.* 1988;28:725.
7. American College of Surgeons, Committee on Trauma: Advanced Trauma Life Support Instructor Course Manual. Chicago, IL: American College of Surgeons; 1997.
8. Talton DS, Craig MH, Hauser CJ, et al. Major gastroenteric injuries from blunt trauma. *Am Surg.* 1995;61:69.
9. Knudson MM, McAninch JW, Gomez R, et al. Hematuria as a predictor of abdominal injury after blunt trauma. *Am J Surg.* 1992;164:482–5; discussion 485.
10. Giannarini G, Grossetti B, Crisci A, et al. Post-traumatic ureteropelvic junction obstruction. *Arch Ital Urol Androl.* 2004;76:100.
11. Mullins RJ, Huckfeldt R, Trunkey DD. Abdominal vascular injuries. *Surg Clin North Am..* 1996;76:813.
12. Chandler CF, Lane JS, Waxman KS. Seatbelt sign following blunt trauma is associated with increased incidence of abdominal injury. *Am Surg.*1997;63:885.
13. Rozycki GS, Shackford SR. Ultrasound, what every trauma surgeon should know. *J Trauma.*1996;40:1.
14. Rhea JT, Garza DH, Novelline RA. Controversies in emergency radiology: CT versus ultrasound in the evaluation of blunt abdominal trauma. *Emerg Radiol.* 2004; 10:289.
15. Brown MA, Casola G, Sirlin CB, et al. Blunt abdominal trauma: screening us in 2,693 patients. *Radiology.* 2001; 218:352.
16. Oyelese Y, Ananth CV. Placental abruption. *Obstet Gynecol.* 2006;108:1005.
17. Livingston DH, Lavery RF, Passannante MR, et al. Admission or observation is not necessary after a negative abdominal computed tomographic scan in patients with suspected blunt abdominal trauma: Results of a prospective, multi-institutional trial. *J Trauma.* 1998;44:273; discussion 280–2.
18. Shanmuganathan K. Multi-detector row CT imaging of blunt abdominal trauma. *Semin Ultrasound CT MR.* 2004;25:180.
19. Udekwu PO, Gurkin B, Oller DW. The use of computed tomography in blunt abdominal injuries. *Am Surg.* 1996; 62:56.
20. Sato T, Hirose Y, Saito H, et al. Diagnostic peritoneal lavage for diagnosing blunt hollow visceral injury: The accuracy of two different criteria and their combination. *Surg Today.* 2005;35:935.
21. Nagappan R, Frank JD. Peritoneal lavage cell count ratio in blunt abdominal trauma—a useful tool in hollow viscous injury? *Crit Care Resusc.* 2001;3:92.

47

Admission Decision Making and Discharge Instructions for a Patient with Abdominal Pain

Charles L. Maddow
Manish N. Shah

HIGH YIELD FACTS

- Diagnostic uncertainty and diagnostic error are unavoidable, even for the most careful and astute clinicians. Disposition should include safeguards that direct patients back to care if and when it is needed.

- In evaluating abdominal pain, the presence or absence of any finding is not sufficient to completely include or exclude serious disease. The only test that can do that is the test of time.

- Disposition decisions should be based on patients' risk profiles for adverse outcomes more than by the results of evaluation. The older the patient, the higher that risk is. Particularly above age 65, older patients with abdominal pain should be discharged from the emergency department (ED) only after great consideration.

EPIDEMIOLOGY

Abdominal pain is the most prevalent single complaint of patients presenting to the ED.[1,2] Roughly 5% of ED visits are for abdominal complaints,[1,3] a statistic that has remained constant for decades,[4] and that remains constant across all age groups.[5,6] One statistic among patients with abdominal pain is immutable: 100% of patients with abdominal pain will require a disposition.

The disposition of patients with abdominal pain is frequently discussed in terms of management of particular diagnoses, or in the incidence of missed diagnoses, which obscures the unique aspects of emergency medicine practice. Emergency physicians assign dispositions in a process coincident with, parallel to, and

to a degree, independent of the diagnostic process. Emergency physicians place equal emphasis upon the diagnosis (or lack thereof) and the risk of adverse outcomes.[7] Determining that risk may be at least as difficult as determining the condition responsible for abdominal complaints, particularly because benign and deadly abdominal conditions often share the same vague and nonspecific features.[8]

In general, 18 % of patients with abdominal pain are admitted to the hospital (either as inpatients or to observation units)[3] on their index ED visit. Up to 10% of patients with abdominal pain require surgery,[3,4] but another 10% to 15% requires admission for nonsurgical, but still urgent interventions (UI), that is, therapies that prevent death or significant disability due to the condition of interest (Table 47-1).[9]

Roughly 25% of patients with abdominal pain may not receive a definitive diagnosis in the ED. Half of them will still not receive a diagnosis upon completion of their follow-up evaluations.[10] Of the 75% of patients who do receive a diagnosis in the ED, over half of those diagnoses may be inaccurate.[9] With these data in mind, the emergency physician is wise to derive an abdominal pain patient's disposition independent of the diagnostic process. This chapter provides a rationale for crafting safe dispositions that ensure that patients with abdominal pain diagnosed with undifferentiated abdominal pain, and those who may have received an incorrect, incomplete, or irrelevant diagnosis, will receive UI if they do require them.

PATHOPHYSIOLOGY

The obvious concern regarding clinical errors is the resultant potential for increased patient morbidity and mortality. Beyond the concern of patient outcome are the issues of physician accountability and litigation. These external forces affect the way physicians make clinical decisions in their attempts to avoid error—the "chagrin factor"—not a source of error in itself, but rather a result of worrying about making errors. The obvious problem with this approach is the inappropriate use of resources. Although some physicians believe that ordering more tests is good risk management, this view is unsubstantiated.[11,3]

Fundamentally, ED patients may receive one of two dispositions: discharge or admission.[*] Although these

---

[*]Although technically and often administratively distinct, admission as an inpatient, admission to an observation unit, and continued evaluation in the ED all share the common feature that the patient has not been discharged and will all be considered under the term "admission."

Table. 47-1. Conditions Causing Abdominal Pain for which Urgent Interventions are Indicated.

Abdominal aortic aneurysm
Aortic dissection
Appendicitis
Bowel obstruction
Cholangitis
Cholecystitis
Ectopic pregnancy
Gastrointestinal bleeding
Intraabdominal or pelvic abcess
Mesenteric ischemia
Obstructive jaundice
Pancreatitis
Perforated viscus
Peritonitis
Vascular or venous thromboembolism

Adapted with permission from Hendrickson and Naparst 2003.[9]

terms refer to the patient's physical destination, either within or outside of the hospital facility, the important distinction between these dispositions is whether the physician who makes the disposition (as with admission), or the patient or caretakers, who are not under the influence of the disposition maker (as in discharge), bears the responsibility for performing and interpreting reassessments and/or therapy.

Using a definition of medical error as the "failure to meet a realistic expectation,"[12] a disposition error is the assignment of a disposition that increases, rather than decreases or leaves unchanged, a patient's risk of morbidity or mortality.[13] Contrary to the belief that "no one was ever wrong for admitting someone, only for not testing or sending a sick person home,"[11] neither an erroneous discharge nor erroneous admissions are benign. The risks attending erroneous discharge are generally intuitive and require little discussion here. These risks are generally adverse outcomes such as perforation or sepsis, whose risk increases as the delay from onset of symptoms to UI lengthens.[8,10,14] Erroneous admission, while less intuitive, may lead to a wide variety of adverse consequences. Three percent to 4% of inpatients suffer adverse events immediately related to their hospitalization. Most are "blame free" complications of tests or therapy, as in prolonged recovery, medication or dye allergy, etc., whereas 30% of adverse events are due to "human errors," such as medication errors and procedures that are performed on the wrong site.[15] Additionally, patients who are erroneously admitted affect the risk profiles of other patients. The average patient with abdominal pain uses 2.9 hours of physician time,[16] which, like nurse and staff time, ED and inpatient bed space, and diagnostic testing access and turnaround time, are all finite and competitive resources. The consumption of a hospital's last inpatient bed in one study, for example, increased the average patient's time from admission order to physical departure from the ED from 1.9 to 2.8 hours,[16] during which that patient's presence in the ED delayed the next ED patients' evaluations, and continued to cost provider time. It is clearly imperative, therefore, to correctly pair limited resources to actual patient needs, both for patients themselves as well as for the sake of patients who require, and are in competition for, UI.

CLINICAL FEATURES

Even the best-trained clinicians, skilled in the scientific basis of medical decisions and aware of their own cognitive biases, will face uncertainty. Their actions in the face of incomplete information and risk may determine their success.[12]

Why do disposition errors happen? Clearly, no practitioner intends to commit an error of any type, much less in assigning patient dispositions, and yet strategies to reduce error that have appeared successful in controlled studies, have not translated successfully to the general population.[17] Physicians base their decision making on data that are derived from patients, whether it is the information obtained from the history, from records, or from the results of the physical exam and diagnostic tests, all of which may yield discordant or contradictory data.[17] Ultimately the physician must decide whether, and to what extent each informational item will influence their decisions,[12] as overconfidence or overreliance on any requisite findings will flaw their decision making.[3] Safe dispositions are more likely when they are derived from decisions based upon the patient's risk profile for adverse outcomes, as well as an understanding of the limitations of physical exam and testing.[3,10,12,17]

Simply put, the single greatest determinant of an abdominal pain patient's risk profile is age,[3,17] acting as a surrogate variable for the presence of comorbid conditions.[18] The incidence of adverse outcomes increase as patients with abdominal pain age beyond their 50s and 60s (Table 47-2).[3,19] The elderly may delay presenting for care because of limited access to transportation, fear of costs, or fear of losing autonomy or independence. Upon presentation their true condition may be masked by medications, by coincident conditions with multiple, distracting symptoms, or by a physiologically limited capacity to generate the usual physical signs, such as fever, tachycardia, or abdominal guarding that are frequently

Table 47-2. Incidence of Adverse Outcome Measures by Age.

Age by Decade	LOS >3 Days	Surgery	Mortality
60s	38%	17%	3%
70s	42%	16%	2%
80s	45%	19%	12%

Adapted with permission from Lewis *et al.* 2005.[19]
Abbreviation: LOS, length of stay.

relied upon to indicate dangerous pathology.[3,10] As a consequence, the increased mortality rates for older patients with abdominal pain are stark. Patients older than 60 who present to the ED for abdominal pain have been reported to have a 5% mortality over the following 2 weeks,[19] and patients with abdominal pain over 80 years of age have a mortality rate 70 times greater than younger adults.[20] Thus it is sage advice that,

> **When dealing with elderly patients, the clinician must have a high index of suspicion, and proceed with caution based on the history and clinical epidemiology, rather than relying on [the results of testing].[3]**

The caveat about an overreliance upon testing applies for all patients, however. All tests are imperfect[1,12,17] and for these purposes the physical exam, in which specific maneuvers are performed in order to yield or not yield specific findings, may appropriately be considered a testing modality. Neither localized pain, tenderness, character of bowel sounds, nor the presence or absence of the traditional "surgical abdomen" are sufficient to justify the diagnosis or exclusion of serious disease.[1] Observing at best only moderate inter-rater agreement in assessment of tenderness, and even less agreement in the assessment of peritonitis, the authors of one study concluded "the classic exam for a surgical exam may not be as stereotypical as was thought. . . ."[21]

Other testing modalities therefore have come to play a significant role in the customary evaluation of abdominal pain. Ancillary testing has been shown to change the pretest probable diagnosis and/or disposition in up to 40% of patients, which may explain why as many as two-thirds of patients with abdominal pain have at least one test performed in their evaluation.[22] The ordering prevalence of each testing modality in that study is shown in abbreviated form in Table 47-3.

Of available tests, abdominal and pelvic computed tomography (CT) has been finding increasing favor among clinicians as the most valuable ancillary testing modality, because it provides the most information at little more cost than plain radiography.[10,22] Computed tomography has been reported as the best predictor of

Table 47-3. Test Utilization by % of Patients

Testing Regimen	% Overall Receiving Testing Regimen
None	2
Urine only	2
Serology only	6
Imaging only	0
Urine + serology	27
Urine + imaging	2
Serology + imaging	15
Urine + serology + imaging	48
Plain radiography as only imaging	11
CT as only imaging	38
Ultrasound as only imaging	25
Imaged by plain radiography + CT	13
Imaged by plain radiography + ultrasound	4
Imaged by CT + ultrasound	10

Adapted with permission from Nagurney *et al.* 2003.[22]
Abbreviation: CT, computed tomography.

the need, or lack thereof, for UI, and has been highly recommended for the ED evaluation of abdominal pain without a clear diagnosis.[9] Computed tomography is most useful, however, when the context and limitations of its use are understood. Similar to the physical exam, the interobserver agreement for radiologic interpretation is moderate and variable, and caution and precision should be used in distinguishing between "normal," "negative," "nondiagnostic," "positive," and "consistent with," particularly in older patients.[13] Only 57% of elderly patients' CTs are diagnostic for conditions requiring UI, though 20% of the remaining patients nonetheless required UI, admittedly for nonradiographic diagnoses.[5]

EMERGENCY DEPARTMENT CARE AND DISPOSITION

Even highly motivated, attentive, and experienced clinicians will occasionally experience slips and lapses that are an inherent part of being human. Systems designed with redundancy, cross-checking, and forcing functions might prevent some of these errors.[12]

Disposition: Understanding that even the best-reasoned decisions, built upon sufficient, albeit fallible data, may be erroneous, this section examines the strategies that may be applied to bolster a safe disposition. The process of crafting a safe disposition, particularly a safe discharge, begins with introspection, asking "What if I'm wrong?" or "What if my plan doesn't happen?" In this circumstance, the measure of a safe disposition is whether the patient will retain the potential of a timely recognition of the need for and access to UI.

Whether admitted or discharged, the patient is likely to be the first person to observe a change in their condition, and it is crucial to ensure, rather than assume, that they comprehend that a decision is being made, how the conclusion was reached and what degree of certainty is involved, and what the options and consequences are.[18] Most importantly, however, they should understand what to, as well as what not to expect of their clinical course. By ensuring this understanding, the patient becomes a redundant safeguard in their own disposition. Inappropriately providing diagnoses (e.g., gastroenteritis or viral syndrome) that are not supported by the evaluation, rather than acknowledging extant uncertainty via a diagnosis of undifferentiated abdominal pain, provides a false sense of certainty and security, obscuring the necessity of, and reducing vigilance in the patient's role as their own safeguard.

Admission: Some patients deserve a low threshold for admission, and should be discharged from the ED with reluctance, if at all. Examples are patients with an unreliable ability to perceive, process, or express changes in their own condition. While this increases risk for the inpatient as well as the outpatient, the risks for this patient population is greater if they are discharged. Likewise, if a patient's complete understanding of their disposition is in doubt or cannot be verified, prudence encourages admission. Indeed, in the United States, non-English speakers are admitted more frequently than English speakers with similar conditions, possibly for this reason.[23]

Except in rare cases, older patients with abdominal pain should be discharged from the ED only after great consideration, even if the evaluation is nondiagnostic and the patient's comprehension intact. Similarly, evaluations that reveal relatively benign and common diagnoses (e.g., urinary tract infection), should not signal the end of an evaluation intended to exclude more serious disease.[24] In both cases, the risk profile an older patient with abdominal pain translates to a high likelihood that nondiagnostic evaluations are erroneous, and common benign conditions mere distractions.[18] The purpose of admission in these cases is essentially for one additional test: the test of time. Observation units are ideally suited for this purpose, but in their absence emergency physicians must learn to convince reluctant admitting physicians of the wisdom of observing elderly patients with abdominal pain "hopefully to watch nothing bad happen." An uneventful 10 to 24 hours of observation can provide substantial, though not complete, reassurance.[10] Indeed, even a full inpatient admission does not guarantee that serious disease will be detected.

Discharge: Every surviving patient will be discharged at some point, either from the ED or the hospital. Neither an ED nor inpatient discharge should suggest more than a measured likelihood of health and safety. Roughly 7% of children and 14% of elders discharged from the ED, and almost 9% of elders admitted to the hospital for abdominal pain, will return to the ED.[6,19] While revisits are not common, and are occasionally for unrelated issues,[25] the 30% to 50% admission rate for repeat patients illustrates several concepts. Clearly, clinical certainty about the absence of disease can, and should, never be 100%. Furthermore, while often designated as an indicator for peer review, ED revisits attest that patients can reassess themselves and seek necessary reevaluation.

It is impossible to place too much emphasis on the importance of follow-up for discharged patients, particularly if their abdominal pain lasts longer than the 3 day median duration for benign undifferentiated abdominal pain.[25] The purpose of follow up is to serve as a backup for

Table 47-4. Recommendations for Discharge Instructions/Re-evaluation within 24 hours.*

Issue	Recommendation
Abdominal pain	Pain that worsens, changes in character, or does not resolve or improve significantly in 24 hours requires re-evaluation.
Fever	Onset of new fever, or fever above pre-evaluation levels that is not expected requires re-evaluation.
Vomiting	Vomiting that does not resolve or the vomiting of blood requires re-evaluation
Rectal bleeding	New bleeding or unexpected bleeding requires re-evaluation.
Blood in the urine	Onset of blood in the urine, or the failure of known hematuria to improve with 24 hours of treatment requires re-evaluation.
Dizziness or fainting	Onset of new dizziness or fainting requires re-evaluation.
Blood in stool, dark stool	Onset of blood in stool or stools turning dark or tar like requires re-evaluation.
Vaginal bleeding	Onset of new unexpected bleeding, or worsening of prior bleeding, or bleeding associated with symptoms of fainting requires re-evaluation.
Jaundice	Yellowing of the skin or worsening of known jaundice requires re-evaluation.
Bowel movements	Cessation of bowel movements requires re-evaluation. Diarrhea, that is associated with profound weakness or passing out requires re-evaluation.
New prescribed medications	Take all medications as prescribed. Patients unable to take medications require re-evaluation.
Prior medications	Take previously prescribed medications unless instructed otherwise.
Over-the-counter medications	Take no over-the-counter medications unless recommended by the emergency physician.
Diet	Clear liquids until abdominal pain resolves, or improves significantly. Avoid alcohol, caffeine, and cigarettes.

*Re-evaluation should be performed by the patient's regular doctor if one exists; if the patient does not have a physician, or the patient cannot get an appointment within 24 hours, the patient should return to the emergency department.

patients' surveillance of their own condition (see Table 47-4). While abdominal physical examination is imperfect, diagnostic accuracy improves with repetition over time, and though usually a feature of inpatient and observation management, scheduled outpatient repeat examination is not intuitively unreasonable.[1] Outpatient follow up is not a certain strategy, however, as in one study only 62% of patients had intended a follow-up visit, only two thirds of whom had actually arranged one.[25] What is not clear is whether the remainder declined follow up because their symptoms resolved, but certainly measures to improve follow-up compliance, such as setting a specific time and place, rather than leaving arrangements unmade, are warranted.[1] Should all else fail, the ED itself may always serve this purpose, and even an unofficial, undocumented reevaluation is likely safer than none at all.

PITFALLS

- Overreliance on testing leads to flawed decision making. High risk patients, especially the elderly, may simply have yet to reveal their serious conditions.

- Trust that patients will make their own follow-up arrangements is misplaced. Less than half will actually do so. Make the arrangements for or with them.

- Admitting a patient does not ensure their safety. Errors happen to inpatients, too, and senseless use of resources risks both the current patient and the next one.

- Failure to take the bounce back patient seriously deprives them of a critical safety measure. Welcome the return visit as simply another type of follow-up.

REFERENCES

1. American College of Emergency Physicians. Clinical Policy: Critical Issues for the Initial Evaluation and Management of Patients Presenting with a Chief Complaint of Nontraumatic Acute Abdominal Pain. *Ann Emerg Med.* 2000;36:406.

2. McCaig LF, Burt CW. National Hospital Ambulatory Medical Care Survey: 1999 Emergency Department Summary. Advance data from Vital Health Statistics of the National Center for Health Statistics. 2001;320:1.

3. Kamin RA, Nowicki TA, Courtney DS, Powers RD. Pearls and pitfalls in the emergency department evaluation of abdominal pain. *Emerg Med Clin N Am.* 2003;21:61.

4. Powers RD, Guertler AT. Abdominal pain in the ED: Stability and change over 20 years. *Am J Emerg Med.* 1995; 13:301.

5. Hustey FM, Meldon SW, Banet GA, Gerson LW, Blanda M, Lewis LM. The use of abdominal computed tomography in older ed patients with acute abdominal pain. *Am J Emerg Med.* 2005;23:259.

6. Scholer SJ, Pituch K, Orr DP, Dittus RS. Clinical outcomes of children with acute abdominal pain. *Pediatrics.* 1996;98(4 Pt 1):680.

7. Hack JB, O'Brien K, Benson N. Pilot study: Concordance of disposition for hypothetical medical patients in the emergency department. *Acad Emerg Med.* 2005;12:562.

8. Newton E, Mandavia S. Surgical complications of selected gastrointestinal emergencies: Pitfalls in management of the acute abdomen. *Emerg Med Clin N Am.* 2003;21:873.

9. Gerhardt RT, Nelson BK, Keenan SK, et al. Derivation of a clinical guideline for the assessment of nonspecific abdominal pain: The Guideline for Abdominal Pain in the ED Setting (GAPEDS) Phase 1 Study. *Am J Emerg Med.* 2005;23:709.

10. Graff LG, Robinson D. Abdominal pain and emergency department evaluation. *Emerg Med Clin N Am.* 2001; 19:123.

11. Kovacs G, Croskerry P. Clinical decision making: An emergency medicine perspective. *Acad Emerg Med.* 1999;6:947.

12. Cosby KS. A framework for classifying factors that contribute to error in the emergency department. *Ann Emerg Med.* 2003;42:815.

13. Hofer TP, Hayward RA. Are bad outcomes from questionable clinical decisions preventable medical errors? A case of cascade iatrogenesis. *Ann Intern Med.* 2002; 137(5 Part 1):327.

14. Graff L, Russell J, Seashore J, et al. False-negative and false-positive errors in abdominal pain evaluation: Failure to diagnose acute appendicitis and unnecessary surgery. *Acad Emerg Med.* 2000;7:1244.

15. Handler JA, Gillam M, Sanders AB, Klasco R. Defining, identifying, and measuring error in emergency medicine. *Acad Emerg Med.* 2000;7:1183.

16. Kyriacou DN, Ricketts V, Dyne, PL, et al. A 5-year time study analysis of emergency department patient care efficiency. *Ann Emerg Med.* 1999;34:326.

17. Flum DR, Koepsell T. The clinical and economic correlates of misdiagnosed appendicitis: Nationwide analysis. *Arch Surg.* 2002;137:799.

18. Hendrickson M, Naparst TR. Abdominal surgical emergencies in the elderly. *Emerg Med Clin N Am.* 2003;21:937.

19. Lewis LM, Banet GA, Blanda M, et al. Etiology and clinical course of abdominal pain in senior patients: A prospective, multicenter study. *J Gerontol.* 2005;60A:1071.

20. van Geloven AA, Biesheuvel TH, Luitse JS, et al. Hospital admissions of patients aged over 80 with acute abdominal complaints. *Eur J Surg.* 2000;166:866.

21. Pines J, Pines LU, Hall A, et al. The interrater variation of ed abdominal examination findings in patients with acute abdominal pain. *Am J Emerg Med.* 2005;23:483.

22. Nagurney JT, Brown DFM, Chang Y, et al. Use of diagnostic testing in the emergency department for patients presenting with non-traumatic abdominal pain. *J Emerg Med.* 2003;25:363.

23. Waxman MA, Levitt MA. Are diagnostic testing and admission rates higher in non-English-speaking versus English-speaking patients in the emergency department? *Ann Emerg Med.* 2000;36:456.

24. Pines JM. Profiles in patient safety: Confirmation bias in emergency medicine. *Acad Emerg Med.* 2006;13:90.

25. Weiner JB, Nagurney JT, Brown DFM, et al. Duration of symptoms and follow-up patterns of patients discharged from the emergency department After presenting with abdominal or flank pain. *Fam Pract.* 2004;21:314.

INDEX

Page numbers followed by italic *f* or *t* denote figures or tables, respectively.